FLIGHT STRESS:
STRESS, FATIGUE, AND PERFORMANCE IN AVIATION

T0179094

Dedicated to the memory of Dr. Fred Hyman, aviator

Flight Stress:

Stress, Fatigue, and Performance in Aviation

Alan Stokes

Kirsten Kite

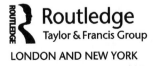

Routledge
Taylor & Francis Group

LONDON AND NEW YORK

First published 1994 by Ashgate Publishing

Published 2016 by Routledge
2 Park Square, Milton Park, Abingdon, Oxon OX14 4RN
711 Third Avenue, New York, NY 10017, USA

Routledge is an imprint of the Taylor & Francis Group, an informa business

British Library Cataloguing in Publication Data

Stokes, Alan
    Flight Stress: Stress, Fatigue, and Performance
    in Aviation
    I. Title   II. Kite, Kirsten
    629.13252019

ISBN 9780291398062 (hbk)
ISBN 9780291398574 (pbk)

Library of Congress Cataloging-in-Publication Data

Stokes, Alan (Alan F.)
    Flight stress: stress, fatigue, and performance in aviation /
    Alan F. Stokes, Kirsten Kite
        p. cm.
    Includes bibliographical references and index.
    ISBN 978-0-291-39806-2 : $55.95 (est.)
    1. Aeronautics—Human Factors.   I. Kite, Kirsten.   II. Title.
    TL553.6.S76   1994
    629.132'52—dc20   94-19176
                                                                                   CIP

Transferred to Digital Printing in 2014

Flight Stress:

Stress, Fatigue, and Performance in Aviation

Alan Stokes

Kirsten Kite

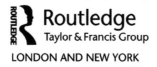

Routledge
Taylor & Francis Group

LONDON AND NEW YORK

First published 1994 by Ashgate Publishing

Published 2016 by Routledge
2 Park Square, Milton Park, Abingdon, Oxon OX14 4RN
711 Third Avenue, New York, NY 10017, USA

Routledge is an imprint of the Taylor & Francis Group, an informa business

British Library Cataloguing in Publication Data

Stokes, Alan
    Flight Stress: Stress, Fatigue, and Performance
    in Aviation
    I. Title   II. Kite, Kirsten
    629.13252019

ISBN 9780291398062 (hbk)
ISBN 9780291398574 (pbk)

Library of Congress Cataloging-in-Publication Data

Stokes, Alan (Alan F.)
    Flight stress: stress, fatigue, and performance in aviation /
    Alan F. Stokes, Kirsten Kite
        p. cm.
    Includes bibliographical references and index.
    ISBN 978-0-291-39806-2 : $55.95 (est.)
    1. Aeronautics—Human Factors. I. Kite, Kirsten. II. Title.
TL553.6.S76   1994
629.132'52—dc20   94-19176
                                                                         CIP

Transferred to Digital Printing in 2014

Contents

Preface

When we are in bed, or floating in water, is the only time when we are
really out of pain. In every other situation there is always some stress.
-- Rose O'Neill, *Garda*

Issues of stress, fatigue, and performance have been addressed in several
books on aviation human factors. These topics are also regularly 'visited'
from time to time in pilots' magazines, various airline company publications, military 'house' journals, and pamphlets and circulars from regulatory agencies. What, then, is the need for a book like *Flight Stress?*

First, some of the available publications treat stress and fatigue anecdotally. There is a role for these, to be sure, since they are intended primarily to be pilots' coping guides more than expository works. *Flight Stress* is
not intended as a coping guide, but as a critical examination of the relevant
research literature.

Second, while there are, of course, a number of other publications that
are expository in approach [and which do make reference to the research
literature], there is a tradition among some of these of citing, in our view
rather uncritically, secondary and tertiary sources -- including each other.
This has led to the perpetuation of various longstanding assertions and folk
assumptions as authoritative. These include, for example, the assertion
that some stress is good for performance, that 'life events' are bad for
performance, that air traffic controllers are not stressed,* that flight anxiety
is merely a (treatable) phobia, that arousal and stress are pretty much the
same, that jet lag is basically sleep loss, and so on. Indeed, the dominance
of received wisdom in this field has dampened if not stifled real debate on
certain topics. We also note that while certain topic areas have become
quite 'fashionable', others are underrepresented in literature targeted to-

---

*At least in publications influenced predominantly by US sources.

ward aviation professionals. For example, cockpit resource management (the coordination of team work on the flight deck) is a topic that has penetrated both the scientific and professional literature very well -- as it deserves to. However, the management of human resources *off* the flight deck (in the airlines or flying schools, for example) is, by comparison, hardly mentioned at all. Thus, organizational factors and adverse union/management relations (which, we have concluded, represent among the most potent stressors and threats to flight safety) receive less than their due share of attention. One reason for writing *Flight Stress*, then, was to highlight some topics that may have been 'skated over' somewhat in the past, to re-open a number of 'settled' issues, and to do so in sufficient detail to provide grist for debate.

A third and related reason for writing *Flight Stress* is to make, or at least reinforce, a point about the centrality of stress, mood, and affect (or 'energetic' factors, as they are sometimes called) in aviation psychology. In most of the aviation literature the subjects of stress and fatigue are usually addressed relatively briefly, in a page or two, a section, or an invited article. It is a rare aviation book that devotes a whole chapter to them. However, the philosophy behind the writing of *Flight Stress* is that stress and fatigue should not be considered as peripheral factors in aviation psychology (or, indeed, in cognitive psychology). Rather, they should be considered as being among the stuff and substance of those enterprises, ingredients of the main course and not a 'side dish'.

To this extent we regard energetic factors as integral elements of human information processing, not as a set of 'junior' phenomena occasionally mediating mainstream cognitive processes. Thus, in our view the role of stress and fatigue in aviation should not be shunted off into a sidebar or section within a longer text on human performance, for it is inseparable from that performance. As Fraser Watts* recently wrote,

> It is unhelpful to regard cognitive and emotional functioning as two parallel, perhaps alternative, psychological systems. This way of thinking is part of the unfortunate inheritance from the debate ... about whether cognition or emotion is primary. The cognitive approach is a general style of theorizing and doing research, within which one can tackle a variety of substantive topics, including emotion. (p. 154)

---

*Watts, F.N. (1992), 'Applications of current cognitive theories of the emotions to the conceptualization of emotional disorders', *British Journal of Clinical Psychology*, vol. 31, pp. 153-67.

The book's focus. Having argued for the centrality of energetic factors, it has to be conceded that stress can be something of an 'exploding' concept. It sometimes appears that the more that is written about it, the more phenomena it seems to encompass. Indeed, as we intimated above (and discuss at length in Chapter 2), there are those who assert that stress (in modest amounts, of course) is a positive and beneficial thing in aviation and elsewhere. Others, as we discuss in Chapter 5, consider even positive life events such as weddings and promotions to be stressful, in the same sense that bereavement, for example, is stressful. There are potential problems in the broadening of the stress concept in these ways. For example, stress could become little more than a rather 'chic' catchall term for almost any factor in experience, aversive or otherwise, that might conceivably influence opinion or sense of ease and well-being, from airline food to hangovers, from promotions to middle-age spread.

Apart from the fact that concepts that can be stretched at will to encompass all phenomena are not scientifically useful, too inclusive an approach would have drawn us into the broadest treatment of aviation medicine and human factors. We have attempted to avoid such an approach, and in so doing have largely centred our discussions around emotional or psychological distress. We wish to distinguish such stress from purely environmental effects, from medical conditions and, in particular, from workload. Occasionally, the aviation human factors literature slips almost imperceptibly back and forth between the concepts of stress and workload, not only as though they were necessarily related, but as though they were near synonyms. In the view developed in Chapter 1, it is only when workload (or any other factor) is perceived by the individual as possibly exceeding his or her coping abilities that it becomes stressful.

Similarly, but to an even greater extent, the literature often slips from the concept of arousal to the concept of stress, as though these terms too were virtually synonymous. This issue is taken up in Chapter 2. While we have attempted to keep the stress/arousal distinction clear, some of the studies we (necessarily) report are rather less clear. For example, an extensive program of research on air traffic controller stress conducted in the USA (and discussed in Chapter 10) relied rather heavily upon physiological measures of arousal, which, as we discuss in Chapters 1 and 2, may or may not index psychological stress.

An overly inclusive view of stress is not the only potential pitfall, of course. There are also drawbacks associated with the opposite tack, the resort to narrow prescriptive definitions of stress. These include the risk of unduly impoverishing the 'everyday' concept and limiting consideration to an artificially truncated set of phenomena (for example, physiological aspects of arousal). If our interest leans in any direction it is toward cognitive and behavioural effects of stress rather than physiological effects per se, for several reasons. First, the aeromedical literature already contains more (and more comprehensive) accounts of physiological problems than of the psychological and performance implications of stress in aviation. Second, modern developments in the design of flight decks, aircraft systems, and air traffic control facilities (e.g., 'glass cockpit' computerized colour displays, advanced automation, and the like) refocus attention upon the role of information processing as a component in the human-machine system. Human cognition is, of course, a system element that humans did not design, and which has very complex failure modes. It is the system component we understand least, and nowhere is our understanding thinner than in the area of emotion and performance, the affective processes of (what is sometimes called) 'hot' cognition. While we cannot provide redress for this, we hope that *Flight Stress* is at least a step in the right direction.

Topics covered. In writing the book we have tried to be more or less true to everyday conceptions of stress and fatigue, and to confine our discussion to those phenomena that can properly be subsumed under these terms as they are commonly understood. This excludes certain topics that might be discussed in a general text on aerospace medicine -- drugs, anoxia, and G forces, for example. This is not to deny the importance of these topics, or to maintain that the sources of poor performance in the real world of flight operations can be easily compartmentalized. It is true, for example, that stress on the job or at home may lead to substance abuse, and that substance abuse can, in turn, have profound effects upon job performance. Occupational or domestic stress may also lead to smoking, overeating, cardiac problems, or ulcers. These conditions and behaviours, like many others, can be significant influences upon performance in the complex web of cause and effect that characterizes life outside the research laboratory. Nevertheless, we considered these sorts of factors to fall outside the scope of this book.

On the other hand, we have decided that the subject of fatigue merits two chapters rather than one, primarily in order to deal adequately with the topic of circadian rhythms -- that is, cyclical changes in physiological functioning. Much of the literature on fatigue in aviation fails to discriminate between the effects of normal undisrupted circadian rhythms upon performance, and the effects of desynchronized rhythms such as those associated with transmeridian flight. This latter is a complex problem in its own right and Chapter 9 is, therefore, devoted entirely to it.

Readership. *Flight Stress* is intended to function as a source book and reference work on the subject of stress as it relates to aviation. As such it is meant to serve a wide audience. Potential readers include practitioners of aviation medicine, aviation human factors specialists in the public sector, private sector, or academia, and other aviation professionals such as pilots, air traffic controllers, and those involved in the work of professional associations. The book should also be of interest to some flight students, to graduate students researching stress related topics, and to persons interested in occupational stress in general.

Text and sidebars. The structure of the book includes both a main text, which necessarily devotes a good deal of space to discussions of theoretical and empirical stress research, and a series of boxed inserts ('sidebars') containing supplementary material. These include, for example, descriptions of actual, stress related events in the operational world of flying. Some of this boxed material is drawn from autobiographical and eyewitness accounts in historical aviation literature; we have also made use of accident reports from the United States National Transportation Safety Board as well as incident/accident reports from the NASA Aviation Safety Reporting System (ASRS). A few words about these are in order here.

The ASRS database contains records of thousands of reports of aviation accidents and incidents (i.e., near accidents), filed in confidence by the aircrew and air traffic controllers involved. As archived on the computer ASRS reports are couched in a condensed telegraphic style with heavy use of abbreviations and technical 'flight speak'. We have, therefore, minimally edited and condensed these into an acceptable form appropriate to a more general readership. By the same token we have compressed certain lengthy NTSB reports. However, in each case we have stayed true to the content and tone of the reports and made no attempt at editorial comment.

It is important to realize that ASRS accounts are not 'objective' reports by detached and dispassionate third parties, as might (with greater justification) be claimed for accident reports from investigating bodies such as the NTSB. They are, rather, accounts by the individuals involved in (and often responsible for) some or all of the difficulties they are reporting --

accounts, moreover, written in the emotional aftermath of sometimes distressing events. Filing an ASRS report confers some immunity from regulatory enforcement action by the Federal Aviation Administration, but the reports may nevertheless gloss over the reporters' own poor planning or performance and focus upon the shortcomings of others. The interest and value of these reports lie more in their status as eyewitness opinions than as factual briefs.

Two other caveats might be made. First, compared to the drama of the events so often recorded in the reports of fatal accidents, the incidents in the ASRS database may appear to be somewhat trivial. It can, however, be quite informative to analyze situations which did not end catastrophically but could have. It is an axiom of accident investigators that 'accidents are a subset of incidents'; that is, the causative factors are likely to be similar, although the actual outcomes may differ. The philosopher Hannah Arendt spoke of the 'banality of evil'; by the same token, the seemingly mundane quality of incidents should not mislead us. Incidents should, perhaps, be thought of as fatal accidents which (providentially) went wrong.

Second, the events described in various personal accounts and in NTSB accident and ASRS incident reports cannot be read as though they were 'factor pure' hypothetical examples of a particular stress or fatigue process. Inevitably, they are 'muddy' real world examples, in which processes we discuss in the narrative are discernible in the multifactor context of actual flight or ATC operations.

Acknowledgements. We wish to acknowledge the invaluable assistance given to us by Vince Mellone, the ASRS Deputy Program Manager, as well as by Stephanie Frank of the ASRS service at Battelle, who conducted searches of the ASRS database and provided us with both printed and computer readable ASRS records. We are also indebted to John Nance for details concerning management practices at Downeast Airlines and the crash of Flight 46. Our brief account in Chapter 11 hardly does justice to the topic, and we commend John Nance's book *Blind Trust* to readers interested in corporate malfeasance. We recognize too the help of Captain Neil Johnston of Aer Lingus, with whom we have had a continuing (if heavily quantized) dialogue at conferences over the past nine years and whose publications also influenced the contents of Chapter 11. We thank Dr. Neville Moray of the University of Illinois for providing access to his collection of papers, and we apologize for keeping it so long. We also thank D. Lenorowitz of CTA Incorporated for granting permission to reproduce his ATC diagram in Chapter 10 and for kindly providing us with an original copy. For their comments on draft chapters, we thank Dr. Gavan Lintern of the University of Illinois and Dr. Frank Webbe and Dr. Jeff Rain of the Florida Institute of Technology. Needless to say, any remaining inaccuracies, inadequacies or infelicities of style are ours alone.

Finally, we owe a debt of gratitude to John Hindley at Ashgate Publishing for his grace, patience, advice, and encouragement.

Introduction

We should not consider stress reactions as exceptional states. On the contrary, they can be thought to be the foundation of behaviour regulatory processes ... required for the survival of all living organisms.
                                                    -- Timsit-Berthier[*]

This is a book about routine everyday reality. It is not about arcane or extraordinary phenomena. Yet stress and fatigue are often thought of as special, esoteric, or occasional factors disrupting the otherwise smooth functioning of our lives -- pathologies interfering with the normal metabolism of experience. In fact, stress and strain, weariness and depletion are integral and universal features of that experience, waxing and waning to be sure, but as much a permanent part of our humanity as fallibility and mortality. This, however, is hardly the central theme of the mythology of aviation, a world of confident young top-gun aces, avuncular silver-haired captains, and ever-vigilant air traffic controllers -- unruffled, unflappable professionals, all. This is not a world in which pilots 'freeze' in emergencies, controllers suffer from 'night shift paralysis', and union disputes culminate in fist fights on the flight deck (see Chapters 7, 10, and 11, respectively).

Notwithstanding mystique or public wishful thinking about aviators' intrepid coolness, rationality, and fortitude, pilots and air traffic controllers are no more a society of Spocks or Stepford Wives than are (for example) chefs, nurses, or attorneys. Like cookery, medicine, and law, aviation takes place within the context of mood, emotion, and disposition -- in a word, 'affect'. Aviation professionals marry and divorce, become involved

[*]Timsit-Berthier, M., Ansseau, M., and Legros, J.-J. (1986), 'Responses to Stress: An Interdisciplinary Approach', in Hockey, G.R.J., Gaillard, A.W.K., and Coles, M.G.H. (eds.), *Energetics and Human Information Processing*, Martinus Nijhoff, Dordrecht.

in management disputes, lie awake at bedtime, feel sleepy at flight time, and share all the myriad petty frustrations and worries of daily life. Some of these (such as speeding tickets or certain medical problems) may represent minor 'hassles' to nonpilots but can be very damaging to a pilot's career. Pilots may also have to cope with, among other things, an unstable airline industry, the threat of unemployment (with few, if any, transferable skills), unsafe weather, bad management, unpredictable schedules, unreliable equipment, and poor maintenance.

In recognizing the human fallibilities and vulnerabilities of aviation professionals, we can better appreciate the remarkable performance achieved daily and routinely by thousands of aircrew and air traffic controllers. Occasionally brief periods of the most acute stress are superimposed upon the humdrum tribulations of everyday service, and while the following chapters are full of examples of failure under these circumstances, we should recognize that quite exceptional presence of mind is shown from time to time. One example that springs to mind is the outstanding performance of the flight deck crew of United Flight 232, the mechanically disabled DC-10 which was nursed back for a (regrettably, spectacular) crash landing at Sioux City, Iowa, in 1989. Similarly, one can only admire the efficiency and quick-wittedness of the cabin attendants of USAir Flight 5050, which also came to grief in 1989 at LaGuardia Airport in New York. The passengers of this flight were, for the most part, evacuated safely after a poorly executed rejected takeoff ran their Boeing 737 off the runway, by night, into the waters of Bowery Bay. Both groups' performance under stress saved hundreds of lives.

There is, of course, something odd about lumping together, under the one umbrella term 'stress', not only the emotional component of traumatic incidents such as the two just referred to, but also the routine 'hassles' of life such as parking tickets and unpredictable schedules, as well as chronic emotional effects such as those that might stem from divorce, insecurity, or bereavement. To make sense of this it is helpful to step back for a moment and start from the beginning, with the term 'stress' itself.

Pilots and damsels: stress versus distress

Stress, viewed as a generic aversive ingredient of life, is in some respects a uniquely modern concept. Obviously, psychological and emotional suffering is hardly an invention of the late industrial age: in Shakespeare's

Stress -- it's the ailment of the '90s. It even has its own jargon, from Type A personality to post-traumatic stress disorder. In some circles, it's acquired cachet: the more stress, the more important the person. Soon you'll be reading about celebrities checking into stress detox centers. But stars and superachievers don't have a monopoly on stress. It affects averyone, from children to the elderly -- and women are often hit the hardest. Managing a house and caring for the kids may be rewarding but they're also major sources of stress. And when you consider that more women are working outside the home, it's no surprise that we begin to feel frazzled.

Despite all this, stress isn't always a bad thing. When present in manageable doses, it can be a great motivator. Deadline pressure at work is what forces you to finish that project. Competition with your peers makes you complete that aerobics class. Too little stress, and life is uneventful; too much and it's overwhelming. The path to stress resiliency is striking a balance -- learning how to push yourself enough so that you're the best you can be, but not so much that you go through life harried and unhappy.

-- From an article in *For Women First* magazine, June 7, 1993

plays, for example, the English language has a body of literature which, like no other, relishes the very epitome of the stressful -- murder, guilt, treason, passion, intrigue, adversity, and the like. Yet in this whole corpus of work, Shakespeare never once uses the term 'stress'. As J.E. Singer[*] has noted, stress became a fashionable buzzword in the 1970s, associated with tabloid newspapers, starlets, and chic clinics. Stress, but not fatigue, has since become a prestigious executive complaint, like ulcers, and bespeaks of responsibility and power.

The word 'stress' is by no means some modern pop neologism, however. In its origin it appears to be no more than a shortened form of the word 'distress', having come about by aphesis (the syllable dropping process that gave us 'plane' from 'aeroplane', for example). Nevertheless, it would be a mistake to assume that 'distress' is an archaic form and con-

[*]Singer, J.E. (1980), 'Traditions of Stress Research: Integrative Comments', in Sarason, I.G. and Spielberger, C.D. (eds.), *Stress and Anxiety*, vol. 7, Hemisphere Publishing Corporation, New York.

cept while 'stress' is a twentieth century form and concept: in point of fact, both forms can be traced back to well before Shakespeare's time and into Middle English. Moreover, in the centuries since then both have been used fairly interchangeably with pretty much the same (enormous) range of meanings that they take today. Indeed, *Webster's New Collegiate Dictionary*, in defining distress, refers to physical or mental stress or strain and gives as examples fear, anxiety, and shame.

It is arguable, however, that the late twentieth century is seeing some subtle divergence of meaning in these terms, although the semantic overlap remains great. This divergence has probably been occasioned in part by the broadening of the concept in the 1970s referred to above, as well as by the leakage of specific postwar technical and scientific usages of the term 'stress' into everyday language. 'Stressed' suggests process and external pressures, while 'distressed' suggests state and internal reaction (issues dealt with at length in Chapter 1). Hence, pilots are more likely to be described as being 'stressed' by an engine fire (they are in the process of coping with time pressure, anxiety, etc.) while the passengers may be described as being 'distressed' (helplessly enduring an emotional state). Be that as it may, it certainly appears that in the late twentieth century stress as a concept has been broadened, popularized, and in some sense, sanitized (of the taint of overemotionality). It is socially acceptable, or as we noted, even chic, to be 'stressed'. These cultural and linguistic changes appear to have left 'distress' as a slightly more marked and 'up-register' form. This retains, perhaps, more of the emotional overtones of duress that befit helpless damsels in need of princely rescue, as opposed to pilots or air traffic controllers managing an emergency. Interestingly, the popular informal American phrase 'stressed out' seems to recapture some of the emotional content and finality of 'distressed',* but appears to function as a socially 'safe' and acceptable term which does not hint at emotionality, unmanliness, or helplessness.

The meaning of stress

St. Augustine once noted that the concept of time is something we all understand -- that is, until we stop to think about it. In some ways the concept of stress is similar. To test this one only has to observe reactions

---

*Perhaps through its reverberation with 'burned out' and 'worn out'.

to such questions as "Is stress an emotion?" "Is stress, by definition, always bad for you?" or "Is anxiety a cause or a result of stress?" In any group of people such questions generally open a Pandora's Box of arguments replete with personal definitions, overlapping concepts, prescriptions, and anecdotes. This is not surprising when one considers that the *Oxford English Dictionary* contains about three full pages of small print under the entry 'stress'. Much of this remains even after eliminating no longer used archaisms, arcane legal usages, and grammatical, prosodic, and phonetic meanings (for example, stress as emphasis, timing, or loudness in an utterance). Among the usages the *OED* records can be found stress as strain, hardship and adversity, suffering, affliction and injury, force, pressure, compulsion, overwork, harassment, and fatigue. There is also engineering stress (e.g., stress cracks in a wing spar), psychological stress, physiological stress, and financial stress.

Amid this profusion of usages an interesting dichotomy can be identified. On the one hand there is stress viewed as an agent, circumstance, situation, or variable that disturbs the 'normal' functioning of the individual; on the other hand there is stress seen as an effect -- that is, the disturbed state itself. Obviously, even without the optimistic concept of a stress free normality, this bifurcation of meaning is highly unusual and potentially confusing. Twentieth century science has, with a few exceptions, done little to reconcile these meanings. On the contrary, as we shall see in the following chapter, the dichotomy has led to divergent schools of thought which, in turn, have had an important effect upon the ways in which stress in aviation is considered.

1 Concepts of stress

*The simplest way to understand human stress is to relate it to the materi-
al strength of an aircraft. The demands placed on it by the pilot or the
environment in which it flies, must not exceed its capacity to meet them.
In relation to the human body too, this is what stress is all about.*
-- Campbell and Bagshaw,[5] *Human Performance Limitations in Aviation*

*Men and their organizations are not machines, even if they have ma-
chine-like aspects, and the analogy breaks down rather too easily.*
-- Cox,[10] *Stress*

As discussed in the Introduction, the word 'stress' as it used in everyday
language is rich, polysemous, and subtly dependent upon context. However, the same qualities that make it a powerful and useful term for common
conversation make it a problem for researchers, who promptly narrow and
redefine the term for the purpose of scientific inquiry. This in turn makes
the relevance of many research results to the 'real world', not least the
operational world of aviation, more difficult to gauge.

We should not think for a moment, however, that science has converged
upon a sharp, generally agreed definition of stress. On the contrary, in the
world of research 'stress' is a word associated with important conceptual
confusions.[16] It has been used as a catchall term for actual or presumed
anxiety eliciting events, for psychological and emotional states, and for
behavioural and physiological responses to particular events or circumstances. Many contemporary stress researchers tend to regard stress not as
a variable itself, but rather as an organizing concept, "a rubric consisting
of many variables and processes", as Richard Lazarus and Susan
Folkman,[44] leading theorists in this area, have put it (p. 22).

This is an important and often misunderstood idea. It does not, of
course, mean that there are no models or theories of stress. There are
plenty to choose from. However, many applied studies, not least those in
the field of aviation human factors, are couched in no coherent model of
stress whatsoever, and fewer still present any kind of model explicitly. We
will describe three basic approaches or philosophies in stress research:
stimulus based models, response based models, and transactional models,[10]

6

and examine how these relate to aviation. Note that the three approaches are not necessarily mutually exclusive. (For example, life events research, as discussed in Chapter 5, integrates elements of both stimulus and response based models.) The three approaches emphasize, respectively, situational variables, generalized responses (especially biochemical responses), and intervening psychological variables -- that is, individual assessment of threat.[23]

Models of stress

Stimulus based approaches

A significant proportion of human factors psychology, not least in aviation, has for many decades tended to work within a simple and often tacit stimulus based conception of stress, one which focusses attention almost exclusively on external events or conditions rather than on the subjective experience itself. This approach was pithily summed up by Sir Charles Symonds, who asserted, in connection with Royal Air Force bomber crews during the Second World War, that "stress is that which happens to the man, not that which happens in him; it is a set of causes, not a set of symptoms."[72] Within such a view, there is a tendency for situational variables that are assumed to be aversive (e.g., workload, time pressure, noise, even 'life events' such as promotion, moving house, or marriage) to simply be labelled *a priori* as stressors.

In keeping with this philosophy, a good deal of applied research has consisted of selecting a given variable, manipulating it experimentally, and terming the manipulation 'stress'. Thus, time restrictions or increases in workload (for example) are sometimes labelled as stressors irrespective of whether the individuals studied actually experience any distress or discomfort whatsoever. This approach (and also the response based approach) has been criticized on the grounds that stress becomes "merely a convenient label and collective noun indicating certain environmental and organismic conditions" (Sanders,[57] p. 62).

Certainly the list of factors that have been named as stressors is impressively long: it features almost every imaginable physical, environmental, and social condition, and includes army food, the weather, poverty, and (in the words of Alvin Toffler) 'future shock' -- the "shattering stress and disorientation that we induce in individuals by subjecting them to too much change in too short a time."[74] The point is not that these factors cannot be stressful, but rather that almost anything that can be named (from fame to average temperatures) can, under some imaginable circumstance or other, induce psychological stress. Simply labelling flight tests, emergencies, noise, g-loading and the like as stressors, therefore, makes no special claims about these factors and, in the absence of some theoretical under-pinning, leaves us none the wiser.

Stress and strain in man and plane.   One variable that has often been suggested as an external stressor is anxiety.[29] An alternative view (and one we shall discuss at length later), is that anxiety is not an external factor causing stress, but is an internal factor (a result, not a cause of stress). This external/internal dichotomy is often expressed in a distinctive way in the stimulus based approach to stress, that is, by using an engineering analogy: the 'stress and strain' model. This model holds that just as stress is an external force -- an aerodynamic or mechanical loading, say, applied to a wing spar resulting in strain within the spar -- so human stress is best viewed as an external factor (Symond's 'set of causes') that produces 'strain' within the person. Hence, as Campbell and Bagshaw[5] state in the epigraph at the head of this chapter, "the simplest way to understand human stress is to relate it to the material strength of an aircraft" (p. 105).

Regrettably, there are a number of serious problems with this otherwise neat and tempting formulation. Wing spars do not, of course, evaluate the stress they are under; thus the 'strain' has no real meaning, that is, no emotional component to it. All wing spars react similarly to stresses, and a spar stressed this week responds identically to when it was stressed last week. This is not an adequate description of human stress response. It is a striking fact that similarly qualified and trained persons may react very differently in identical circumstances. (A stark example of this, in the context of a rejected takeoff emergency, is described in Chapter 7 in the discussion of stress induced inaction.)

In human stress response, individual differences are important: individuals do not react identically,[27,28] even at the most basic physiological level, as research on endocrine responses has shown.[56,71] Moreover, not only is it true that what stresses Captain Smith may not stress First Officer Brown, it is equally true that what Captain Smith interpreted as stressful last week she may not regard as stressful this week. In short, two major shortcom-ings of the stimulus based approach in general and the engineering analogy in particular is that they ignore individual differences and simply omit the emotional component of the experience that is the very hallmark of the everyday concept of human stress.

Response based approaches

In contrast to stimulus based views of stress, response based approaches focus not on the external circumstances assumed to induce stress reactions, but on the reactions themselves. In fact, within this model the responses (or patterns of responses) displayed in a given situation are considered to be the defining parameter of stress. In other words (to invert Sir Charles Symonds's phrase), stress is viewed as a set of symptoms rather than as a set of causes.

In theory, this conception of stress could incorporate many different categories of responses -- behavioural, affective, cognitive, and possibly others. In actuality, this has not been the case to any great extent. Historically, the most extensively studied type of stress response has been the physiological. In part, this emphasis has its roots in investigations conducted early in the twentieth century by Yerkes and Dodson.[78] (This research and its impact on subsequent thinking about stress is discussed in Chapter 2.) However, perhaps the most often cited body of work is that of Hans Selye, whose work has exerted a profound influence on response based approaches to stress, and, indeed, on popular conceptions of stress in general.

Selye, who was studying physiological responses to injury, emotion, and other intense stimuli, observed that while some of these reactions were clearly linked to particular stimuli, others seemed to be less specific and tended to appear in a wide variety of aversive or demanding situations. This latter group included increases in heart rate, respiration, adrenalin output, and a number of other metabolic and endocrine functions associated with autonomic nervous system activity.[59]

This generalized, 'nonspecific' physiological reaction is typically considered to represent an increase in 'arousal', a hypothetical construct usually taken to mean the basic energetical state of an organism. There are important problems with this construct, but for the time being it is sufficient to note that various biochemical and psychophysiological measures have been proposed as indices of arousal. Selye's importance does not stem from this, however (he was by no means the first to observe and describe the phenomenon of physiological arousal, which can be traced back to Cannon's work in 1915).[6] Rather, Selye's influence comes from

---

Frequently used measures or indices of stress

Subjective: *Ratings and protocols of how the person feels, how well he believes he is doing. Confidence/anxiety reports.*

Behavioural: *Objective measures of performance change on 'real world' tasks or specialized performance tests, including computerized test batteries and instrumented flight simulators.*

**Psycho-
physiological:**   *Objective measures of variables such as heart rate, muscle tension, galvanic skin response (skin conductance), respiratory rate, etc.*

Biochemical: *Objective measures of neurotransmitters and their metabolites, e.g., serotonin, epinephrine, norepinephrine, dopamine.*

As we move down the list from subjective to biochemical measures, the techniques tend to become more and more intrusive, ultimately involving costly (and for potential volunteer subjects, intimidating) urinalysis and blood analysis. And yet it should not be assumed that progression toward ever more complex and intrusive techniques is in some sense more scientific, or brings us closer to measuring 'real stress'. Cognitive appraisal theorists might argue exactly the converse, in fact. Certainly, psychophysiological measures and biochemical measures sometimes do not correlate at all. Likewise there can be dissociation between psycho-physiological or biochemical measures and subjective measures of stress.

---

the way in which he associated arousal with the idea of 'stress', using a construct which he popularized with the term 'General Adaptation Syndrome', or GAS.[59] He referred to it as *general* because he believed it to represent a systemic, nonspecific reaction common to many different categories of stimulus. He regarded it as a form of *adaptation* to the extent that its function is to prepare the individual to respond to an external threat, presumably either by warding off the attack or escaping -- the so-called 'fight or flight' reaction.

However, Selye's description of the process as a *syndrome* (a term more commonly associated with pathology) hints at the fact that he did not regard it as universally adaptive. First, it is not without metabolic cost to the organism; in other words, it consumes energy. Second, it has been Selye's contention that repeated or long term activation of the arousal response can lead to depletion of the very neurochemicals and other physical resources that give rise to it in the first place. This will consequently leave the individual ill equipped to cope with further threats that arise. He or she may also become subject to feelings of exhaustion and, possibly, a compromised immune system with increased vulnerability to opportunistic diseases. While Selye's model of stress is no longer tenable (and we return to this later), these latter insights do seem to represent an important and enduring contribution to stress theory.

Nevertheless, following Selye's model, a good deal of empirical research on stress responses, not least in aviation, has assumed that physiological arousal is essentially a measure of psychological distress. This kind of approach is evident, for example, in much of the literature on air traffic controllers cited in Chapter 10.[48,62] Carlton Melton, a researcher at the Civil Aeromedical Institute of the US Federal Aviation Administration, has published several studies based on physiological monitoring, and summarizes his working view of stress as follows:

> 'Stress,' commonly called 'tension' by flight instructors, is difficult to define. The indicators of it are many ... usually a battery of measurements is employed, encompassing biochemical estimates of adrenomedullary, adrenocortical, and other glandular outputs into the blood and urine together with physiological appraisals of the condition of the nervous system as reflected in the heart rate, blood pressure, respiration, and skin resistance. Additional measurements sometimes employed include the electro-oculogram, electroencephalogram, and electromyogram.[49]

In the realm of flight, for example, putative 'stress related' endocrine effects observed include elevations in plasma phospholipids in Boeing 737 pilots facing a simulated birdstrike emergency,[61] heightened urinary catecholamine excretion in trainee fighter pilots[40] and in student pilots practicing spins,[41] elevated testosterone in F-16 fighter pilots during simulated emergencies,[75] and increased adrenalin output under conditions of emotional stress.[15] Other physical processes also show marked changes: increases in heart rate, for example, have been observed in combat pilots during takeoff and bombing runs,[45,55] in student pilots and helicopter pilots undergoing checkrides,[4,50] and in parachutists prior to jumps.[54,58] Similar elevations have been documented in respiration rate and skin conductance.[22]

The approach adopted in such studies has the cachet of objective, quantitative, 'hard' science. The difficulty, however, lies in deciding what it is that these various results actually tell us about flying or stress. After all, similar symptoms of adrenergic arousal (the adrenalin 'rush') are associated with exhilaration, illness, effort, keen anticipation, and sexual activity. (We would expect to find similar physiological changes in, for example, thrilled teenagers enjoying hectic fairground rides -- but we have not seen this, or, indeed, any equivalent control condition used in most aviation experiments!) Certainly, among stress theoreticians the (physiological) response based approach to stress has come under a good deal of criticism, insofar as it suffers from the same shortcomings as the stimulus based approach. Both tend to consider stress effects purely in terms of a simple stimulus-response or direct cause-and-effect relationship, essentially bypassing the role of the individual as a thinking, reflective, purposive, emotionally engaged participant in the process.[43]

In this sense both stimulus and response based approaches are curiously nonpsychological. They acknowledge little or no role for cognitive appraisal or mediation between stimulus and response. Neither view of stress has anything to say about the *perception* of threat, a perception presumably influenced by the individual's (or crew's) purposes, goals, and hypotheses about (and interpretations of) events in particular situational contexts. As a consequence, these approaches, although very widely used, in fact have very limited usefulness as conceptual frameworks for stress research in many military and civilian contexts, including many aspects of flight operations. British stress theorist Tom Cox[11] has pointed out that "from reading the popular literature on stress, the researcher believes that [a simple physiological index unarguably related to stress] exists." He adds, "alas, it is a myth borne out of hope rather than understanding" (p. 1155).

Transactional approaches

In recent years, a number of influential stress researchers have gone beyond stimulus and response based views to develop transactional models of stress.[13,23,47,77] This approach has, in fact, been described as a radical redirection in stress research.[14] Transactional models conceptualize stress as inhering neither in the person nor in the environment as such, but rather in the transaction between the two -- in the nature of the *encounter*, as Lazarus, an important theorist, has put it. These encounters have affective meaning because the individual has beliefs, goals, hopes, and fears, while the environment imports threats, challenges, opportunities, and risks. The process of evaluating these factors in the light of personal motivations or agendas lies at the core of the stress experience and of coping with stress. As Hamilton[30] has stated, "an event does not become a stressor until a cognitive processing system has identified it as such on the basis of existing long term memory data" (p. 117).

Transactional approaches, then, emphasize the role of cognitive appraisal in the human stress response. Rather than focussing exclusively either on precipitating factors (stimuli) or on responses to these factors, the concern is with the interpretation or appraisal of situations in terms of their demand and the individual's perception of his coping resources. Transactional models must, of course, recognize the importance of stimulus events and of physiological and behavioural responses, but in an important sense they are more 'psychological' than either of the two earlier approaches to stress, in that they acknowledge the subjective nature of stress and emphasize the mental processes which mediate the individual's reactions.

Transactional models have been used widely in studies of workplace stress, as well as in a range of 'high stress' contexts, from civil disasters and terrorism to surgery and skydiving.[2,9,20,37] Indeed, the transactional view represents an emerging consensus among psychologists specializing in such research.[12] However, the influence of this approach is only just beginning to be felt among aviation psychologists and human factors specialists, many of whom were schooled in the earlier stimulus or response based models of stress. As Hammond has recently pointed out in a comprehensive review of the literature on stress and judgement, human factors researchers have tended not to cite the stress literature from personality research, clinical studies, or social psychology; however, this is where most theoretical progress in the transactional approach has been made.[31]

Perhaps one reason that applied human factors research has lagged behind theoretical advances lies in the fact that transactional models of stress are more complex than their stimulus and response based predecessors, and are therefore more difficult to operationalize experimentally. It can be done, however, as is evident from such transactionally oriented stress research as does exist in the field of aviation. These include a series of simulation based experiments on pilot decision making conducted at the University of Illinois,[67-70] as well as a number of applied studies in the field of military operations. One of these, a joint Australian and Swedish study, examined cognitive appraisal and coping processes in the brief time before ejection from fast-jet fighters.[42] Another, a German Army study of stress in actual low altitude night helicopter operations, systematically evaluated on multiple dimensions three elements: the pilot, the situation, and the interaction between the two.[32] To provide an idea of the range of variables scrutinized, the physical and psychological parameters that the study examined within the three components of analysis are presented in Table 1.1.

Cognitive appraisal. As cognitive appraisal is an integral aspect of many transactional approaches to stress, a few words are in order concerning the nature of this process. Dylan Jones[38] has written that "the analysis of perceptions of ... stressful settings is potentially an extremely powerful one" (p. 72). The key word here is 'perceptions'. While one view of stress might be to consider it as resulting from a mismatch between the demands of a situation and the individual's ability to meet those demands, the notion of cognitive appraisal introduces the element of subjectivity. Within this framework, stress is viewed as the result of a mismatch between an individual's *perception* of the demands of the task or situation, and his *perception* of the resources he has to cope with them. What this means is that an individual who, for example, *over*estimates her resources (e.g. flying skill, fuel, time, altitude, and so forth), or *under*estimates the demands of the task (complexity, distance, etc.) will continue unstressed until something -- some feature of a deteriorating situation, say -- prompts a reevaluation of demand or resources. Likewise, an individual who either overestimates demand or underestimates his coping ability may respond negatively, irrespective of the 'objective' circumstances. Such an appraisal can result in feelings of helplessness and resignation in situations which could, in fact, be mastered. There is certainly evidence that such misperceptions can lead directly to stress and error in flight decision making:

> Analyses of aircraft accident and incident reports have shown that some cases of misjudgment by pilots after encountering nonroutine situations are clearly due to misassessment of the seriousness of the event. This misassessment can occur even when the nature of the event is correctly identified, and will frequently result in an incorrect course of action. Underassessment of potential consequences will result in failure to take timely or appropriate action. Overassessment of the consequences of an event, on the other hand, creates a strong situational stressor, often culminating in the rapid deterioration of judgment and performance.[60]

Edward Simmel and his colleagues give the example of a pilot whose aircraft suffered an alternator failure by night, leaving perhaps twenty min-

Table 1.1
The transactional approach as operationalized in a helicopter study
(adapted from Harss,[32] p. 6)

PERSONAL CHARACTERISTICS (independent variables)
　　　　Objective　　　　　　　　　　　　　　Subjective

PHYSICAL	PSYCHOLOGICAL (quasi-objective)	PSYCHOLOGICAL
EKG	Behaviour observation	Interviews
EMG	(experts)	Questionnaires
PGR	Achievement tests	Scales
Blood Pressure (Baselines)	Peer ratings	Self-evaluation

SITUATIONAL CHARACTERISTICS (independent variables)
　　　　Objective　　　　　　　　　　　　　　Subjective

PHYSICAL	PSYCHOLOGICAL (quasi-objective)	PSYCHOLOGICAL
Terrain	Expert ratings of difficulty	Individual perception Difficulty
Humidity	Controllability	Controllability
	Situation demands	Situation demands
	Coping possibilities	Coping possibilities
	etc.	etc.

INTER- (OR TRANS-) ACTION CHARACTERISTICS (dependent variables)
　　　　Objective　　　　　　　　　　　　　　Subjective

PHYSICAL	PSYCHOLOGICAL (quasi-objective)	PSYCHOLOGICAL
EKG	Observational	Stress/strain
EMG	stress data	Emotions
PGR	Behaviour	(anger, fear, etc.)
Blood Pressure	Calmness, etc.	Cognitions, etc.

EKG = electrocardiogram EMG = electromyogram

---

utes of battery power -- easily sufficient to fly to his well-lit destination airfield. Overestimating the situation, and underestimating the resources available to him, the stressed pilot attempted to land immediately on a short unlit runway beneath him -- and died in a fiery collision with trees at the far end of the runway.[60] An interesting parallel is evident in the fate of Air Illinois Flight 710 in 1983. This aircraft, too, suffered complete loss of generator power by night, and ended up flying on the battery. Initially the departure airport was close enough to make a safe return possible. This time, however, the pilot underestimated the seriousness of the situation and overestimated his ability to cope with it, electing to press on, through deteriorating weather, to the distant destination airport. Flying at low level in instrument weather by the light of a handheld flashlight, the pilot continued, with remarkable nonchalance, until the aircraft hit rising ground, killing all ten persons on board.[51]

A framework for considering such events is provided in the diagram in Figure 1.1, which presents a model of stress suggested by Cox and Mackay. In this model, the situation's actual demands, as well as the individual's actual capabilities, are each evaluated through the filter of perception and then compared against one another in the process of cognitive appraisal. An imbalance between the two perceptions results in stress, which itself can be analyzed in terms of various manifestations (e.g., psychological, physiological, cognitive, behavioural). While this model is more comprehensive than many, there are additional variables that researchers have identified as being relevant to the appraisal process. McGrath, for example, has defined stress in terms of *three* elements: perceived demand, perceived ability to cope, and perception of the importance of coping -- that is, the extent to which the demands of the situation threaten the goals or aspirations of the individual.[47] This makes intuitive sense: it seems unlikely that stress is proportional to the perceived mismatch between demand and capability irrespective of how critical that mismatch is. Even a modest imbalance may be very stressful if life is at stake, as in flying. Conversely, a profound skill deficit may be of little import if the situation is one in which the individual has no need or expectation of excelling (consider, for example, a beginning private pilot who, for the fun of it, attempts to fly a jet simulator).

Another variable that has been related to stress is uncertainty.[76] This may well constitute a significant fourth element in cognitive appraisal models since small demand/resource imbalances may also create stress through the increased uncertainty of the outcome where success is impor-

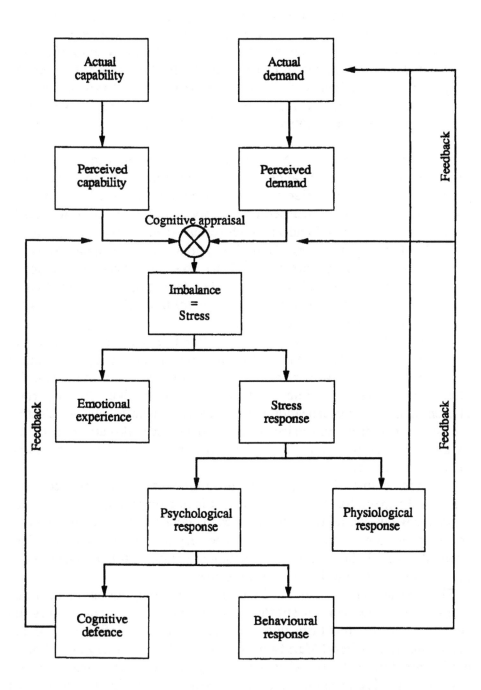

Figure 1.1 Transactional model of stress *(from Cox and Mackay[13])*

tant. Indeed, it seems likely that stress may also occur where ability to cope is perceived as positive but marginal, risks are perceived to be high, and success is therefore deemed to be vital (as in a low hour IFR pilot flying down to minimums in bad weather). By the same token, an ill-prepared flight student who is convinced that she will fail her ground school examination may actually experience less stress and anxiety than someone who has studied intensively but feels that success is a 'toss-up'.

Conservation of resources. S.E. Hobfoll has advanced a model of behaviour in stressful circumstances based on the notion of conservation of resources.[33] It, too, reflects a transactional approach, but it differs somewhat from those discussed previously, which focus predominantly upon cognitive appraisal and in which resources are viewed primarily as task related coping resources. Hobfoll's approach focusses upon losses, be they actual, potential, or threatened. Thus, stress is defined as "a reaction to the environment, in which there is either *(a)* the threat of a net loss of resources *(b)* the net loss of resources, or *(c)* the lack of resource gain following investment of resources" (p. 25).

The resources referred to here are defined very broadly -- financial resources, security, affection, reputation -- in fact, almost anything valued by an individual. However, resources also include all of the means for attaining these assets -- time, skills, power, and the like. An important element in this conceptualization is summarized in item *(c)* above. That is, the notion that stress may arise not via actual or even threatened loss, but by a simple failure to gain despite the investment of perhaps substantial personal resources.

Given the nature of flying and flight training (expensive, time consuming, highly specialized, and so forth), it is not surprising that there are various obvious and all too real instances of 'failure to gain' in aviation. A friend of the authors, for example, became very distressed when, after four years of costly flight training, the aviation job market all but collapsed and her next most saleable skill was as a waitress.

Time, effort, and money are by no means the only losses in such circumstances, however. A subtler feature of this stress reaction is the component of loss that turns upon self esteem and self definition. As the pioneering aviator Beryl Markham[46] pointed out half a century ago, "for all professional pilots there exists a kind of guild, without charter [or] by-laws" (p. 11). Expulsion from this privileged society or 'guild' has its own psychological trauma: the loss or threatened loss of personal identity that can be entailed in such circumstances can be highly stressful.[21,33] Both unemployed pilots and unemployed (fired) air traffic controllers, for example, report embarrassment, shame, and feelings of worthlessness and uselessness.[26] Medically grounded aviators sometimes exhibit symptoms of outright grief, while others, especially younger males, sometimes even equate the loss of flight status with loss of virility.[25]

Another feature of Hobfoll's approach is that it specifies the positive behaviours of the stressed individual. That is, it recognizes not only that coping strategies come into play when the individual is faced with the loss or potential loss of resources, but also defines the general direction of those strategies: the individual will attempt to conserve resources, minimizing overall loss and maximizing overall gain, by investing further resources. This entails a particular action sequence which may or may not succeed. For example, the waitress-aviator could endure poverty for two years, saving her money for more advanced flight training, or she might sacrifice her weekends to 'build hours' flying a glider tug. Hobfoll even gives an example of 'spending' some personal pride by pleading with parents for financial help.

Anxiety

The phenomenon of anxiety has been mentioned several times in the preceding discussion, generally in conjunction with references to stress. Perhaps a few words are in order concerning the relationship between these two phenomena. Some theorists have tended to use the words 'stress' and 'anxiety' more or less interchangeably,[64] while others have, as noted previously, debated as to whether anxiety constitutes a cause of stress, an effect of stress, or, perhaps, a form or manifestation of stress.

Anxiety is not so much a reaction to an actual, present danger as an *expectation* of harm, the source of which may be real or imagined. One text on the subject[3] characterizes anxiety as an "intense dread and foreboding, conceptualized as internally derived and unrelated to external threat" (p. 3). This view originated with Freud, who further defined anxiety as having both a psychological and a physiological component, the latter consisting of what has been called arousal.[24]

This bipartite model (nonspecific feelings of apprehension combined with physiological arousal) is still accepted by many modern psychologists,[64] and is also reflected in the lay definition offered by *Webster's*

Dictionary: "an abnormal and overwhelming sense of apprehension and fear often marked by physiological signs (as sweating, tension, and increased pulse)".

State and trait

All of the descriptions given above refer to anxiety as a transitory condition, one which varies in intensity from one point in time to another, depending on the individual's perceptions of the external circumstances. In recent decades, however, the term has also been used to describe a more stable and enduring personality characteristic. The first type of anxiety is known as state anxiety, or A-State, while the second is referred to as trait anxiety, or A-Trait. Charles Spielberger, a noted anxiety researcher at the University of South Florida, has suggested that the failure to distinguish between these two types of anxiety has resulted in much conceptual and empirical confusion in research on the subject.[63-65] Moreover, since many studies of pilots and controllers referred to in later chapters distinguish between state and trait anxiety, it will be useful to clarify these terms here.

The concepts of state and trait anxiety were first introduced in the late 1950s by Cattell and Scheier, who identified them as separate phenomena based on an review of multivariate analyses of anxiety factors.[7,8] The distinction was further developed by Spielberger,[63] who has summarized the two types as follows:

> Anxiety is perhaps most commonly used in an empirical sense to denote a complex reaction or response -- a transitory state or condition of the organism that varies in intensity and fluctuates over time. But the term anxiety is also used to refer to a personality trait -- to individual differences in the extent to which people are characterized by anxiety states and by prominent defenses against such states. (p. 12)

In other words, state anxiety can be defined as an emotional reaction to a specific, perceived threat. As it is marked by autonomic nervous system activity coupled with negative affect (tension, apprehension, nervousness), its presence is determined both by self report and by physiological measures of, for example, heart rate, blood pressure, and galvanic skin response. It is the type of reaction most commonly associated with the word 'anxiety' (see, for example, the dictionary definition given above). State anxiety is by its nature a transitory, acute condition.

Trait anxiety, in contrast, can be described as chronic. Because this kind of anxiety is not a reaction to specific external circumstances, it tends not to fluctuate over time. Rather, it represents a stable, relatively un-changing personality characteristic. This is not to suggest that individuals with high levels of trait anxiety go through life in a permanent state of unbearable dread; rather, as Spielberger[65] puts it, "A-Trait dispositions are reactive and remain latent until activated by the stress associated with a specific danger situation" (p. 136). In other words, the trait anxious person is more likely both to perceive a given situation as threatening, and to react to this apparent threat with higher levels of state anxiety. Trait anxiety has also been described simply as 'anxiety proneness' and as 'the tendency to respond with A-State under stress'.[17]

In fact, it would be more accurate to define trait anxiety as 'the tendency to respond with A-State *under some kinds of stress*'. Research in this area has particularly focussed on two distinct categories of threat: concrete physical dangers, and what are sometimes referred to as ego threatening conditions: that is, situations involving social risk, the possibility of per-sonal failure, or damage to self esteem. Response to physical threat is largely unaffected by the presence or absence of trait anxiety.[1,66] For example, experiments involving the threat of electric shocks have, not surprisingly, been shown to increase state anxiety, but these changes do not correlate with the levels of trait anxiety observed in the test subjects.[35,36,39] However, so-called ego threatening conditions have typically been found to elicit higher levels of state anxiety in individuals who are trait anxious than in those who are not.[34,52,53]

Some variation has been observed in this pattern, possibly occasioned by differences between the various personality tests used to assess trait anxie-ty.[17] Most studies have used either the Taylor Manifest Anxiety Scale[73] or Spielberger's State-Trait Anxiety Inventory[66] to identify trait anxious sub-jects. However, one study that used the somewhat more elaborate S-R Inventory of Anxiousness[18] found no consistent differences in the reactions of high and low trait anxious subjects either to physical or to ego threats.[19] In evaluating the many stress studies in aviation that have used the state and trait constructs it is obviously important to bear these findings in mind.

Summary

Three broad approaches to stress have been discussed here: stimulus based, response based, and transactional models. The stimulus based approach has had a long history within aviation psychology and in laboratory and performance research, and has served to highlight the role of external (usually aversive) factors such as vibration, heat, high G, and so forth in pilot performance. Nevertheless, the emphasis on stimuli has become an overemphasis, a preoccupation with external conditions, with 'stressors' presumed to effect 'strain' in the individual -- in any individual, at any time. The list of putative stressors grows ever longer, with factors such as time pressure, life events, and workload drawn in and subsumed under the same general model. This model is inadequate, disregarding as it does the human being for whom the events have meaning. External events or conditions can represent either opportunities or threats, challenges or obstacles, and to ignore the crucial role of human appraisal of these events or conditions is to impoverish the concept of stress and to hamstring the operational usefulness and generalizability of much research right from the outset.

The response based approach to stress warrants similar criticism. It, too, has been a very popular model in aviation research, especially in operational or field studies. The response based model has most often manifested itself as the physiological monitoring of individuals during various activities. There are serious limitations inherent in defining stress soley in terms of heart rate, catecholamine excretion, galvanic skin response, or any other psychophysiological or biochemical function -- not least because such variables need not co-vary, and may actually be associated with a wide range of affective states, both positive and negative. (Chapter 2 will address in more detail the traditional confusion between stress and arousal.) Physiology aside, to define 'stress' solely in terms of a general set of effects or responses is to ignore both the circumstances that elicit the responses and the person who experiences them.

Transactional views -- in particular, cognitive appraisal models -- represent a more insightful and, in general, more psychologically oriented way of looking at stress. Rather than focussing exclusively either on supposed causes or effects of 'stress', such models view stress as a function of the interrelationship between external circumstances and human reactions to them. This kind of approach permits a more substantive consideration of such issues as individual differences in stress reactions. It also provides better conceptual clarity for assessing the interactions (and distinctions) between stress, arousal, and workload; the role of fatigue and sleep deprivation; the differing effects of acute situational stressors, minor but iterative daily 'hassles', and traumatic life events; and responses to physical versus social 'threats'.

References

1. Auerbach, S.M. (1973), 'Trait-state anxiety and adjustment to surgery', *Journal of Consulting and Clinical Psychology,* vol. 40, pp. 264-71.

2. Ayalon, O. (1983), 'Coping with Terrorism: The Israeli Case', in Meichenbaum, D. and Jaremko, M.E. (eds.), *Stress Reduction and Prevention,* Plenum, New York.

3. Basowitz, H., Persky, H., Korchin, S.J., and Grinker, R.R. (1955), *Anxiety and Stress,* McGraw-Hill, New York.

4. Billings, C.E., Gerke, R.J., Chase, R.C., and Eggspuehler, J.J. (1973), 'Stress and strain in student helicopter pilots', *Aerospace Medicine,* vol. 44, pp. 1031-5.

5. Campbell, R.D., and Bagshaw, M. (1991), *Human Performance Limitations in Aviation,* BSP Professional Books, Oxford.

6. Cannon, W.B. (1915), *Bodily Changes in Pain, Hunger, Fear, and Rage,* Appleton, New York.

7. Cattell, R.B., and Scheier, I.H. (1958), 'The nature of anxiety: a review of 13 multivariate analyses containing 814 variables', *Psychological Reports,* Monograph Supplement, vol. 5, pp. 351-88.

8. Cattell, R.B., and Scheier, I.H. (1961), *The Meaning and Measurement of Neuroticism and Anxiety,* Ronald, New York.

9. Cohen, R.E., and Ahearn, F.L., Jr. (1980), *Handbook for Mental Health Care of Disaster Victims,* Johns Hopkins University Press, Baltimore.

10. Cox, T. (1978), *Stress,* Macmillan, London.

11. Cox, T. (1985), 'The nature and measurement of stress', *Ergonomics,* vol. 28, pp. 1155-63.

12. Cox, T. (1987), 'Stress, coping and problem solving', *Work and Stress,* vol. 1, pp. 5-14.

13. Cox, T., and Mackay, C. (1976), 'A Psychological Model of Occupational Stress', paper presented to the Medical Research Council meeting, 'Mental Health in Industry', London, November.

14. Coyne, J.C., and Lazarus, R.S. (1980), 'Cognitive Style, Stress Perception, and Coping', in Kutash, I.L., Schlesinger, L.B., and Associates (eds.), *Handbook on Stress and Anxiety,* San Francisco, Jossey-Bass, pp. 144-58.

15. Debijadji, R., Perovic, L., and Varagic, V. (1970), 'Evaluation of the sympatho-adrenals activity in pilots by determination of urinary catecholamines during supersonic flight', *Aerospace Medicine,* vol. 41, pp. 677-9.

16. Elliott, G.R., and Eisdorfer, C. (1982), 'Conceptual Issues in Stress Research', in Elliott, G.R. and Eisdorfer, C. (eds.), *Stress and Human Health: Analysis and Implications of Research,* Springer, New York.

17. Endler, N.S. (1975), 'A Person-Situation Interaction Model for Anxiety', in Spielberger, C.D. and Sarason, I.G. (eds.), *Stress and Anxiety,* vol. 1, John Wiley & Sons, New York.

18. Endler, N.S., Hunt, J. McV., and Rosenstein, A.J. (1962), 'An S-R inventory of anxiousness', *Psychological Monographs,* vol. 76, (17, whole no. 536), pp. 1-33.

19. Endler, N.S., and Shedletsky, R., (1973), 'Trait versus state anxiety, authoritarianism, and ego threat versus physical threat', *Canadian Journal of Behavioural Science,* vol. 5, pp. 347-61.

20. Epstein, S. (1983), 'Natural Healing Processes of the Mind: Graded Stress Inoculation as an Inherent Coping Mechanism', in Meichenbaum, D. and Jaremko, M.E. (eds.), *Stress Reduction and Prevention,* Plenum, New York.

21. Erikson, E.H. (1968), *Identity: Youth and Crisis,* Norton Press, New York.

22. Fenz, W.D., and Epstein, S. (1967), 'Gradients of physiological arousal in parachutists as a function of an approaching jump', *Psychosomatic Medicine,* vol. 29, pp. 33-51.

23. Fisher, S. (1983), 'Memory and search in loud noise', *Canadian Journal of Psychology,* vol. 37, pp. 439-49.

24. Freud, S. (1936), *The Problem of Anxiety,* Norton, New York.

25. Geeze, D.S. (1987), 'Grief in the grounded aviator', *Aviation, Space, and Environmental Medicine,* vol. 58, pp. 799-801.

26. Girodo, M. (1988), 'The psychological health and stress of pilots in a labor dispute', *Aviation, Space, and Environmental Medicine,* vol. 59, pp. 505-10.

27. Glass, D.C., and Singer, J.E. (1972), *Urban Stress: Experiments on Noise and Social Stressors,* Academic Press, New York.

28. Grinker, R.R., and Spiegel, J.P. (1945), *Men Under Stress,* McGraw-Hill, New York.

29. Hamilton, V. (1980), 'An Information Processing Analysis of Environmental Stress and Life Crises', in Sarason, I.G. and Spielberger, C.D. (eds.), *Stress and Anxiety,* vol. 7, Hemisphere Publishing Corporation, New York.

30. Hamilton, V. (1982), 'Cognition and Stress: An Information Processing Model', in Goldberger, L. and Breznitz, S. (eds.), *Handbook of Stress: Theoretical and Clinical Aspects,* Free Press, New York, pp. 105-20.

31. Hammond, K. (1990), *The Effects of Stress on Judgment and Decision Making: An Overview and Arguments for a New Approach,* University of Colorado, Boulder.

32. Harss, C., Kastner, M., and Beerman, L. (1991), 'Personality, Task Characteristics, and Helicopter Pilot Stress', in Farmer, E. (ed.), *Stress and Error in Aviation,* Avebury Technical, Aldershot, Hants.

33. Hobfoll, S.E. (1988), *The Ecology of Stress,* Hemisphere Publishing Corporation, New York.

34. Hodges, W.F. (1968), 'Effects of ego threat and threat of pain on state anxiety', *Journal of Personality and Social Psychology,* vol. 8, pp. 364-72.

35. Hodges, W.F., and Spielberger, C.D. (1966), 'The effects of threat of shock on heart rate for subjects who differ in manifest anxiety and fear of shock', *Psychophysiology,* vol. 2, pp. 287-94.

36. Hodges, W.F., and Spielberger, C.D. (1969), 'Digit span: an indicant of trait or state anxiety?' *Journal of Consulting and Clinical Psychology,* vol. 33, pp. 430-4.

37. Janis, I. (1983), 'Stress Inoculation in Health Care: Theory and Research', in Meichenbaum, D. and Jaremko, M.E. (eds.), *Stress Reduction and Prevention,* Plenum, New York.

38. Jones, D.M. (1991), 'Stress and Workload: Models, Methodologies and Remedies', in Farmer, E. (ed.), *Stress and Error in Aviation,* Avebury Technical, Aldershot, Hants.

39. Katkin, E.S. (1965), 'The relationship between manifest anxiety and two indices of autonomic response to stress', *Journal of Personality and Social Psychology,* vol. 2, pp. 324-33.

40. Krahenbuhl, G.S., Marett, J.R., and King, N.W. (1977), 'Catecholamine excretion in T-37 flight training', *Aviation, Space, and Environmental Medicine,* vol. 48, pp. 405-8.

41. Krahenbuhl, G.S., Marett, J.R., and Reid, G.B. (1978), 'Task-specific simulator pretraining and in-flight stress of student pilots', *Aviation, Space, and Environmental Medicine,* vol. 49, pp. 1107-10.

42. Larsson, G., and Hayward, B. (1990), 'Appraisal and coping processes immediately before ejection: a study of Australian and Swedish pilots', *Military Psychology,* vol. 2, pp. 63-78.

43. Lazarus, R.S., DeLongis, A., Folkman, S., and Gruen, R. (1985), 'Stress and adaptational outcomes: the problem of confounded measures', *American Psychologist,* vol. 40, pp. 770-9.

44. Lazarus, R.S., and Folkman, S. (1984), *Stress, Appraisal, and Coping',* Springer, New York.

45. Lewis, C.E., Jones, W.L., Austin, F., and Roman, J. (1967), 'Flight research program: IX. Medical monitoring of carrier pilots in combat -- II. *Aerospace Medicine,* vol. 38, pp. 581-92.

46. Markham, B. (1942), *West with the Night,* Houghton Mifflin, Boston.

47. McGrath, J.E. (1976), 'Stress and Behaviour in Organizations' in Dunnette, M.D. (ed.), *Handbook of Industrial and Organizational Psychology,* Rand-McNally, Chicago.

48. Melton, C.E. (1982), *Physiological Stress in Air Traffic Controllers: A Review,* FAA Office of Aviation Medicine Report No. AM-82-17.

49. Melton, C.E., McKenzie, J.M., Kelln, J.R., Hoffmann, S.M., and Saldivar, J.T. (1975), 'Effect of a general aviation trainer on the stress of flight training', *Aviation, Space, and Environmental Medicine,* vol 46, pp. 1-5.

50. Melton, C.E., and Wicks, S.M. (1967), *In-Flight Physiological Monitoring of Student Pilots,* FAA Office of Aviation Medicine Report AM-67-15.

51. National Transportation Safety Board (1983), *Aircraft Accident Report: Air Illinois Hawker Siddley HS 748-2A, N748LL near Pinckneyville, Illinois, October 11, 1983,* National Technical Information Service, Springfield, Virginia.

52. O'Neil, J.F., Spielberger, C.D., and Hansen, D.N. (1969), 'The effects of state anxiety and task difficulty on computer-assisted learning', *Journal of Educational Psychology*, vol. 60, pp. 343-50.

53. Rappaport, H., and Katkin, E.S. (1972), 'Relationships among manifest anxiety, response to stress, and the perception of autonomic activity', *Journal of Consulting and Clinical Psychology*, vol. 38, pp. 219-24.

54. Reid, D.H., Doerr, J.E., Doshier, H.D., and Ellerton, D.G. (1971), 'Heart rate and respiration rate response to parachuting: physiological studies of military parachutists via FM/AM telemetry -- II', *Aerospace Medicine*, vol. 42, pp. 1200-7.

55. Roman, J., Older, H., and Jones, W.L. (1967), 'Flight research program: VII. Medical monitoring of navy carrier pilots in combat', *Aerospace Medicine*, vol. 38, pp. 133-9.

56. Rose, R.M. (1980), 'Endocrine responses to stressful psychological events', *Advances in Psychoneuroendocrinology*, vol. 3, pp. 251-76.

57. Sanders, A.F. (1983), 'Towards a model of stress and human performance', *Acta Psychologica*, vol. 53, pp. 61-97.

58. Schane, W.P., and Slinde, K.E. (1968), 'Continuous ECG monitoring on civil air crews during free-fall parachuting', *Aerospace Medicine*, vol. 39, pp. 597-603.

59. Selye, H. (1956), *The Stress of Life*, McGraw-Hill, New York.

60. Simmel, E.C., Cerkovnik, M., and McCarthy, J.E. (1987), 'Sources of Stress Affecting Pilot Judgment', *Proceedings of the Fourth International Symposium on Aviation Psychology*, Ohio State University, Columbus.

61. Sive, W.J., and Hattingh, J. (1991), 'The measurement of psychophysiological reactions of pilots to a stressor in a flight simulator', *Aviation, Space, and Environmental Medicine*, vol. 62, pp. 831-6.

62. Smith, R.C. (1980), *Stress, Anxiety, and the Air Traffic Control Specialist: Some Conclusions from a Decade of Research*, FAA Office of Aviation Medicine Report No. FAA-AM-80-14.

63. Spielberger, C.D. (1966), 'Theory and Research on Anxiety', in Spielberger, C.D. (ed.), *Anxiety and Behavior*, Academic Press, New York.

64. Spielberger, C.D. (1972), 'Anxiety as an Emotional State', in Spielberger, C.D. (ed.), *Anxiety: Current Trends in Theory and Research*, vol. 1, Academic Press, New York.

65. Spielberger, C.D. (1975), 'Anxiety: State-Trait Processes', in Spielberger, C.D. and Sarason, I.G. (eds.), *Stress and Anxiety*, vol. 1, John Wiley & Sons, New York.

66. Spielberger, C.D., Gorsuch, R.L., and Lushene, R.E. (1970), *Manual for the State-Trait Anxiety Inventory*, Consulting Psychologists Press, Palo Alto, California.

67. Stokes, A.F., Barnett, B., and Wickens, C.D. (1987), 'Modeling Stress and Bias in Pilot Decision Making', *Proceedings of the Human Factors Association of Canada XXth Annual Conference*, pp. 45-8.

68. Stokes, A.F., Belger, A., and Zhang, K. (1990), *Investigation of Factors Comprising a Model of Pilot Decision Making, Part II: Anxiety and Cognitive Strategies in Expert and Novice Aviators*, University of Illinois Aviation Research Laboratory, Urbana-Champaign.

69. Stokes, A.F., Kemper, K.L., and Marsh, R. (1992), *Time-Stressed Flight Decision Making: A Study of Expert and Novice Aviators*, University of Illinois Aviation Research Laboratory, Urbana-Champaign.

70. Stokes, A.F., and Raby, M. (1989), 'Stress and Cognitive Performance in Trainee Pilots', *Proceedings of the Human Factors Society 33rd Annual Meeting*, Human Factors Society, Santa Monica, CA.

71. Strelau, J. (1989), 'Individual Differences in Tolerance to Stress: The Role of Reactivity', in Spielberger, C.D., Sarason, I.G., and Strelau, J. (eds.), *Stress and Anxiety*, vol. 12, Hemisphere Publishing Corporation, New York.

72. Symonds, C., cited in Cox, T. (1978).

73. Taylor, J.A. (1953), 'A personality scale of manifest anxiety', *Journal of Abnormal Psychology*, vol. 48, pp. 285-90.

74. Toffler, A.W. (1970), *Future Shock*, Random House, New York.

75. Vaernes, R.J., Warncke, M., Myhre, G., and Aakvaag, A. (1988), 'Stress and Performance During a Simulated Flight in an F-16 Simulator', in AGARD Conference Proceedings No. 458, *Human Behaviour in High Stress Situations in Aerospace Operations*, NATO, Neuilly-sur-Seine, France.

76. Warburton, D. (1979), 'Physiological Aspects of Information Processing and Stress', in Hamilton, V. and Warburton, D. (eds.), *Human Stress and Cognition*, John Wiley & Sons, New York.

77. Welford, A.T. (1973), 'Stress and performance', *Ergonomics*, vol. 15, pp. 567-80.

78. Yerkes, R.M., and Dodson, J.D. (1908), 'The relation of strength of stimulus to rapidity of habit-formation', *Journal of Comparative and Neurological Psychology*, vol. 18, pp. 459-82.

2 Stress and arousal

Stress usually signifies something unpleasant and, when associated with flying, tends to imply danger.
-- Alan Roscoe,[25] *Stress and Workload in Pilots*

Accidents are caused by lack of stress, as well.
-- Aircraft Owners and Pilots Association, *Stress and the Pilot*

Notwithstanding the second epigraph cited above, we do not usually think of accidents as being caused by an *absence* of stress, much less by insufficient amounts of 'danger' or 'unpleasantness'. What is apparently meant by AOPA's remark is that accidents can stem from a lack of alertness, attention, or arousal. The concepts of stress, arousal, and performance will arise repeatedly in the following chapters, and it would be a mistake to proceed as though the relationships between these often vague categories were somehow intuitive or obvious. Indeed, the aviation literature abounds with curious statements like the one above, which seem to require explanation rather than providing it.

Such statements are hardly confined to aviation, however. Indeed, it is fair to say that the general scientific literature concerning the relationships between stress, arousal, and performance has for the last ninety years been a confusing conceptual and terminological quicksand, with merging, overlapping, and intermingling notions of aversion, stimulation, drive, motivation, arousal, anxiety, and stress. Many of these concepts have also changed subtly over time with theories or fashions in psychology. Terms such as motivation, arousal, and stress are sometimes used interchangeably, as though one were tantamount to the other. The upshot of this is that, rather than clarifying (or at least stating the limits of) our knowledge of stress and performance, too much of the literature on aviation psychology (and virtually all popularized accounts in flying journals) merely perpetuates certain received notions of stress, arousal, and performance that are simplistic and misleading at best. There is no more important an example of this than the unquestioned dominance of the 'inverted U' curve representation of stress effects on performance.

The ubiquitous 'U'

There is scarcely a text on aviation human factors -- indeed, hardly a discussion of stress and performance in any context -- that does not reprint some version of the famous 'inverted U' curve graph plotting the claimed relationship between stress and performance. An important insight said to be expressed in such graphs is that while high levels of stress are bad for performance, so are low levels of stress (equally so, in some symmetrical versions of the graph). In other words, the central claim derived from 'inverted U' theory is that intermediate or moderate levels of stress result in the best performance.

The nature of that performance is not generally made explicit, and the reader is usually left to guess as to whether it refers equally to aircraft control, cockpit resource management, planning and risk analysis, fault diagnosis, map reading, weapons delivery, or any of the other myriad functions that can make up a pilot's job. Moreover, many commentators appear to be undaunted by the fact that there is little or no evidence that the performance of any of these tasks really is optimal under moderate levels of 'real world' stress. Brecke,[2] for example, writing on aircrew judgement and decision making, asserts (without supporting data) that "stress will affect judgment performance in a non-linear fashion: *positively* up to an individual maximum and negatively beyond that" (p. 954).

Some versions of the U curve are rather idiosyncratic. For example, Thomas, in his book *Managing Pilot Stress,* divides his symmetrical version of the curve (Figure 2.1) into two mirror image lobes, labeled "positive stress" on the left and "negative stress" on the right.[30] This modification effectively adds the puzzling claim that pilot performance does not immediately deteriorate but rather continues at its highest level when 'positive stress' suddenly switches to 'negative stress'. Figure 2.2 reproduces a version of the U diagram as it appeared in a paper entitled "Stress for success: how to optimize your performance".[6] The title of the paper itself implies that stress (like business suits and country club memberships, perhaps) may be a positive career asset, while the diagram goes so far as to posit (among other things) fatal consequences from too little stress!

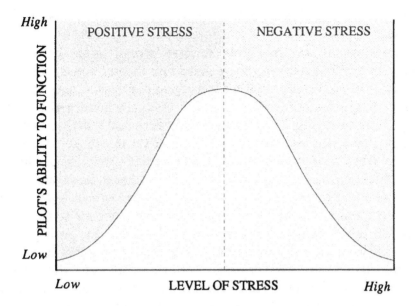

Figure 2.1 Positive and negative stress *(from Thomas,[30] p. 31)*

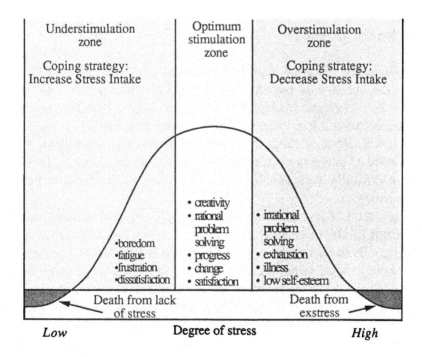

Figure 2.2 Stress and performance *(from Gmelch,[6] p. 11)*

Even disregarding individual eccentricities, the central claim derived from these graphs does not seem to comport with intuition, everyday experience, or the way in which the term 'stress' is used in ordinary speech. As the first epigraph that opened this chapter noted, "to the man in the street stress usually signifies something unpleasant, and, in the case of flying, dangerous" (Roscoe,[25] p. 630). Certainly pilots and controllers don't go around saying, "I've had a bad week: wasn't stressed enough". Similarly, those who use the inverted U diagram to counsel in favour of moderate stress do so only in theoretical terms and rarely explain how this is to be operationalized in practice. As far as we know, not a single author goes on to recommend (in the interest of optimal human performance) *moderately* strained employee-management relations for air traffic controllers, *mildly* upsetting preflight arguments for aircrew, or, perhaps, *somewhat* bothersome aircraft unreliability. The fact that, in this context, it is impossible to cite some quite probable 'real world' stressors without sounding tongue-in-cheek should alert us to the fact that something is not right. The oddity of the claim that moderate levels of stress are beneficial should pique our interest in the nature and origin of the claim.

Stress versus arousal

The inverted U diagram emerged from experiments performed near the turn of the century by two American psychologists referred to briefly in Chapter 1, Yerkes and Dodson[32] (see sidebar on p. 37). Over the intervening nine decades it has been widely accepted as a model for performance under stress, albeit without the benefit of much critical scrutiny.[10] Indeed, the inverted U curve is even referred to as the Yerkes-Dodson *Law* and has become virtually an iconic symbol for stress, as the front cover of this book testifies.

In fact, the U curve idealized from the original Yerkes and Dodson data relates not to stress at all, but to arousal, a very different hypothetical construct. Even where the inverted U graph is labelled and presented as a claim about arousal rather than stress (e.g., in Figure 2.3), there frequently follows 'slippage' in the interpretation and conclusions reached. This can be seen, for example, in a recent book on human performance in aviation: the familiar U graph appears with the X axis labelled 'arousal' (Figure 2.4); however, on the same page the authors extrapolate from this that "an optimum amount of *stress* is needed for us to function efficiently in flying

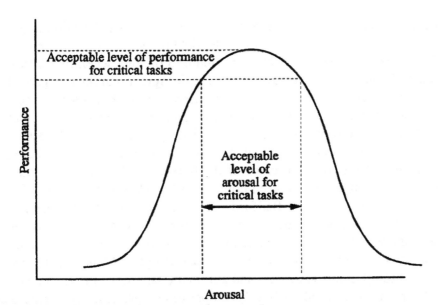

Figure 2.3 A hypothetical relationship between arousal and performance after Yerkes et al. *(from Hawkins,[9] p. 35)*

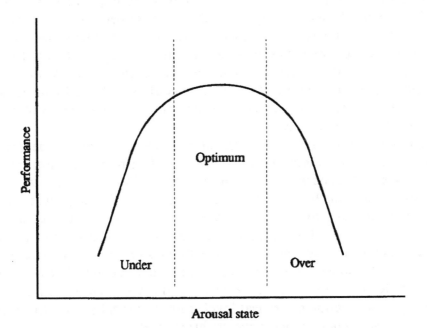

Figure 2.4 Performance and arousal *(from Campbell and Bagshaw,[3] p. 106)*

operations" (Campbell and Bagshaw,[3] p. 106). Similar transitions can be found in a number of other works in the field of aviation human factors.

What we are seeing, in fact, is a tribute to the overwhelming influence of Hans Selye's biochemical/psychophysiological response approach to stress,[27] an influence which has even filtered through academia and into business journals, pilot advisory circulars, and other professional aviation literature. Arousal has come to be regarded by many as all but a synonym for stress. It is, of course, no such thing: the former is far from being an adequate and accurate indicator of the latter. Evidence for this may be seen, for example, in research conducted by Alan Roscoe at the Royal Aircraft Establishment in Bedford. Roscoe selected what is perhaps the most widely used physiological measure in stress research -- heart rate -- and monitored this variable in pilots performing a variety of demanding flight tasks, including ramp takeoffs in Harrier fighter bombers, supersonic flights through monsoon rains, and automatic landings in fog. As expected, heart rate increased during these operations, particularly during busy periods such as the landing phase. This was not in itself a novel finding; however, Roscoe also sought to determine whether this effect arose from tension and anxiety concerning the outcome of the flight, or simply from the high demands placed on the pilot during these periods. He therefore collected data not only on the pilots who actually manipulated the controls but on those who were merely observing, the assumption being that the latter group would experience emotional involvement but not workload effects. His conclusion was that while arousal, as indexed by heart rate, did correlate with cockpit workload, it was not an accurate index of actual emotional stress or anxiety.[25]

Another indication that stress and arousal are not identical phenomena can be seen in the observation that humans often find some low arousal conditions such as boredom and sensory deprivation* very unpleasant and aversive; they usually try to avoid such conditions. Equally, a wide variety of high arousal activities are regarded as pleasant and desirable, and are actively sought out. These observations have been systematized in a model of the relationship between arousal and stress proposed by Michael Apter of University College, Cardiff, who suggests that individuals have a preferred state of arousal at any given time.[1] In this view, stress does not vary directly as a function of arousal level; rather, it results when the actual level of arousal does not match the preferred level.

---

*The removal of almost all external sensory stimuli by, for example, being placed in blacked out conditions, in total silence, in water at body temperature.

Of Mice and Men: Yerkes, Dodson and the Inverted U Curve

It is no fault of Yerkes and Dodson that their experimental findings have been overgeneralized by subsequent researchers. This is what their study did and did not do. First, it did not use humans, but mice. Second, it was a study of simple mouse learning, not of complex multitask cognitive performance appropriate to flight decks or air traffic control. Third, the experimenters did not measure stress or even arousal in the mice, but merely administered electric shocks at five different strengths. (It is not even known how different, as the shocks were poorly calibrated.) Subsequently a one-for-one correspondence in changes in the animals' arousal level has simply been inferred. The shape of the U curve reflects this assumption.

The mice had to learn to discriminate a white from a black passageway. Traversing the black one earned an electric shock. 'Performance', the vertical axis of the inverted U graph in Figure 2.5 (overleaf), actually represents the number of attempts the mice made before they learned not to venture down dark alleys. The values for 'stress' (or arousal), the horizontal axis in Figure 2.5, were not derived from any direct assessment of the animals themselves, but simply reflected the varying strengths of the electric shocks.

It was found that the most rapid learning occurred at shock intensities other than the highest and lowest levels. This finding was to metamorphose into the first and most reported Yerkes-Dodson principle, that performance is best at some optimum level of stress. A second finding was that the more difficult the discrimination task, the lower was the optimal level of shock: that is, as the animals were confronted with increasingly difficult discriminations, shocks of lower and lower intensity produced the fastest learning. This became the second Yerkes-Dodson principle: that the optimum level of stress is inversely related to the difficulty of the task.

Hancock and Scallen[7] have reviewed the original Yerkes-Dodson experiments and point out a significant number of flaws. In addition to methodological inadequacies, they also note that subsequent attempts to replicate the Yerkes-Dodson results (for example, with chickens and kittens[4,5]) were largely unsuccessful. Another researcher, Rob Neiss[22] has reviewed a large number of studies of arousal and human performance, many of which also used electric shock as the stressor. However, no studies were found which provided clear support for the inverted U hypothesis, and many actually contradicted it. "Current support for the inverted-U hypothesis," Neiss has concluded, "is psychologically trivial" (p. 353).

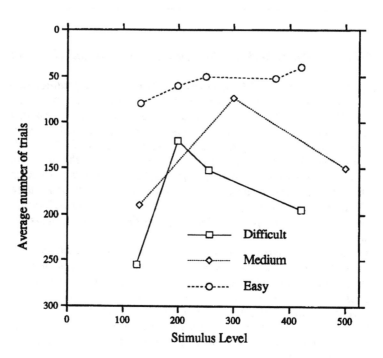

Figure 2.5 Original Yerkes and Dodson data *(from Hancock and Scallen,[7] p. 65)*

Thus, stress can be experienced in both low and high arousal states. The theory specifies the circumstances under which an individual will be stressed by invoking the concept of two different motivational states. One (which Apter terms the 'telic' state, but which we might call 'wanting a bit of peace and quiet') is characterized by the avoidance of arousal: thus, in this state low arousal is experienced as pleasant relaxation, while high arousal is experienced as tension and anxiety. However, in the opposite state (the 'paratelic' state, or 'wanting kicks, a bit of action, etc.'), high arousal is actively sought and is experienced as pleasant excitement, while low arousal is experienced as boring or unpleasant. (The issues of underarousal, stress, and boredom are discussed further in Chapter 12.)

If more evidence were needed that arousal and stress are not synonymous, one could cite the fact that physiological or visceral cues are meaningless until interpreted in the light of psychological expectations. An anecdotal example of this is provided by one of the authors, who, en route to demonstrate a flight simulator to Federal Aviation Administration officials, noticed an increase in heart rate and began to feel somewhat clammy and shaky. Mildly perplexed, this moderately intrepid aviator ascribed these symptoms to stage fright or to unaccustomed preflight nerves. However, over the course of the day the symptoms developed into an impressive bout of influenza, occasioning a reappraisal of what had initially been taken as somatic symptoms of anxiety.

Melton[21] has asserted that "like fatigue or pain, stress leaves no doubt in a person's mind when he is experiencing it" (p. 4). Actually, however, it appears to be quite possible to be mistaken about stress, that is, to misattribute one's own feelings. This is important because it suggests that stress, and other affective states, are better viewed as the conjunction of two factors, arousal and a cognitive appraisal of the situation, rather than as arousal alone. (This model, too, has limitations, but does represent an improvement over the simplistic equation of arousal with stress.)

Empirical evidence for a two-factor theory of emotion may be found in the now famous experiment by Schachter and Singer,[26] in which subjects were unknowingly administered adrenalin, placed in what was ostensibly a waiting room, and given what they were told was a pretest questionnaire. In the room was another 'subject' (actually a confederate), also filling out a questionnaire. This individual repeatedly expressed considerable and vociferous annoyance at the overly personal nature of some of the questionnaire items, ultimately throwing the questionnaire to the floor and leaving the room. The real subject, when subsequently asked to describe his emotional state, would typically reply that the questionnaire made him so angry that he felt physically agitated and that his heart was racing. Needless to say, these symptoms were actually caused by the adrenalin, but the subjects, not knowing this, attributed their reactions to external cues.

In an alternative condition, the stooge would behave in a highly exuberant manner, crumpling paper into balls and throwing them across the room; in this case the subject would attribute his increased heart rate to 'high spirits'. Interestingly, control subjects who had been informed of the physiological reactions they would experience tended not to be 'infected' by the confederate's behaviour and showed no particular changes in mood.

Certainly if arousal and stress were identical, it would be impossible to misinterpret one's own arousal as being due to illness, excitement, or some other state. In fact, however, arousal is a biochemical and psychophysiological construct that excludes such cognitive appraisals. As such the construct has been described as "unduly reductionist ... a holdover from the era of behaviorism" (Neiss,[22] p. 346).

The nature of arousal

A further problem connected with equating arousal and stress concerns the nature of arousal itself. For many years arousal was regarded as the general level of activation of an organism, a single, unidimensional continuum of excitation or 'energy' which would have coma or hibernation near one end and some extreme manifestation of frenzied cognitive and endocrine activity near the other. It has also been defined as the notional state of activation that would remain if specific effects (such as loud noises, threat, drugs, and time of day variations) were removed.[13,24] In this view arousal is analogous to the famous and much disputed *g* factor in general intelligence, and it is this single, unidimensional, and hypothetical phenomenon that is plotted against (some equally undifferentiated notion of) performance in the ubiquitous U.

It has become increasingly recognized, however, that the unidimensional notion of arousal is too simplistic, global, and all inclusive,[13] and that it just does not seem to fit the observed facts.[8] Even in the 1960s, when general activation theory was at its most popular, Lacey[15] showed that "arousal of the hand, the heart, and the head" had little in common, meaning that various ways of indexing arousal give different results (cited in Revelle and Loftus,[24] p. 211).

More recent research has confirmed that various biochemical and psychophysiological measures usually taken as indices of arousal do not correlate particularly well.[14,28] Some theorists would assert that there is no reason why they should. Cognitive appraisal theorists, for example, have argued that particular (stress related) cognitive appraisals do not elicit a simple, diffuse, generalized, arousal reaction, but, rather, provoke specific and distinct patterns of arousal.[16,18] This clearly brings the theory even further from Selye's notion of a General Adaptation 'Syndrome'.

Some arousal theorists have taken a componential approach to the problem. Thayer identified two dimensions of arousal (one a continuum from energetic to tired, the other a continuum from tense to calm).[28] These are said to correlate positively at low levels of psychological demand, but negatively at high levels of demand. This two dimensional model would 'explain' why it is, for example, that a period of intense pressure (a long frantic ATC shift, for example) can leave an individual 'stressed out' in the sense of feeling both fatigued *and* tense. The traditional unidimensional model has difficulty combining an apparently low arousal condition such as fatigue with a high arousal condition such as tenseness.

Pribram and McGuiness, on the basis of a review of some two hundred studies, propose a model consisting of three separate but interactive 'energetical systems': arousal, activation, and effort.[23] Arousal consists of the individual's immediate responses to external influences. Activation refers to 'readiness', or the ability to respond with arousal. The effort component is a control system that coordinates the first two. It has also been suggested that the first two elements, arousal and activation, are differentiated both by brain hemisphere and by neurotransmitter.[31] According to this view, arousal from immediate external sources (e.g., inflight emergencies) is associated with activity of the right hemisphere and parietal region, and is controlled by the secretion of adrenalin and noradrenalin. Activation, on the other hand, is "internally oriented, associated with the left hemisphere and frontal regions, and controlled by dopaminergic transmission" (Neiss,[22] p. 353).

There is certainly experimental evidence suggesting that these hypotheses are closer to the truth than unidimemsional theories. Consider, for example, the work of McClelland and his colleagues.[19] These researchers point out that many laboratory studies invoke what McClelland refers to as "power arousal" (p. 52) by using challenge or threat stressors such as electric shock, other physically aversive stimuli, or examinations, tests, and the like. Typically such stressors are associated with arousal dominated by increased adrenalin production (the result of which the subject is likely to be aware, as in Schachter and Singer's experiment). "Affiliative arousal", by way of contrast, is said to be associated with the stress arising from divorce, bereavement, adolescent romantic tribulations, and the like. It has been demonstrated that such arousal is characterized not by elevated adrenergic activity but by increased dopamine levels.[19] Different stress and motivational states appear, therefore, to be underpinned by different neuroendocrine systems.

It is useful to recall these results when considering the 'Life Stress' studies examined in Chapter 5. Many life stresses are of the affiliative type, while most inflight incidents and emergencies involve acute threat of the 'power' stressor type. Attempts to predict response in the latter from experiences in the former may rest upon the tacit assumption that a unitary dimension of arousal can incorporate both acute reactive stress and 'life' stress. What is more, equivalent assumptions that life stress and acute reactive stress are simply additive fall at the same hurdle. In arousal terms, certain studies could be described as exercises in predicting apples from oranges or adding apples to oranges.

The shape of the curve

Assuming, for the sake of argument, that both arousal and performance *are* unidimensional variables that can usefully be plotted one against the other, would an inverted U curve be a satisfactory description of the likely relationship of arousal to performance in the 'real world'? The U curve is frequently represented as a tall symmetrical bell shape that is remarkably (indeed, suspiciously) similar to the familiar 'normal distribution' curve found in statistics books (see, for example, Figures 2.1-2.3). The left hand tail of the curve suggests that increased stress (or arousal) has little or no initial effect upon performance. The right hand tail suggests that the final few increments of stress (the 'straws on the camel's back') also leave performance relatively unaffected. The operational world of aviation gives little reason to believe that performance and arousal (not to mention stress) are really related either in this way or in other kind of any 'inverted U' curve relationship.

As a matter of fact, decades of laboratory research using a wide variety of stressors and performance measures have generated a very mixed picture of findings, including curves of various shapes and dimensions, monotonically sloping straight lines, flat straight lines, and so on. Even where the stressor has taken the form of electric shocks, as in the original Yerkes and Dodson experiment, a number of studies have been unable to demonstrate any significant deterioration in performance whatsoever.[22] The 'curve,' if we can call it that, is in these instances flat. These results do not appear so strange in the light of what we now know of multiple dimensions of arousal and the importance of endogenous opioid secretion (endorphins) in inhibiting sympathetic nervous system reactivity during stress.[20]

There is no reason to assume that the anxiolytic effects of these natural opioids (including the blunting of pain and the elevating of mood) are confined to the laboratory. Indeed, Idzikowski and Baddeley, in a well-known paper on fear in dangerous environments, have made the important observation that even persons who appear to be 'highly aroused' and frightened do not always exhibit much, if anything, in the way of a performance decrement.[11] In these situations, various biochemical compensatory adjustments (nonadrenergic arousal), together with cognitive coping strategies (as discussed in later chapters) probably help to maintain performance or, at least, permit it to degrade very gradually and gracefully, in a controlled fashion.

Of Curves and Triangles: Is the 'U' Scientific and Useful?

Looked at overall, research supports, at best, a correlational, but not a causal interpretation of the U curve relationship between arousal and performance.[22] *This is very weak, the equivalent to merely observing that a number of aircraft have vanished in an area called the 'Bermuda Triangle', without ascribing their loss to the infamous triangle. The analogy can be driven a little further. The Bermuda Triangle is any triangle you care to draw. Its parameters, size, shape, even duration, apparently vary from author to author, depending upon which disappearances each author wishes to include and 'explain' by the Triangle's malign, but unspecified power. The reason that the Bermuda Triangle is not a useful explanatory concept is because it (a) accounts for everything and cannot be refuted, and (b) because it provides no causal mechanism for the events associated with it.*

Similarly, the inverted U curve is pretty much any inverted U curve that can be drawn. Its parameters are not specified in advance or anchored. 'Optimal arousal' varies from task to task and person to person and is never predicted in absolute terms. Virtually all data potentially fit the curve (if they don't, it can usually be argued that the data are merely **part** *of some larger curve). The claim that performance will be best at some level of arousal between complete coma and uncontrolled frenzy, is as irrefutable as it is trivial. Finally, as Robert Hockey has noted, there is nothing in U curve theory itself which provides any causal mechanism for the claimed relationship of arousal to performance.*[10]

An alternative to the inverted U curve model comes from the literature on critical events sometimes termed 'catastrophe theory'.[29] This literature describes a mathematical model applicable to many systems in which smooth continuous inputs result in abrupt discontinuous responses. It has been applied to seismic events, for example, chemical reactions and, more controversially, to prison overcrowding and subsequent riots. The model predicts a gradual, incremental change until a certain critical point is reached, at which juncture there ensues a major, sudden, and 'catastrophic' alteration in system state. Thus, the notional stress/performance 'curve' may be discontinuous: flat for most of its length (when performance is resistant to change) until a critical stress level or 'break' point is reached, whereupon the plot plunges downward as performance collapses. In this

conception the final few 'increments of stress', far from leaving performance relatively unaffected, as in many idealized 'U curves', would in fact
represent the last 'straw on the camel's back.'

Finally, the performance that we are often most interested in is crew
performance, not individual performance. There is no evidence that crew
performance under stress accords with the 'inverted U' model. What
evidence there is, and it is slim enough, suggests more of a linear impairment of performance.[17] Crew performance introduces significant new
variables into the equation, such as group cohesion (discussed in Chapter
7) and communications (discussed in Chapter 4). Therefore, although this
limitation of 'U curve' theory is not a fair *technical* criticism of the
Yerkes-Dodson 'Law' (since the latter makes no claims about teams), it is
nevertheless a relevant observation with significance for the operational
world of flying. If the uncritical acceptance of the 'inverted U' relationship between stress and performance is questionable for individual pilots or
controllers, it is doubly so for teams or crews.

The notion of an optimum: stating the obvious?

Both literally and metaphorically, the middle portion of the 'inverted U'
curve lies at the centre of traditional arousal theory, because the entire
edifice is built upon the notion that there exists a single, optimal arousal
level. This assumption alone could be queried on a number of levels. For
example, one of the implications of Apter's intuitively plausible model,
discussed earlier, is that there is not one optimum arousal level but two,
one for each motivational state.[1] However, as Jones[12] points out, there is a
much more fundamental problem with the optimal arousal concept:

> As with other approaches embodying an optimum, the difficulty of circu-
> larity has yet to be countered. This means that the optimum can be
> specified only *post hoc*. The problem of the optimum is further compli-
> cated by the dynamic nature of the stress response, that is, not only do
> models of stress need to specify the optimum in advance, they also need
> to account in advance for changes in the optimum. (p. 73)

Ironically, despite the associated difficulties, it is probably the very notion
of an optimum which has had so much appeal as to lead to the overgeneral-
ization of the original Yerkes-Dodson findings. Noted British stress researcher Robert Hockey suggests that this probably occurred because the
'inverted U' relationship between performance and arousal (or, with a little

conceptual slippage, stress) is intuitively satisfying.[10] It is, after all, a matter of common sense that optimal performance will neither be associated with extreme lethargy nor with highly emotional states. Similarly, it feels intuitively appropriate that anxiety and nervousness will tend to have a stronger adverse effect on the performance of difficult tasks than of comparatively simple ones. As Hockey states, we might have no particular difficulty changing a car tyre while in an emotionally agitated state, but we would probably not want to try to repair a watch mechanism.

However, if the 'inverted U' is claiming no more than this, is it merely a trivial formalization of our intuitions? If it embodies substantive claims that go beyond this, what are they, and to what extent are they true? Certainly, as Hockey points out, the Yerkes-Dodson Law does not explain how or why performance changes occur, why high arousal would have an adverse effect on performance, or what specific aspects of a task make it difficult to perform under conditions of high arousal. Failure to address these issues has, according to Hockey,[10] left many researchers content with "circular reasoning and naive operational definitions" (p. 144).

Summary and implications

From the perspective of the studies reviewed above, stress and arousal are not only not identical constructs, they are not even similar -- although they may be related in more or less complex and systematic ways. Stress cannot be said to cause or to be caused by generic unidimensional arousal; rather, various cognitive, biochemical and psychophysiological functions are likely to be influenced differentially depending upon the eliciting conditions. These changes, however, need not necessarily be associated with *any* general alteration in performance. Similarly, pilot or controller performance is inadequately and misleadingly represented when depicted as a single continuum on a graph, even if team performance variables are excluded. Cognitive performance is made up of many elements, and the nature of any stress related change in cognitive performance will obviously depend upon the specific cognitive 'structure' or requirements of tasks as complex as flying an aircraft or controlling air traffic.

Each flight or ATC task can be thought of as a specific suite or profile of cognitive demands or components (e.g., memory, inference, judgement, motor control, and so forth). The profile for any single task is not necessarily fixed across individuals, however, because of individuals' preferred strategies and styles. Consider this very simple example: for the student pilot who has yet to realize the advantages of trimming the aircraft properly, many manoeuvres have an important psychomotor element merely because the pilot is continuously 'fighting' an out-of-trim aircraft. However, for his instructor, who trims the aircraft correctly, very little psychomotor control input may be needed to perform the identical manoeuvres.

This is not just a matter of experience, however, but also of individual differences in problem solving strategies. As a second example, consider Pilot Smith, who, as a personal style, is uncomfortable with approximations, 'guesstimates', and the like. He is always calculating courses, intercept angles, ground speed, and so forth. For him many instrument flight operations have an important mathematical component. Pilot Brown, in contrast, is less comfortable with mathematics and has evolved a variety of strategies which successfully avoid many calculations by using various 'rules of thumb', approximation plus progressive fine tuning, instrument 'tricks', and the like. For Brown the same instrument flight operations primarily involve scanning and visuospatial skills.

The particular cognitive demand profile of a flight task or situation acts in conjunction with the particular stress characteristics of the situation, and with the biopsychological predispositions of the individual. These interactions determine the pattern of performance changes (possibly increments as well as decrements) that result. From the viewpoint of individual differences interacting with a broad range of multifactor situations, we would anticipate that these interactions are complex but nevertheless lawful. The task of modelling stress effects upon individual performance would, from this perspective, involve identifying these systematic relationships, rather than depending upon the reflexive invocation of the Yerkes-Dodson 'Law'.

References

1. Apter, M.J., and Svebak, S. (1989), 'Stress from the Reversal Theory Perspective', in Spielberger, C.D., Sarason, I.G., and Strelau, J., (eds.), *Stress and Anxiety*, vol. 12, Hemisphere Publishing Corporation, New York, pp. 39-52.

2. Brecke, F.H. (1982), 'Instructional design for aircrew judgment training', *Aviation, Space, and Environmental Medicine*, vol. 53, pp. 951-7.

3. Campbell, R.D., and Bagshaw, M. (1991), *Human Performance Limitations in Aviation,* BSP Professional Books, Oxford.

4. Cole, L.W. (1911), 'The relation of strength of stimulation to rate of learning in the chick', *Journal of Animal Behavior,* vol. 1, pp. 111-24.

5. Dodson, J.D. (1915), 'The relation of strength of stimulus to rapidity of habit-formation in the kitten', *Journal of Animal Behavior,* vol. 5, pp. 330-6.

6. Gmelch, W. (1983), 'Stress for success', *Theory into Practice,* vol. 22, pp. 7-14.

7. Hancock, P.A., and Scallen, S. (in press), *Stress and Human Performance.*

8. Hartley, L., Dunne, M., Schwartz, S., and Brown, J. (1986), 'Effect of noise on cognitive strategies in a sentence verification task', *Ergonomics,* vol. 29, pp. 607-17.

9. Hawkins, F.H. (1987), *Human Factors in Flight,* Gower Technical Press, Aldershot, Hants.

10. Hockey, G.R.J. (1979), 'Stress and the Cognitive Components of Skilled Performance', in Hamilton, V. and Warburton, D.M. (eds.), *Human Stress and Cognition,* John Wiley & Sons, New York.

11. Idzikowski, C., and Baddeley, A.D. (1983), 'Fear and Dangerous Environments', in Hockey, R. (ed.), *Stress and Fatigue in Human Performance,* John Wiley & Sons, Chichester, pp. 123-44.

12. Jones, D.M. (1991), 'Stress and Workload: Models, Methodologies and Remedies', in Farmer, E. (ed.), *Stress and Error in Aviation,* Avebury Technical, Aldershot, Hants.

13. Jorna, P.G.A.M. (1992), 'Spectral analysis of heart rate and psychological state: a review of its validity as a workload index', *Biological Psychology,* vol. 34, pp. 237-57.

14. Krahenbuhl, G.S., and Harris, J. (1984), *Biochemical Measurements of the Human Stress Response*, AFHRL-TR-83-40, Air Force Human Resources Laboratory, Williams AFB, Arizona.

15. Lacey, J.I. (1967), 'Somatic Response Patterning and Stress: Some Revisions of Activation Theory', in Appley, M.H. and Trumbull, R. (eds.), *Psychological Stress*, Appleton-Century-Crofts, New York.

16. Lazarus, R.S., and Folkman, S. (1984), *Stress, Appraisal, and Coping*, Springer, New York.

17. Lowe, R, and McGrath, J.E. (1971), *Stress, Arousal and Performance: Some Findings Calling for a New Theory*, Air Force Office of Scientific Research, Technical Report AFI 161-67.

18. Mason, J.W. (1975), 'Emotion as Reflected in Patterns of Endocrine Integration', in Levi, L. (ed.), *Emotions, Their Parameters and Measurement*, Raven, New York.

19. McClelland, D.C., Patel, V., Stier, D., and Brown, D. (1987), 'The relationship of affiliative arousal to dopamine release', *Motivation and Emotion*, vol. 11, pp. 51-66.

20. McCubbin, J.A. (1993), 'Stress and endogenous opioids: behavioral and circulatory interactions', *Biological Psychology*, vol. 35, pp. 91-122.

21. Melton, C.E., McKenzie, J.M., Kelln, J.R., Hoffmann, S.M., and Saldivar, J.T. (1975), 'Effect of a general aviation trainer on the stress of flight training', *Aviation, Space, and Environmental Medicine*, vol 46, pp. 1-5.

22. Neiss, R. (1988), 'Reconceptualizing arousal: psychological states in motor performance', *Psychological Bulletin*, vol. 103, pp. 345-66.

23. Pribram, K.H., and McGuinness, D. (1975), 'Arousal, activation and effort in the control of attention', *Psychological Review*, vol. 82, pp. 116-49.

24. Revelle, W., and Loftus, D.A. (1990), 'Individual differences and arousal: implications for the study of mood and memory', *Cognition and Emotion*, vol. 4, pp. 209-37.

25. Roscoe, A.H. (1978), 'Stress and workload in pilots', *Aviation, Space, and Environmental Medicine*, vol. 49, pp. 630-6.

26. Schachter, S., and Singer, J.E. (1962), 'Cognitive, social and physiological determinants of emotional state', *Psychological Review*, vol. 69, pp. 379-99.

27. Selye, H. (1956), *The Stress of Life*, McGraw-Hill, New York.

28. Thayer, R.E. (1989), *The Biopsychology of Mood and Arousal*, Oxford University Press, New York.

29. Thom, R. (1975), *Structural Stability and Morphogenesis*, Addison-Wesley, Reading, Massachussetts.

30. Thomas, M. (1989), *Managing Pilot Stress: What Causes Pilot Stress and What Can Be Done About It*, Macmillan, New York.

31. Tucker, D.M., and Williamson, P.A. (1984), 'Assymetric neural control in human self-regulation', *Psychological Review*, vol. 91, pp. 185-215.

32. Yerkes, R.M., and Dodson, J.D. (1908), 'The relation of strength of stimulus to rapidity of habit-formation', *Journal of Comparative and Neurological Psychology*, vol. 18, pp. 459-82.

3 Pilot performance and stress

The aviation industry does include a cocktail of stressors which is unique when combined with a critical need for a high level of performance.
--Frank Hawkins, *Human Factors in Flight*

I have yet to see any problem, however complicated, which, when looked at in the right way, did not become still more complicated.
-- Poul Anderson, *New Scientist*, 1969

This chapter does not set out to be an encyclopaedic review of the research on human performance and stress. Rather, its focus is on the effects of stress on specific psychological functions important in aviation. The research that will be discussed here includes both 'real world' accounts of pilots engaged in actual air operations, and more generalized laboratory assessments of human psychological functioning in the presence of a variety of aversive conditions. From the researcher's point of view, studies of the latter type do of course have certain advantages: they provide easily quantifiable results, for example, and control the number of variables considered at one time. One issue addressed in this chapter concerns the ways in which the findings from such studies can shed light on performance in the complex, dynamic, multistressor environment of an aircraft cockpit. After identifying some of the psychomotor and cognitive functions that characterize various aspects of the pilot's task (see Table 3.1), the chapter goes on to explore what is known of the effects of stress upon these performance variables. These discussions are also relevant to the controller's task, insofar as there is significant overlap in the cognitive requirements of ATC and flight tasks.

What pilots do

When we ask what pilots do (in this chapter at least), it is a psychological rather than a behavioural question. What we mean by it is, what is involved *cognitively* in flying an aircraft; what information processing opera-

Table 3.1
Information processing interpretation of some flight tasks
(adapted from Braune and Wickens,[14] p. 10)

FLIGHT TASK	*PROCESS*
Preflight:	
a) collect weather and mission information	visual and auditory perception
b) interpret weather and mission information within the framework of intended flight	decision making based on probabilistic data
c) based on interpretation decide on necessary actions to complete mission successfully	problem solving
d) preflight aircraft for malfunctions	visual and auditory perception, decision making
Takeoff:	
e) observe changes in instrument readings and external sources	visual perception
f) rotate aircraft at predetermined airspeed and establish climbout	decision making based on absolute data, visual perception
g) anticipate location and direction of aircraft movement (flight path)	imagery, mental rotation
Cruise:	
h) maintain constant monitoring of flight instruments and external sources	visual and auditory perception
i) identify inputs quickly and accurately and act appropriately	signal detection (perception), decision making
j) maintain information for immediate processing	short term memory capacity and retrieval speed

tions are entailed? Obviously, operating an aircraft (or performing ATC duties) involves extensive training, 'ground' schooling, and many competencies highly specific to aviation -- for example, knowledge of regulations, systems, and procedures. There is some evidence that this kind of aviation specific 'book' knowledge tends to be fairly resistant to stress;[98] in other words, it is not readily forgotten, even under difficult or extreme conditions. However, pilots also depend upon a number of more general cognitive abilities that are, to varying extents, independent of specialized aviation knowledge. These, as we shall see, can be far from 'stress proof'.

For example, the most obvious function carried out by the pilot is that of controlling the aircraft, in the sense of maneuvering it accurately. (Before the advent of flight deck automation, of course, this was perhaps the defining function.) While 'stick and rudder' control is, of course, a learned skill, there are also certain underlying psychomotor processes involved, which may well contribute to the difference between a 'hot shot' aerobatic pilot and a more average one. These fundamental skills can degrade significantly under stress.

Memory functions are also very important in aviation. To be able to use clearances, call signs, advisories, briefings, and so forth, it is obviously necessary to be able to remember them, at least for as long as they are needed. Any compromising of this short term (working) memory function would be likely to render a pilot's performance inefficient, dangerous, or both. In addition, impairment of working memory has the potential to affect visual-spatial processes, among them orientation in three-dimensional space. This function is critical to many aspects of situational awareness, such as the ability to 'see' airports and associated traffic in the mind's eye, and to visualize a scene from different perspectives.

Another important cognitive skill is the ability to integrate a broad range of incoming cues in order to 'make sense of' or interpret a situation. Such cues may be visual (e.g., instrument readings), auditory (e.g., the quality of engine noise), or even kinaesthetic, 'seat-of-the-pants' sensations. Not all of these cues come from the aircraft and its environment, of course: some are also derived from preflight briefings, weather forecasts, and flight planning. Thus, information retrieval skills are also important -- not least the ability to recall apt prior experiences from long term memory (see Chapter 4), and to recognize which elements are relevant to the present situation and which are not.

No less significant than psychomotor and memory functions are attentional processes. One faculty within this category is that of focussed attention, or the ability to concentrate, when necessary, upon the most important aspects or features of a situation without being unduly distracted by extraneous stimuli. Indeed, this ability is often used as a screening criterion both in military and civilian aviation: in the United States, for example, pilots undergoing selection for airline jobs by the Flight Safety Foundation are required to interpret graphs while attempting to ignore irrelevant and distracting ATC radio exchanges played over their headsets. Of equal importance, however, is the conceptually opposite quality of *divided* attention, which is the ability to 'timeshare' between multiple tasks without allocating all mental resources to a single activity or information source. Pilots, of course, have multiple information sources to monitor (see, for example, the sidebar on p. 67, which lists the controls and indicators on the F/A-18 Hornet), and many can recall their instrument flight instructor's stern admonition not to fixate upon one instrument at the expense of the others: "Don't stare! Keep your instrument scan going!"

Another important attentional skill is prioritization, or the ability to plan ahead and rank tasks according to importance, and to avoid the type of priority confusion epitomized by flight instructors as "dropping the aeroplane and flying the microphone". In other words, pilots must be able to allocate attention in efficient, task driven ways, rather than becoming preoccupied with low priority or off-task intrusions (however salient these might appear). Examples of the latter include nonurgent radio calls, 'self referential' thoughts (e.g., worrying or fretting about one's performance), and idle conversation with other crew members.

The dangers of such intrusions should not be underestimated: for example, distractions caused by non-task related crew dialogue have been implicated in a number of accidents, leading the Federal Aviation Administration to impose the so-called 'Sterile Cockpit' rule (Federal Air Regulation 121.542), which prohibits casual conversations or any other distracting off-task activity in critical flight phases below 10,000 feet. Even with this rule, a number of major accidents (and many lesser ones) have been attributed in part to the crew's engaging in distracting, low priority activities; examples include the crash of Delta Airlines Flight 1141 in Dallas in 1988,[9] and the collision of a USAir 737 with a SkyWest Metroliner in Los Angeles in 1991.

Yet another attentional skill that should be mentioned here is vigilance. A vigilance task is one that requires consistent monitoring without lapses in attention. This can become a challenge if the task is a monotonous one with little variation (for example, staring at a radar display for long periods of time). Vigilance has always been important in aviation, of course; pilots need to be constantly aware both of their instrument readings and of the surrounding airspace (the so-called 'see and avoid' principle). However, the need for vigilance skills has arguably never been as great as today. The skies are more crowded than ever, and advances in flight deck automation have increasingly emphasized the pilot's role as a system monitor (see Chapter 12). Air traffic control also requires high levels of vigilance, and this, too, may be affected by the automated systems of the future (see Chapter 10). Vigilance performance under stress or fatigue has been the focus of many laboratory studies, as we shall see.

One final cognitive function that is obviously of great importance in aviation is that of judgement and decision making. More than one study has shown that many (or even most) accidents involving pilot error can be traced at some level to suboptimal decision making,[43,60,61,85] a problem that can be profoundly exacerbated by stress. Training programs have been developed which attempt to provide pilots with direct instruction in decision making strategies;[19,25,89] in addition, the more general field of decision theory has seen considerable advances in the past decade or so. Because of its importance, this topic will be discussed separately in Chapter 4, along with the subject of stress effects on communication.

Stress and manual control

On the night of 30/31 January, 1944, Lieutenant Ron Munday's bomb laden Lancaster was on its way to Berlin when it was attacked by a German night fighter. As Mr. Munday[75] recalls,

> We went into a diving turn to port but, at the changeover point, on the climbing turn to port which was the next phase of the corkscrew, I yanked the control column back a bit hard in my heightened state of anxiety ... One wing went down and we found ourselves on our back. All the blind flying instruments toppled. The packets of Window [tinfoil anti-radar 'chaff'] stored behind my seat all went floating freely up to the inverted roof, along with the flight engineer -- who was known as 'Upside-down Simmonds' for the rest of his tour. I don't think the whole thing took longer than a minute or a minute and a half, though the pulse rate and adrenalin levels took a little longer to achieve normality. (pp. 252-3)

Lieutenant Munday's brave account is so good humoured and understated that the bloodchilling nature of the episode is almost lost. Such encounters usually had only one ending. In this case, however, the Lancaster lost 10,000 feet (thereby evading the fighter) as a result of a control input that was, as Munday put it, "a bit hard" -- sufficient, in fact, to roll the unwieldy and fully laden four-engined bomber onto its back.

There is no doubt that extremes of emotion can be associated with poor perceptual-motor coordination, as well as other, similar impairments of motor control[30] (see, for example, the sidebar below). Indeed, the English language is replete with phrases such as 'shaking with anger', 'quaking with fear', and the more general 'trembling with emotion'. There has, however, been very little research that examines the effects of these high stress states on aircraft control. Such studies as do exist have mostly addressed the relationship between tracking performance and the presence of so-called 'stressor' variables such as heat,[48] carbon monoxide concentration,[44] or G forces.[39] However, there is also some evidence that impairment of motor control can be induced by levels of psychological stress that fall short of the very extremes, such as those encountered during the normal execution of (admittedly high risk) activities.

For example, Alan Baddeley and his colleagues reported, in a series of studies of divers, that manual dexterity became more impaired the more dangerous the dive.[57] Similarly, a study of British paratroopers showed that

---

Richmond, Virginia, October, 1991: I left Richmond in marginal VFR. I looked down at my clipboard, looked up, and was in a cloud. I panicked and pulled up on the elevator. Apparently I pulled up and to the left as my gyroscope spun. I was disorientated although I was only in the cloud for approximately three to five seconds. When I came out there were clouds below me with only occasional glimpses of ground. I was afraid of not being able to see the runway and also of descending through the clouds as there might be be obstacles. I then called Norfolk Approach who instructed me to squawk 7700. In retrospect I should not have looked at my clipboard until cruising altitude. Also, as this was my first encounter with a cloud, it was incredibly dangerous to panic and pull up hard on the yoke, as this could have resulted in the plane stalling. Had it done so, recovery would have been difficult because of my disorientation. I found it very reassuring to speak with air traffic controllers, given my anxiety level.

-- NASA Aviation Safety Reporting System (Accession No. 191317)

tracking task performance deteriorated immediately prior to a parachute jump.[47] Interestingly, experience and training appear to have afforded some protection from this effect, as army regulars did better than army trainees, who, in turn, did better than Territorial Army trainees (a National Guard-like militia).

There are also a number of studies which have used less ecologically valid ('real world') contexts, but which have nevertheless been conducted within aviation relevant domains. An early study of radar tracking, for example, found that tracking accuracy was adversely affected by five different 'stress' variables: distractions, secondary tasks, extended time on task, speed, and workload.[42] Another study conducted in Scandinavia examined the performance of military recruits tracking (simulated) guided missiles.[11] The 'stressor' used was electric shock; the introduction of shock increased both heart rate and the average rate of errors. With time, however, a habituation process appeared to assert itself, as evidenced by error rates declining to preshock levels and even heart rate slowing appreciably.

It should be pointed out, by the way, that while electric shock is the archetypal laboratory stressor, it is actually not a very good analogue of stress or fear in real life. It consists merely of varying degrees of pain (a known element), and is more aversive than threatening as such. It need not, for example, provoke anxieties about coping ability. Despite these qualifications the results of this study are interesting. (As an incidental observation, no optimum level of performance was observed for intermediate levels of arousal, although this is what would have been predicted on the basis of the Yerkes-Dodson 'Law' -- see Chapter 2).

Another study, conducted by Stokes, Belger, and Zhang, attempted to create a functional simulation of an aircraft cockpit in terms of workload and cognitive activities.[83] Although the primary purpose of the study was to examine flight decision making processes both in experienced and inexperienced pilots (see Chapter 4), it also provided some data on the effects of stress on a computerized tracking task. The task involved tracking a target using a joystick with first-order (i.e., velocity or rate) dynamics rather than simple zero-order (position) control, and thus provided some representation of aircraft control dynamics.

In the stress manipulation, subjects were exposed to 90 dBa of white noise (a condition thought to simulate the effects of anxiety[53]), and were also required to maintain a concurrent Sternberg memory search task intended to simulate necessary cockpit workload. This (putative) stress condition is certainly mild compared to the stress associated with (for example) diving, parachuting, or night fighter attack; however, the idea was not to provoke an extreme stress reaction but rather to simulate the increased workload and anxiety associated with a somewhat critical (but not completely hair-raising) inflight episode. In this way it was hoped to provide some realistic indication of the degree of stress related impairment likely to occur in routine flight operations.

The results showed that in this condition, tracking accuracy was impaired by about 15 percent; the amount of time spent 'off-target' (analogous to the amount of time the needle is 'out of the doughnut' in VOR tracking or on an ILS approach) increased by about 20 percent. This was true both for experienced and inexperienced flyers, although in real life operational circumstances the greater efficiency of experienced pilots in coping with cockpit workload would most likely reduce the impairment in tracking performance. (In this study, for purposes connected with the decision making component, the tracking task and its concurrent memory search task were deliberately made domain independent -- that is, abstract and stripped of any specific flight or cockpit features which might favour the greater knowledge possessed by experienced pilots.)

In sharp contrast to this experiment, Dutch researchers examined trait rather than state anxiety in a very domain specific study of tracking behaviour.[62] In this study pilots with high and low trait anxiety scores flew a standard traffic pattern or circuit in a flight simulator. The tracking data were then subjected to spectral analysis, that is, the pilots' control inputs were broken down by frequency and amplitude. The researchers expected high time pilots to make more control inputs at the low frequency end of the spectrum, to the extent that experience facilitates anticipation of future system states. Lower time pilots may, in this view, be obliged to correct excursions from the intended flight path only after the deviation has occurred, that is, in a reactive, compensatory mode. Thus, expert control was expected to reflect a 'pursuit tracking' strategy, while novice control was expected to reflect a compensatory tracking strategy consisting mainly of high frequency, low amplitude stick inputs. A prime performance effect of trait anxiety, it was suggested, might be to 'simulate' lower skill by provoking a regression to these high frequency, low amplitude control inputs.

A significant difference was indeed found in the control behaviour of the two groups. Highly trait anxious pilots showed smaller standard deviations in aileron control. However, this was a difference which was observable right across the frequency spectrum. While such a result is compatible with the view that mental load limits control activity in trait anxious individuals, it falls short of demonstrating the hypothesized regression to a compensatory tracking mode. This interesting hypothesis is certainly worth further scrutiny, however.

In summary, then, it must be recognized that there is, to date, very little solid information that clarifies the nature of performance changes in tracking and similar manual control exercises under realistic stresses. We know of no study which, for example, separates error due to increase in tonic tremor from impairment due to 'overcontrol' inputs over and above the tremor component. Over a decade ago, Idzikowski and Baddeley made the observation that it is difficult to specify whether tracking impairments are due to the effects of stress primarily upon perceptual or upon sensorimotor processes;[57] it remains just as difficult today.

Similarly, it is still not known how cognitive resources are parcelled out when aircraft control competes with aeronautical decision making in actual fear provoking environments (as opposed to laboratory dual task situations). Likewise, it is not understood why some stressed or anxious pilots 'fight' the aircraft, overcontrolling and creating appreciable additional workload, while in other individuals, undercontrolling or even 'freezing' is observed (see Chapter 7). Although speculative answers can, as ever, be formulated, there exists at present no model capable of predicting the specific control behaviour of individual pilots in conditions of emotional stress. Such a model would have value for both selection and training.

Memory

A simplifying analogy likens the human memory system to an office desk: incoming materials are taken from the 'in' tray (perception) and placed on the desk top (working memory) to be worked on, while more permanent knowledge not in current use is stored in the file drawers (long term memory, or LTM). Desktop materials eventually go either to the wastebasket (i.e., they are forgotten), or, if they are likely to remain useful in the future, to the file drawers. Later, if circumstances require, information can be taken from the file drawers and placed on the desk top again along with any new incoming material.*

---

*Computer users may prefer to substitute 'input buffer' for 'in tray', 'RAM' for 'desk top', and 'hard disk' for 'file drawer'.

When considering the effects of stress, persistence with the desk analogy generates some odd but entertaining 'Alice in Wonderland' images. For example, the effective working area of the desk top may shrink, accompanied by selective jamming of the file drawers. Likewise, the 'in' tray may suddenly get ideas above its station and begin to drastically screen and filter incoming information, becoming increasingly selective about just what it will permit to pass on to the desk top. In fact, of course, while the desk analogy is picturesque and to some extent helpful, it is too mechanistic to illustrate the full range of stress effects on memory (for example, on cognitive strategy), and it is necessary to consider the evidence more directly.

Working memory

For any given flight there is a good deal of specific information to be acquired and retained (albeit temporarily) -- for example, step down fixes, decision heights, and the call signs of other aircraft. In monitoring the flight this information must also be integrated with instrument readings of navigational position, attitude, altitude, speed, direction of flight, and so forth, as well as with the status of various system variables such as fuel state and cabin pressure. All of these calculations go into an overall mental model of the progress of the flight, which is, moreover, constantly being updated. For inexperienced pilots in particular, the sheer number of things to be kept in mind can seem overwhelming. Even a more seasoned aviator, however, may experience difficulties if stress has a significant impact on his cognitive abilities.

Anxiety, stress, and fatigue have all been demonstrated to affect working memory functions.[28,66,92] Indeed, one researcher, Hamilton,[46] has even *defined* stress in terms of working memory degradation: "By definition, cognitive stressors are those cognitive events, processes, or operations that exceed a subjective and individualized level of average processing capacity" (p. 109). The mechanisms by which this occurs are not perfectly understood, however, and it may reasonably be asked what is meant by 'processing capacity', and how this should be measured. In considering the issue it is useful to conceptualize working memory as a system consisting of two separate components: an information storage function and an information processing function.[27] Available evidence indicates that stress affects both of these processes, which can also be termed memory *capacity* and memory *strategy*.

Capacity. Many models of working memory have traditionally been based on the idea of a finite storage capacity which, under stress, becomes even more constrained. According to one influential theory, for example, stress effects on working memory can be explained as a process whereby anxious persons divert part of their working memory capacity into worrying about irrelevant matters, and hence have less available capacity to allocate to the task.[33,34] The working memory test known as the digit span task, in which subjects are shown sequences of numbers which must then be recalled, is a good example of an assessment tool that addresses primarily the storage component of working memory. Performance on this test tends to deteriorate when the individual is in an anxious state. This was true, for example, in the study by Stokes, Belger, and Zhang cited earlier (in which the stress manipulation consisted of a combination of noise and added workload): in this study, scores on a computerized digit span test dropped by over one-third in the 'stressed' condition.[83]

In the majority of studies, however, performance decrement on the digit span task has tended to be only moderate and not entirely consistent.[35,93,94] One possible explanation is that the digit span task for the most part leaves the *processing* function of working memory untaxed.[6] In support of this hypothesis it may be noted that the effects of anxiety are more pronounced with tasks that require the subject not only to memorize information but also to manipulate it in various ways.[26,27] In the case of the study cited here, it is possible that a test that had incorporated a larger processing component would have shown even greater performance decrements.

Strategy. If stress influences attention allocation in part by channelling attentional resources into conscious monitoring of stressors, autonomic activity, and the preparation of coping strategies, it is possible that the limited capacity of the human cognitive system predisposes it toward strategies that reduce or simplify memory load under stress. There is in fact experimental evidence to the effect that humans under stress do restructure information to make it easier to assimilate. This is accomplished by 'chunking' and integrating information more, and by reducing the number of discriminations made and categories used.[64] This phenomenon is sometimes referred to as the 'simplification heuristic', and, it appears, can be triggered both by physical threat and by social threat (i.e., fear of failure or threat to the ego). Whether or not this effect of stress is negative in its implications for performance depends upon the circumstances. On the one hand, it may create a tendency to overgeneralize, to prefer stereotypes, to ignore important distinctions. The accidental destruction of friendly aircraft in wartime ('blue on blue' or 'home goal' accidents) probably owes something to this tendency, as individuals in a heightened state of tension engage any target resembling the enemy.

In terms of signal detection theory, then, stress may encourage 'riskier' (more 'trigger happy') responses, with both more hits and more false positives identified.[97] For example, an anxious crew may land at the wrong airport, when some, but (of course) not all the cues are consistent with it being the correct destination. The rationalization or self persuasion often involved in these types of errors is known as confirmation bias. Whether confirmation bias is affected differentially by workload and nonworkload stressors has not been addressed experimentally.

In many cases, however, simplification strategies probably work as nature presumably intended, reducing the wasteful processing of situational information that it is not necessary to know. For example, a pilot making discriminations about aircraft attitude or instrument functioning might well find that simple classifications such as 'right way up' versus 'upside down', or 'working' versus 'not working' are, in some stressful circumstances, more helpful than the many intermediate discriminations of attitude or instrument function that could be made.

Another important strategic shift is known as the speed/accuracy tradeoff. In stressful circumstances, individuals may attempt to maintain the speed of their responses (at the possible expense of accuracy), or they may, alternatively, slow down to maintain correct performance. Available research indicates that the former tradeoff is the more common: both in domain independent laboratory investigations[53] and in behavioural studies of aircrew decision making,[83,98] response accuracy has decreased under stress while speed has remained relatively unaffected.

This may not, however, represent the optimal strategy: evidence from simulation research conducted at the University of Illinois suggests that superior flight decision makers appear to be the ones who take their time under stress.[83] Any tendency of stress to accelerate action at the expense of greater error is probably also more marked in impulsive personalities. The effect may at times be the result of 'premature closure' (a feature of overly hasty decision making discussed in Chapter 4) and of 'intolerance of ambiguity' (see Chapter 6).

Spatial decrements. To the extent that working memory capacity is reduced by stress, we might expect to see stress related performance decrements in tasks involving spatial processes in working memory, such as orienting oneself at an unfamiliar airport (see sidebar). Experimental evidence for this is inconclusive, however. For example, Stokes and his colleagues were unable to provoke impairments of performance on a computerized hidden figures test, even when the test was given in a condition that required pilots to mentally rotate the target figure. On the other hand, stress did appear to increase the time it took pilots to solve screen presented mazes. In a speed/accuracy tradeoff contrasting with that discussed previously, pilots seemed to invest the time necessary to maintain accuracy at very high levels.[83]

The effect of stress upon maze performance is all the more interesting when it is known that cognitive maze tracing ability has been shown in one flight simulation study to be linked to pilots' ability to detect relevant decision cues from their environment.[84] This may be because both abilities involve the right parietal lobe of the brain.[82]

Cognitive maze tracing involves no physical tracking through the maze, so the measure is not confounded with manual control. It is an intriguing fact that cognitive maze tracing scores fall dramatically under the effect of alcohol and, sometimes, depression.[82] Thus, stress, depression, and alcohol may not be so very different in some of their performance effects, especially where the processing of visual-spatial cues is concerned.

Buchanan Field, Concord, California, January, 1991: I was on my way to my third solo flight. I spent about five to seven frustrating minutes to get ground clearance to taxi. (It could have been a radio problem). Finally the controller responded. The active runway was changed from 1 Left, a familiar runway, to runway 19 Right, a runway I had not taxied to before. Not being too familiar with the layout of the airport I started to taxi in the wrong direction. Being completely nervous and disoriented, I flipped open a map of the airport, which didn't seem to help. I crossed an active ruway without knowing it was active. However, I had looked before crossing the runway and no traffic was in sight (the traffic must have been at least seven miles out). About two seconds later the controller started yelling at me. That of course magnified my nervousness and at that time I was completely lost. The controller helped me taxi back to the hangar and the flight was terminated.

-- NASA Aviation Safety Reporting System (Accession No. 169360)

Finally, a study by Wickens and his colleagues examined the decision performance of pilots in such a way that performance on visual-spatial problems could be distinguished from performance on other types of in-flight problems. A variety of stress manipulations were used, including low volume irritating noise, time pressure, and financial risk. The results showed that problems with a high demand for spatial operations in working memory were particularly sensitive to the degrading influence of the stress manipulations.[98] In contrast, performance on problems dependent upon declarative knowledge retrieved from long term memory was unaffected by stress.

Long term memory

Although a great deal of research has been conducted on the effects of stress upon processes in working memory, very much less has been published which addresses long term memory (LTM) effects. A few important effects have been identified in two areas, however: the encoding of information into LTM (that is to say, learning), and the retrieval of information from LTM when it is needed.

Encoding: the effects of stress on learning. Stress has a negative effect upon the transfer of information from working memory to LTM. In other words, stress may be bad for learning. Many aviation organizations (Air Forces, for example) believe in 'realistic' training, in which students are exposed to stresses similar to those that they will later encounter in actual operations. This will, it has been suggested, increase training effectiveness by reducing uncertainty and fear of the unknown.[23,96] Other theorists have argued, however, that the presence of intense criterion-like stress may seriously impair the learning of skills the training is supposed to teach; some even suggest that what trainees actually learn in these circumstances is fear, emotional sensitivity, or even despair.[45,58,65]

Flight instructors, of course, love to argue about this over beer, a process greatly helped by the paucity of aviation research on the topic. Indeed, few studies of any sort have actually examined training under stress. One that did was reported in 1984 by Keinan and Friedland, who set out to determine the effectiveness of training (in this case, of a laboratory visual search task) in which different levels of electric shock were used as the 'stressor'.[63] While the methodology is obviously similar to that of the original Yerkes-Dodson experiment discussed in Chapter 2, in this case it was concluded that training was most likely to be effective when conducted with *minimal* interference from exposure to stressors (and not with intermediate levels of exposure, as the Yerkes-Dodson 'inverted U' would predict). Nevertheless, these researchers went on to suggest that benefits might yet accrue from trainees' familiarity with the stresses they were to encounter in the (post training) criterion situation.

This hypothesis has been tested in a recent and more sophisticated investigation by the same researchers.[40] The basis for this study was a comparison of three training approaches, called 'graduated intensity training', 'phased training', and 'customized training'. Graduated intensity training involved exposing trainees to stress which gradually intensified. (This strategy is derived from the concept of stress inoculation, which holds that it is possible to become inured to certain kinds of (otherwise) stressful circumstances through a process of progressive 'acclimatization'.[72,73,76]) Phased training separated skill acquisition and exposure to stressors into separate segments of the training process. Customized training attempted to maximize the trainee's familiarity with criterion stressors and to minimize any negative effects of stressed training, by varying stress intensity on an individual basis according to the personal characteristics of each trainee.

In the study, these three approaches were used on subjects whose task was to learn to locate a target digit within a display of digits; the 'stressor' used was again electric shock. The results indicated that phased training (involving the separation of the skills aquisition and the stress exposure elements of training) was the most promising approach of the three, at least for military instruction. The researchers also considered this kind of strategy to be the most useful for tasks requiring mastery of complex skills, such as those involved in piloting an aircraft. Customized training was also very effective, and was recommended for small, specialized units and for individual instruction. However, it was judged to be too costly and impractical for implementation on a large scale.

The results achieved with graduated intensity training were not greatly encouraging. Perhaps surprisingly, the graduated intensity approach impaired training effectiveness more than any other procedure. It was also associated with serious practical difficulties: as the researchers observed, more often than not it is difficult or impossible to quantify or calibrate 'real world' stressors along a continuum.[40] (Even if this were feasible, transactional views of stress would have us pay attention to a good deal more than putative external 'stressors': see Chapter 1.) Thus, it may not be realistically possible to manipulate stress intensity 'to order' for the purposes of training. As Friedland and Keinan[40] concluded,

> Our results indicate that training under constant high-intensity stressors and training that involves no stress are likely to prove counterproductive: The former interferes with the acquisition of skills that are relevant for task performance, and the latter does not sufficiently acquaint the trainee with criterion stressors. (p. 172)

While this study is without doubt a useful contribution to the database, it is not yet clear to what extent it can be generalized to other circumstances -- for example, to the mastery of more complex tasks, to genuinely threatening experiences rather than simple aversive stimulation, or to subjects with different learning styles and stress response characteristics. Additional research is needed to fill in the gaps in our understanding of training for highly skilled performance in stress inducing circumstances.

Retrieval: the effects of stress on recall. Generally speaking LTM retrieval processes appear to work well under stress, which seems to be one reason why high time pilots (who operate on the basis of experience) make better decisions than do low time pilots (who have to 'figure things out' in stress prone working memory). As this issue is considered at length in the following chapter, the present discussion will be confined to the phenomenon of stress related regression: that is, the observation that individuals under stress are prone to revert to behaviours, strategies, and schemata learned earlier, often many years earlier. They also tend to manifest simpler or cruder responses -- which in many cases, of course, *are* the earlier learned responses.[1,10,104]

This effect itself can lead to inappropriate allocation of attention and incorrect prioritization of actions. However, it can be difficult to gauge the everyday significance of the effect because, while such regressions are sometimes obvious (as in the 'earthmover' sidebar overleaf), they can also be subtle and difficult to detect. One low hour flight student, for example, experienced a door open emergency at cruise altitude just prior to descent and landing. He could have remained high and tried to secure the door, or ignored it and continued with the landing procedures. Instead, he immediately dived the aircraft to low level and began 'fighting' with the door while the aircraft bucked and reared close to the stall. Diving the aircraft was obviously not a previously learned response to this never-before-experienced event; however, it was possible to ascertain later (from careful debriefing) that under stress the student had reverted to an earlier, inappro-

---

Frederick, Maryland, January, 1993: I was taxiing with a three hour student. He has had problems taxiing due to past experiences operating earth movers. In an earth mover when you step on the right pedal you turn left and vice versa, the opposite control inputs of taxiing a small aircraft. We practiced slow turns on the taxiway. We began to come within five feet of the left side of the taxiway while steering left. He panicked and reverted back to his initial steering methods. He heavily applied left rudder while applying the brake and locked up his leg. In an effort to get away from the grass quickly he applied full throttle. I couldn't fight him on the rudder, and realizing we were going off the hard surface taxiway I pulled the mixture. The left wheel settled into a hole and the nose came down with the propeller striking the dirt twice until it continued to free spin, stopping due to the mixture.

-- NASA Aviation Safety Reporting System (Accession No. 231117)

---

priate nonpilot's schema, one in which 'high' represents danger and 'low' represents safety. This is, of course, the exact opposite of the proposition internalized by all trained pilots. However, just as one might come down a ladder before retying a shoelace, so the student had descended before trying to close the door.

Stress and attention

Attention is a very limited mental resource that can only be allocated to, at most, a few cognitive processes at a time. The more frequently that processes have been practiced, the less attention they require ... Processes that are highly practiced and require little or no attention are referred to as *automatic*. Processes that require attention are called *controlled*. (Anderson,[2] p. 36)

To someone who had never heard of money, merely describing it as a 'financial resource' would not lead to immediate enlightenment. Similarly, labelling attention a 'mental resource', as most psychologists do, leaves us little the wiser. In recognition of this, various metaphors have been suggested in an attempt to clarify the concept. Attentional resources may, for

---

The F/A-18 Hornet: A Challenge to Memory and Attention[88]

7 switches on the stick

*9 switches on the throttles**

19 switches on the 'up-front control'

59 indicator lights

6 auditory warning tones

675 CRT screen acronyms

40 multi-function display formats

177 CRT symbols

200 filmstrip data frames, plus maps on the horizontal situation MFD

73 CRT threat, warning, caution and advisory messages

22 head-up display formats

*Multiple function switches -- of course

---

example, be likened to a finite supply of energy, such as electricity, or water in a reservoir -- energy which may be channelled to do work in one or two, but by no means all locations. A more ramified version holds that there are multiple resources of attention -- different reservoirs, as it were -- specializing in certain functions.[97]

For example, functions with separate resource pools might include auditory attention and visual attention. Within this conception, flying an approach while trying to read the approach plate might overload the available supply of visual attention (in the the electrical metaphor) or drain it (in the water reservoir metaphor), but flying the approach while listening to ATC should be easier, to the extent that each activity draws on its own reservoir of attentional resources.

If attention is a resource which is allocated to different activities, it is legitimate to ask how it is allocated, and what stress does to that allocation. A brief answer would be that attention is allocated to matters on the basis of their perceived importance -- that is, by their psychological centrality or *salience*. Stress appears to influence which elements of information are considered to be central, and to decrease attention to anything assigned to the status of peripheral or secondary information by the cognitive system. It has been suggested that this occurs because stress restricts the range of environmental cues that the individual processes. The 'cue utilization hypothesis', propounded by Easterbrook in a much cited 1959 paper,[31] argues that "the number of cues utilized in any situation tends to become smaller with increase in emotion" (p. 197). It should be cautioned that the paper does not offer any actual mechanism for this process, and that Easterbrook's conception of emotion as a 'drive state' is not consistent with more recent conceptions of stress or arousal.[*] Nevertheless, the cue utilization hypothesis is consistent with some accounts of reaction to stressful events, in which aircrew have apparently become focussed upon one small part of their environment at the expense of all others.

We may also consider a 1974 finding by Bacon, who demonstrated experimentally that shock induced arousal can indeed restrict the range of perceptual cues considered by the individual. Bacon speculates that this occurs via a 'tuning down' of responsiveness to those features of the situation that were *originally* paid less attention.[4] (This hypothesis is not, by the way, consistent with reports of dramatic switches of attention from task related to threat related thoughts, as discussed below and in Chapter 7.) An alternative suggestion made by Bacon is that this effect may come less from attenuating sensory impressions than from the effect of arousal on processes in working memory (discussed earlier).

Perceptual and cognitive tunnelling

In keeping with the tradition of attention metaphors, perceptual attention has been likened to a searchlight beam.[91] Within this analogy, those elements of the environment falling within the beam are processed by the brain, and those outside are not -- sometimes irrespective of our wishes. As with some adjustable flashlights, the attentional beam may be narrow or broad, 'illuminating' (for example) many instruments on a display panel or merely a single instrument. There is some evidence that stress has the effect of narrowing this attentional beam -- a phenomenon often called 'tunnelling'. Tunnelling is thought to occur in several psychological contexts,[16,50] and is regarded by many psychologists as very much a 'real world' and not merely a laboratory phenomenon. For example, combat stress (discussed in Chapter 7) and the combination of 'life stress' with workload (see Chapter 5) have both been reported as causing 'cognitive' tunnelling (a phenomenon discussed below).[32,101]

---

[*]Indeed, Easterbrook's hypothesis has been used to account for the claimed relationship between arousal (unidimensional, of course) and performance expressed in the Yerkes-Dodson 'inverted U' curve.

Perceptual tunnelling may apparently involve an actual narrowing of the field of vision as measured by visual angle, and has been associated both with emotional stress[50] and cognitive workload.[77,105] Baddeley's review of over twenty research papers suggests that perceptual narrowing is a source of performance impairment in dangerous environments.[5] Actually, perceptual tunnelling may occur in visual and nonvisual sensory channels, as when attention is focused on the most salient elements in the perceptual field -- the loudest, brightest, or most quickly moving cues -- to the exclusion of those that are less salient. There is some preliminary evidence that individuals may differ in their 'baseline' tendency toward salience bias, and that psychological stress and workload have differing effects upon that baseline. Stokes and his colleagues reported a study in 1990 in which individuals played 'Air Attack', a kind of 'space invaders' game featuring both salient and nonsalient targets. Individual players showed stable tendencies toward salience bias, repeatedly exhibiting high bias scores or

Reading, Pennsylvania, March, 1992: I was just south of Pottstown VOR, I saw three or four large dark bird shapes pass just over the windshield. Simultaneously, I heard a WHUMP! and felt an impact to the plane. I pushed the button and said, "Just had a birdstrike, nearest aiport please." The controller said there were two airports and a lot of other stuff I didn't hear -- I was too busy hyperventilating, pumping adrenalin and being scared. I noticed that the controls were unbalanced and that my airspeed was down to 105 from 125. "Say the airport information again," I asked. This time I heard, "two airports ... eight miles ... sixteen miles," but that's all -- my cognitive bandwidth was severely constricted. "I want the eight mile one, what direction is it again?" She told me, I turned towards it and saw the beacon. "Sorry, my cage is a bit rattled," I said. I realized that the airport they had sent me to was dark, except for the beacon. "How long is that runway? Is there a controlled airport nearby?" "Yes," said Approach, "Reading Airport, 330 and sixteen miles." I turned through north and all the way to about 290 degrees and then I saw it and turned back on course. "I have the REILS (runway end indicator lights) and the beacon," I said. "We have all the lights turned up for you," she said. "If I haven't said it yet, I'd like to declare an emergency," I said. "I've determined that I've got a goose hanging from my right wing."

-- NASA Aviation Safety Reporting System (Accession No. 203448)

low bias scores. However, the workload increase represented by an additional memory task had no effect upon this baseline salience bias, while noise (which otherwise simulates the effects of anxiety on performance[53]) was associated with a marked increase in salience bias.[83] Among other things, these findings underscore the desirability of discriminating between the performance effects of workload and of psychological stress. Cognitive tunnelling also represents a salience based narrowing of the attentional field, but one in which the bias is defined in psychological rather than perceptual terms. A pilot attempting to reach a decision under stress, for example, may ignore information about alternative hypotheses and select from a more restricted field of options.

Theoretically, both cognitive and perceptual tunnelling ought (at least some of the time) to result in positive benefits -- i.e., by helping pilots or controllers to focus attention upon the particular task at hand without being distracted by extraneous or peripheral matters. Laboratory evidence is consistent with this. Consider, for example, the Stroop test: this is the famous test in which colour terms are presented in type of some different colour -- the word 'red' printed in blue, for example, or 'blue' printed in yellow.[86] Subjects asked to name the colour terms as rapidly as possible normally find that the need to 'tune out' the print colour slows down their responses; under stress, however, responses may if anything speed up, which suggests that stress may help individuals to focus their attention.[54,83]

Narrowing of attention in the operational world. Does 'real world' stress have analogous positive effects outside the benign confines of the laboratory, in complex operational circumstances? There is room for scepticism. Certainly both cognitive and perceptual tunnelling are suggested by accounts of various types of perseveration under stress: pilots, for example, may become fixated on or 'obsessed with' one equipment item, one response possibility, or one thought (see the sidebar by Saint-Exupery), often despite the operational ineffectiveness of the approach. Despite Bacon's speculation (that whatever originally received most attention attracts even more under stress) there seems to be little operational evidence that stress increases attention to previously central tasks, such as controlling the aircraft or communicating with the crew. Indeed, what becomes psychologically salient or central may be features or symbols of the threat. Consider, for instance, the case of the crashed airliner whose crew (as the voice recorder tape reveals) devoted considerable resources to vocalizing their increasing concerns about terrain clearance, but apparently made no

> *Without any warning whatever, half a mile from Salamanca, I was suddenly struck straight in the midriff by the gale off that peak and sent hurtling out to sea... I tried to climb, as soon as I became conscious of my disastrous mistake: throttle wide open, engines running at my maximum, my plane hanging sixty feet over the water, I was unable to budge. I hung on to the controls of my heavy transport plane, my attention monopolized by the physical struggle and my mind occupied by the very simplest thoughts. I made a discovery that horrified me: my hands were numb. My hands were dead. They sent me no message. Probably they had been numb a long time and I had not noticed it. I began to chant a silly litany which went on uninterruptedly. A single thought. A single image. A single phrase tirelessly chanted over and over again: "I shut my hands. I shut my hands. I shut my hands." All of me was condensed into that phrase and for me the white sea, the swirling eddies, the sawtoothed range ceased to exist. There was only "I shut my hands."*
>
> -- Antoine de Saint-Exupery (1939), *Wind, Sand, and Stars*

effort to actually arrest their descent, the single critical action that could have saved them.[67] (See also the discussion of 'stress induced inaction' in Chapter 7.)

This example illustrates how easy it is, with a little hindsight and post-hoc guesswork, to generate psychological descriptions of what 'must have' happened in an accident or incident.[*] Thus, there is never any shortage of (putative) cases of perceptual and cognitive tunnelling in aviation mishaps. The present authors would be the last to condemn such after-the-fact 'psychologizing', which after all virtually amounts to an international sport among aviation psychologists. Nevertheless, it has to be acknowledged that the confident extrapolation of laboratory research to the operational environment of flying is not without its difficulties. Take for example, the crash of an Eastern Airlines L-1011 in the Miami Everglades in 1972, an accident that has become a commonly cited (indeed, a somewhat hackneyed) example of cognitive tunnelling. The crew of the L-1011 focussed a great deal of attention on a nonfunctioning landing gear extension light

---

[*]However, the reader might like to try this for the Air Virginia accident described in the sidebar on p. 75 -- a complex multistressor event referred to again later.

and failed to notice that the altitude hold had been inadvertently disengaged. The aircraft descended into the swamp, with the GPWS (ground proximity warning system) whooping and commanding 'PULL UP'. There was no intervention by the crew.

The Everglades crash is certainly a good example of distraction and the power of a mental model (in this case, a belief that the aircraft was locked at a safe altitude), but is it a good example of stress induced attentional tunnelling? After all, everyone on the flight deck believed themselves to be quite safe for the time being -- indeed, that very conviction was arguably the problem. Contrast the example of the Everglades crash with the (rarely cited) crash of a Lockheed Electra in Reno, Nevada in 1985. The crew of this aircraft flew into the ground while apparently focussing all their attention upon a vibration which, they erroneously believed, signalled mortal danger and imminent catastrophe (see sidebar).

Task shedding. Task shedding refers to the abandonment of certain tasks (in favour of others) when stress or workload makes it difficult to maintain performance on all tasks at once. In a sense task shedding is tunnelling carried to its logical conclusion: not only are certain sources of information ignored (for example, radio calls), but entire tasks are abandoned (for example, communication).[81] This phenomenon may be more likely to occur under increasing workload rather than during distress, as the introduction of additional tasks makes prioritization necessary. It can also be adaptive if tasks are shed in an optimal sequence, with the least important tasks abandoned first.

However, anecdotal evidence from the operational world of flying suggests that it does not always work this way: as we have noted elsewhere, central tasks may often be disregarded in favour of trivial and peripheral activities (again, see the discussion of action paralysis in Chapter 7). Pilots, for example, are commonly instructed to attend first to the physical operation of the aircraft, secondarily to their position, and then, and only then, to controllers and others ("aviate, navigate, communicate"), but flight instructors routinely observe their students reverse these priorities when shedding tasks under stress or workload. This is most likely an example of a psychological salience effect -- for flight students the radio is an insistent, intrusive and authoritative voice as well as the medium by which their own stumbling efforts are broadcast for the world to hear. The radio seems to be very important and very central; also, it requires slow, deliberative 'controlled' processing to formulate calls. Thus it often claims

Reno, Nevada, 21 January, 1985: Galaxy Airlines Flight 203, with a crew of six and sixty-five passengers on board, departed runway 16 Right bound for Minneapolis, Minnesota. Upon climbout, however, the crew was alarmed by a severe vibration throughout the aircraft. The captain ordered a reduction in power on all four engines. This did not reduce the vibration, and the flight engineer noted that all four engines were performing well. Nevertheless, the throttles remained retarded. The crew, in audible distress, requested a turn left downwind to return to the airport "to get outta here, to get it back on the ground" (Cockpit Voice Recorder tape). The tower controller cleared the flight to turn left downwind into the traffic pattern, but thirty seconds later the aircraft crashed in an orange fireball about one and a half miles from the end of the departure runway. One passenger was thrown well away from the aircraft and survived.

The accident investigation showed that the vibration was caused by a small air start access door which ground handlers had failed to close properly and which was fluttering in the slipstream against the wing. This, however, had no negative effect upon the flyability of the aircraft. Moreover, the sky was clear with some twelve miles of visibility at the time of the accident. The NTSB concluded that "the airplane could have been controlled and flown safely had the flight crew responded appropriately to the perceived emergency" (p. 30). The Board determined that the probable cause of the accident was the captain's failure to control and the copilot's failure to monitor flight path and airspeed. The report cited the effects of acute stress as contributing to the accident, especially in the crew's preoccupation with the vibration and failure either to notice the deterioration in the aircraft's performance or to develop alternative courses of action.

-- Condensed from NTSB Report AAR-86/01

the student's attention, while other tasks, which may appear to the student to be arcane and optional workload increasing rituals (e.g., pre-landing checks), are simply 'shed'.

Prioritization and attention allocation bias

Prioritization: a distinct ability. The ability to prioritize communications data, positional and other flight progress information, and control actions has long been recognized as a distinct skill within air traffic control and among flight training professionals. For example, we have already noted the difficulties that beginning pilots experience with the maxim "aviate, navigate, communicate"; the need to provide auditory and visual cues to priorities within future ATC systems has also been explicitly pointed out.[90]

Evidence from neurological studies suggests, moreover, that the ability to sequence information and actions, to modulate and organize behaviour toward some objective, may be a distinct and separate ability, independent of working memory -- in fact, an 'executive' function of the frontal lobes of the brain. Damage to these areas (by stroke, accident, or disease, for example) appears to impair prioritizing ability while leaving intact many of the faculties most studied by human factors specialists and aviation psychologists: complex visual and spatial processing, language communication functions and recall.[7,8,70]

Despite this, very little is known to date about the practical implications of these findings in applied settings such as aviation, and human factors psychologists have seldom addressed prioritization as a distinct and deserving topic in its own right. One study that at least touches on the subject is that of Raby and Wickens,[80] who examined the scheduling behaviour of student pilots flying simulated ILS approaches under varying degrees of workload. The purpose of the study was to examine the effect of workload on task scheduling and time estimation, and to determine whether increased workload might disrupt pilots' ability to rank tasks according to their level of importance, as well as to accurately estimate the time needed to complete each task. The researchers found that task shedding did indeed occur as workload increased, but that this occurred in appropriate ways: pilots first abandoned the optional 'could do' tasks (which were secondary tasks assigned by the flight instructor), and then, if necessary, the 'should do' tasks (reviewing checklists and calling ATC), in order to allow adequate time to complete the 'must do' tasks (map reading, setting of instruments, and responding to ATC communications).

Since the level of task workload appears to have been well within the capabilities of these pilots, these data do not, by themselves, tell us much about prioritization under *stress*. However, a rather interesting effect was observed in the initial practice session, when the subjects were familiarizing themselves with the task prior to actual data collection. Task prioritization at this stage was noticeably poorer than subsequently: there was, for example, a tendency to overcomply with ATC instructions. The authors attribute this to novelty (the subjects were relatively unfamiliar with simu-

Raleigh-Durham, 1988: On January 15 Air Virginia (later renamed AVAir) filed for Chapter 11 bankruptcy protection from its creditors and ceased operations. It resumed on February 3. On February 19 AVAir Flight 3378 departed runway 23 Right at Raleigh-Durham for Richmond with two aircrew and ten passengers on board. The aircraft, a Fairchild Metro, climbed into low cloud, turned right, and overbanked to 45 degrees. Seconds later the aircraft crashed into a reservoir, killing all on board. No mechanical fault contributed to the accident.

The captain of the aircraft was suffering from sinus congestion and gastrointestinal problems, and the first officer conducted the takeoff. Both pilots had a record of difficulties in flying at AVAir, but those of the first officer were particularly acute, including a history of deficiencies in basic aircraft control and piloting skills. The Safety Board concluded that an examination of her difficulties suggested that her performance tended to deteriorate under stress. This was unfortunate because the circumstances of the flight itself (the visually restrictive conditions) and the first officer's recent history (a four and a half week layoff) created a highly stressful situation for her. Additional stressors included a last-minute change in ATC clearance, ATC pressure to initiate the turnout prematurely, and a Piedmont jet taking off behind AVAir 3378.

The Safety Board added that the AVAir management created extraordinary conditions for the company which included misjudgements of financial and operational planning. These extended to the failure to exercise proper supervision of the first officer. AVAir's management had been informed that the first officer's performance was marginal, but it failed to respond to progress and evaluation reports. The Safety Board concluded that this failure is accounted for, in part, by the turmoil AVAir was experiencing at the time and must be counted as a contributing factor in the accident, in addition to inadequate FAA surveillance of the company.

-- Condensed from NTSB Report AAR-88/10

lators), and to an excessive desire to comply with the demands made by the experimenter. In other words, there was both situational and social uncertainty, and some degree of anxiety may well have been present.

Attention allocation bias. Evidence from the study of clinically anxious patients suggests that anxiety can bias attention toward very specific and significant types of information, e.g., emotionally threatening stimuli.[102]

This evidence emerges from experiments which examined responses to the semantic content of screen presented words, some emotionally threatening and some emotionally neutral. The lexical design of the experiments is important because the results cannot be interpreted as an example of perceptual narrowing or of a physical salience effect. It is, of course, important to know whether these results mean that anxiety in nonclinical individuals (normal pilots or air traffic controllers, for example) also tends to shift attention toward the presumed source of the threat, whether or not it is physically salient (and thus, perhaps, away from truly diagnostic information or appropriate control inputs). Follow-up research conducted on normal subjects does suggest that the effect is not confined to clinical patients.[17]

One factor that appears to contribute to allocation bias is trait anxiety: individuals who are anxious by nature are more likely to focus upon threatening matters, while state anxiety does not appear to elicit the effect on its own in nonanxious or mildly anxious persons. Even the trait effect is weak, however, except in very trait anxious individuals, although there may be a tendency for the bias toward threatening data to be magnified in a 'vicious circle': the highly anxious pilot in a stressful situation may well attend disproportionately to the threatening features of the situation, which, in turn, will cause him to focus yet more exclusively upon just those features, and so on.

An important caveat to bear in mind is that the Spielberger Trait Anxiety Scale primarily indexes potential response to social threats and is a somewhat weaker predictor of response to physical threats.[37] Therefore, the stressful situations with which we might associate these attentional shifts are more likely to be certification checkrides, employee/management conflicts, threat of unemployment, personality or other social conflicts on the flight deck, marital problems, and, indeed, many of the circumstances described in the chapters on organizational and life stress.

The results found for highly trait anxious individuals should not be taken to imply that their low trait anxious counterparts are a homogeneous group of well-adjusted people who suffer from no attention allocation biasses. Actually, low trait anxious individuals may fall into one of two groups, those 'naturally' or 'authentically' low in anxiety, and those who repress their anxiety (but who exhibit high adrenergic arousal).[3] Recent work carried out by New Zealand researcher Elaine Fox essentially confirms this point, but differentiates between these two groups: in the study, genuinely nonanxious individuals remained unaffected by the emotionality of the stimuli, while repressors shifted attention *away* from emotionally threatening material.[36] This 'cognitive defence' (which will be discussed at greater length in Chapter 6, in the discussion of psychological defence mechanisms, and also in Chapter 7) stands in marked contrast, of course, to the responses of highly anxious individuals who shift attention *toward* threatening stimuli.

Despite the contribution of these interesting studies it must be conceded that the phenomenon of bias in attention allocation has yet to be thoroughly researched; discussion of this topic must perforce take the form of questions rather than answers. It remains to be determined, for example, whether cues are processed in actual order of their importance, or whether (apart from the tunnelling hypothesis) stress can cause a temporal 'rescheduling' of cues (for some speculation on mechanisms which could bring this about, see the section on paralysis of action in Chapter 7). It is also unclear to what extent the objective importance of a task influences attention allocation: it may be that stressed individuals are less likely to respond appropriately to minute-by-minute changes in task priorities and are more apt to adhere to a particular activity or strategy irrespective of changes in the nature of the task.

Vigilance

A third class of task often used in laboratory studies of attention is the vigilance task, which involves monitoring a situation for occasional signals of some kind. Although the signals occur only intermittently (and unpredictably), the subject must remain alert and ready to respond at all times. Performance of vigilance tasks has long been known to decrease substantially the longer the task is performed, even in the absence of any actual fatigue. Vigilance improves, however, with the use of amphetamines or with the introduction of an interrupting stimulus (for example, a telephone call) midway through the task;[71] this has been interpreted as suggesting that the performance decrement is linked to decreased arousal or motivation.[52]

In fact, performance on vigilance tasks is influenced by a variety of external factors, including lack of sleep,[99,100] heat,[78] and circadian rhythms.[12,24] Reviews of the effects of various putative stressors on vigilance have been compiled by Davies and Tune,[29] Poulton,[79] Broadbent,[15] and Hockey,[51] and can be summarized as follows. Vigilance is generally enhanced by moderate levels of 'stress' (where 'stress' is interpreted as heightened adrenergic arousal). Vigilance is decreased by fatigue and loss of sleep (thought to reduce such arousal). Noise and heat, which are assumed to increase arousal, may either improve or impair vigilance; in experiments the effect varies with task difficulty and 'stress' level (again, almost always operationalized as adrenergic arousal or simple workload). Within these restrictions, the results of vigilance research are consistent with the second precept of the Yerkes-Dodson 'Law' (see Chapter 2). Noise in particular has received considerable attention, as its relationship to vigilance is a somewhat complicated one. The presence of noise typically improves performance of complex vigilance tasks (for example, tasks in which the cues come from more than one source), but impairs performance of simpler tasks.[50] The task confronting researchers is to identify specific conditions associated with either greater or reduced efficiency.

Of course, signal detection theory considers not only the frequency with which cues are accurately detected, but also the number of *false* reports made. Typically, tasks with high event or signal rates are associated with numerous false alarms, while those with low signal rates are not. Broadbent and Gregory found that the detrimental effect of noise on performance was mainly confined to tasks with high signal frequency; performance of tasks with low signal rates was sometimes even enhanced.[18] This effect was interpreted not as a stress related change in visual acuity but as a difference in the level of decision confidence: when performing tasks with low signal rates, subjects were more cautious in deciding whether a signal was present, and when signals came frequently (a more 'stressful' task only in the workload sense), a less conservative, 'risky' criterion was apparently adopted, which had the effect of maximizing detection rates. Interestingly, recent research using self reported fatigue and motor activity measures of stress has demonstrated that while event rate influences vigilance performance, it may have no effect at all upon restlessness and sense of well-being.[41] In short, high event rates cannot be assumed to be stressful per se, even though performance is indeed impaired.

In discussing the effects of stress on vigilance it is sometimes easy to overlook the fact that vigilance tasks may be experienced as stressful in their own right.[49] Such tasks have been associated with increased negative affect, reported tiredness, and depressed mood states.[41,55,95] Even standard physiological 'measures of arousal' such as muscle tension and catecholamine excretion have been observed to increase during tedious vigils.[38,55] However, there is evidence that visual monitoring is experienced as being more stressful than auditory monitoring,[41] a finding which may have implications for display design in some cases.

Before leaving the subject of vigilance, the potentially confusing term 'hypervigilance' should be mentioned. Hypervigilance refers to a phenomenon described by Irving Janis and his colleagues.[59] In its most acute forms, the phenomenon consists of "an extremely agitated state of panic or near panic ... characterized by indiscriminate attention to all sorts of minor and major threat cues as the person frantically searches for a means of escaping from the anticipated danger" (p. 2).

Pilots in this condition may be hyperventilating and can be expected to show impaired judgement and poor decision making, often exhibiting a pattern of 'dithering' punctuated with impulsive choices. Thus, if vigilance means sustained attention, hypervigilance is something of a misnomer, insofar as it suggests *excessively* sustained attention. In fact, it means the opposite. Moreover, vigilance is a cognitive function affected in various ways by stress, but hypervigilance is not such a function but one of those effects itself.

Generalizability to complex multistressor environments

It is always safe to advise that a little humility and caution be exercised in extrapolating the results of laboratory studies in a simplistic way to complex 'real world' situations. However, the point is rarely better justified than in the case of stress research and aviation. Consider the crash of AVAir 3378 in 1988 (see sidebar on p. 75). As in so many cases, the possible contributing causes of this accident run the gamut of topics discussed throughout this book, and, as such, illustrate the 'muddiness' of causality in actual operational contexts. The stress and anxiety experienced by that unfortunate crew probably originated from a number of sources, both individual and corporate, as well as from time pressure, self doubt, and other variables.

However, as discussed in Chapter 1, many stress studies, not least those relevant to aviation, are simplistic experiments in the tradition of stimulus based or physiological approaches to stress.* Hardly any studies have examined complex multistressor circumstances such as those that prevailed in the AVAir mishap (and probably most aviation mishaps), let alone crew performance under these conditions. This lack of demonstrated operational

---

*And, to be fair, often intended to be controlled tests of various theoretical hypotheses, and not 'applied' research at all, which even today has low status connotations in many university departments.

relevance has been called one of the worst kept secrets of stress research in aviation: many aviation psychologists acknowledge that a high proportion of the available laboratory research findings have only a tenuous and, often, speculative connection with the interdependent performance of pilots, crews, dispatchers, and controllers operating long hours in a complex international airspace system.

Threats versus 'stressors'

Part of the research problem appears to lie in the time-honoured adherence to older models of stress. As noted in the opening chapter, (physiological) response based models have informed much of the field research that has been reported in both flight and ATC contexts, while laboratory and simulator research has very often been based in a tacit stimulus based model of stress. Thus, a significant proportion of the extant research literature is concerned more with putative 'stressors' rather than with perceived threat per se.

Aviation studies rarely discriminate between the performance effects of a given variable (workload, for example), and the performance changes due to any distress associated with that variable (workload that threatens success, for example). However, from the perspective afforded by cognitive appraisal models, stress does not inhere in the experimental manipulations or conditions themselves (e.g., noise, vibration, workload, or electric shock), but in the meaning that is ascribed to them. This is not to say that noise, vibration, and so forth have no performance effects worthy of study, merely that these should not be confused with the performance effects of *stress*.

The crash of Flight 203 in Reno (see the sidebar on p. 73) is a good case in point. In this instance, the crew became stressed by the presence of considerable airframe vibration and noise, which probably led to defective performance and, ultimately, tragedy. What provoked whatever reactions there were, however, appears not to to have been the noise or vibration itself, but the mortal threat that it signified.[*] Had the crew encountered similar conditions in a laboratory experiment, or even in a flight simulator study, it is unlikely that they would have experienced identical feelings and made the same responses as on the crash flight, however realistic the presentation. The vibration could have been reproduced. The noise could

---

[*]Compare, too, the role of the 'rumbling noise' in the crash of Flight 5050 at LaGuardia, discussed on p. 114.

have been reproduced. The threat, however, could not have been. Perhaps it is not surprising, then, to find that (methodologically easy) studies of vibration, noise, heat and suchlike variables are numerous, while (methodologically difficult) studies of threat are rare. Yet, as the accident and incident reports cited in this book testify, poor performance, incidents, and accidents due purely to noise, heat, cold, and the like are relatively rare in mainstream aviation, while problems due to anxiety, fear, and fatigue are common.

Control: a built-in experimental bias

Of all the methodological problems afflicting the research reported in this chapter (as elsewhere), there is one which is as important as it is intractable -- the role of individual control over events. For example, the crew of a flight simulator exposed to a 'Reno-like' event would know that they were going to walk away from the laboratory, not only perfectly safely, but with the experimenter's profuse thanks (not to mention a token payment for participating). In fact, any test subject can walk out whenever he or she pleases. The subject has ultimate control. This represents a nontrivial weakness inherent in virtually any laboratory or simulator based stress research.

Animal studies have amply demonstrated that the aversiveness of conditions do not by themselves explain the severity or duration of stress reactions. When the subject is unable to control or avoid the stimulus, stress reactions appear to increase. When the subject has control over the stimulus (or even perceived control), stress reactions are much less severe. For example, corticosterone levels in rats become elevated following exposure to electric shock, but return to normal relatively quickly (within ninety minutes) if the shock is escapable. However, if conditions are such that shock cannot be avoided, levels remain elevated for several hours following exposure.[87]

Humans, too, are more stressed by aversive events when they cannot control them.[13,20,74] The perception of control over events has a profound effect upon experienced stress levels, and also, presumably, on the nature and severity of any stress related performance changes. (Chapter 11 gives the example of female pilots 'trapped' on the flight deck for long duty days with abusive and sexist captains.)

Needless to say, ethical considerations preclude experiments in which humans are subjected to inescapable stress conditions. All human subjects are, for example, required to sign consent forms which usually state explicitly (among other things) that they are free to terminate the experiment at any time. Even if this were not the case, adults in this (increasingly litigious) society are not so naive as to believe that any experimenter would knowingly allow them to come to harm, and readily assume -- correctly, of course -- that any apparent threats they encounter are 'only part of the experiment' and represent no real cause for alarm. Thus, as Yates[103] has put it, "it seems quite plausible that although individuals might adopt sensible strategic responses to mild stresses in the laboratory, they would find themselves caught up in radically different reactive responses in severe, naturally occurring stressful situations" (p. 17).

Natural stress laboratories. The difficulties and limitations associated with conventional 'stress' research do not, of course, invalidate the database that exists, but they do invite us to attempt to supplement these studies (at least to replicate their findings) in more 'ecologically valid', i.e., realistic settings. The task of designing empirical, controlled studies of genuine human stress reactions may appear to be a difficult and daunting one. Indeed it is, but it is by no means impossible.

One quite promising approach, which has not been utilized nearly to the extent that it could be, involves the use of what have been called 'natural stress laboratories' -- that is, real-life situations in which the potential threat is both quite genuine and uncontrollable. Examples of this kind of research include the parachute and diver studies cited earlier in the chapter. The natural laboratory approach presents few ethical problems, insofar as the threat is an inevitable part of the circumstances and not a condition imposed by the experimenter. Naturalistic settings that have been used in this way include medical school examinations and cancer surgery (i.e, involving contrasts between students taking important versus unimportant exams, and patients undergoing either diagnostic or actual operative procedures).[56]

Other situations that represent possible settings for stress research include bomb disposal operations, hostage crises, flight checkrides, spin training, and forced landing training. While some of these situations have been explored in the context of stress and personality research (for example, bomb disposal -- see Chapter 7), few studies have been conducted that make use of aviation operations in the design of natural stress laboratories. However, this is not, of course, necessary in order to obtain results applicable to aviation.

Conclusion

The research evidence discussed in this chapter certainly suggests that under stress a range of cognitive functions important to piloting and air traffic control exhibit potentially important changes. These changes appear to be overwhelmingly in the direction of impairment, although increased adrenergic arousal may well improve vigilance and, in the laboratory at least, focussed attention. From the aviation perspective, the human factors/stress research 'coverage' appears to be rather patchy, however, leaving significant gaps in our knowledge. Some of this is probably due to the reluctance on the part of stress researchers in human factors and engineering psychology to utilize the findings in other stress literatures, such as those from clinical and personality research.

Many human factors stress studies are tacitly stimulus based. Because of this, the crucial role of the individual has often been overlooked, effectively resulting in poorly controlled experiments. For example, test subjects are often not evaluated for trait anxiety, or for chronic stress backgrounds, self efficacy, locus of control, or tolerance of ambiguity, all variables which have important effects upon stress reactions (see Chapters 5 and 6). Thus it is, for example, that in the area of psychomotor control, no studies have addressed the issue of which pilots under stress will overcontrol and which will undercontrol, and in what circumstances. In the area of attention allocation, no studies have attempted to predict which pilots will 'tunnel' on the primary flight task and which will focus exclusively upon the threat. The research that comes closest to doing so is perhaps the Scandinavian research involving the Defence Mechanism Test[68,69] (see Chapter 6, pp. 175-7).

The notion of threat, whether situational or perceived, is curiously absent from many human factors 'stress' studies. The operational relevance of the psychological database on stress would be improved significantly if more research focussed on perceived threat rather than on 'stressors'. The increased use of 'natural laboratories' may be helpful in this; in any case there is also a need for more studies which search for and elucidate the nature of synergisms -- that is, potent *combinations* of factors. Among these are:

1. Cognitive and personality variables among crew members. These include such factors as cognitive style, individual biasses, trait anxiety, and other factors pertaining to individual characteristics. The perform-

ance under stress of persons with particular cognitive and personality 'profiles' may vary greatly, depending upon whether they are paired with individuals of like or dissimilar profiles.

2. Multiple sources of performance degradation, such as chronic distress factors (life events, perhaps), combined with fatigue and acute threat (for example, inflight emergencies). It has been suggested that human factors researchers have tended to neglect chronic stress factors;[21,22,103] performance research addressing these factors would hence be especially welcome.

There is also a need for greater research on the effects of stress upon higher level 'open ended' problem solving. Most laboratory stress studies in human factors seem to have concentrated on well-defined 'low level' tasks, such as target search, tracking, and the like. However, as Yates and colleagues have pointed out in a report on human factors research needs, many real crises involve novel 'free form' tasks, especially for individuals with organizational responsibility.[103] The influence of stress upon such tasks may be even greater than upon the traditional, well-defined tasks so often studied. Nevertheless, as the report indicates, "There has been practically no direct study of such influences. So our 'understanding' of them is little more than speculation" (p. 10).

In particular, there is a need to increase research in the area of long term memory effects of stress, a subject which has been neglected somewhat in favour of studies of working memory. If the consensus on expert decision making is correct, and retrieval from long term memory is a major component of decision making,* then stress effects upon retrieval also deserve greater study. This is particularly the case where novel situations are concerned, since so little is known about the effects of stress upon selecting analogue information from long term memory.

There is, then, a need for basic performance data on stressed individuals in interaction with others, on the effects of multiple acute and chronic stress factors, and on higher level organizational, decision making, and communication skills in conditions of real threat. Without this, human factors stress research must remain modest in its claims to authority on issues of performance in the muddy waters of everyday flight operations and air traffic control.

---

*As opposed to analytic decision making in working memory (see Chapter 4).

References

1. Allnut, M. (1982), 'Human Factors: Basic Principles', in Hurst, R. and Hurst, L.R. (eds.), *Pilot Error*, Aronson, New York, pp. 1-22.

2. Anderson, J.R. (1985), *Cognitive Psychology and Its Implications*, W.H. Freeman & Co., New York.

3. Asendorpf, J.B., and Scherer, K.R. (1983), 'The discrepant repressor: differentiation between low anxiety, high anxiety, and repression of anxiety by autonomic-facial-verbal patterns of behavior', *Journal of Personality and Social Psychology*, vol. 45, pp. 1334-6.

4. Bacon, S.J. (1974), 'Arousal and the range of cue utilization', *Journal of Experimental Psychology*, vol. 102, pp. 81-7.

5. Baddeley, A.D. (1972), 'Selective attention and performance in dangerous environments', *British Journal of Psychology*, vol. 63, pp. 537-46.

6. Baddeley, A.D., and Hitch, G. (1974), 'Working Memory', in Bower, G. (ed.), *Recent Advances in Learning and Motivation* (vol. 8), Academic Press, New York.

7. Banich, M., Stokes, A.F., and Elledge, V. (1987), *Cognitive Function Evaluation in the Medical Certification of Airmen: A Literature Review*, University of Illinois Aviation Research Laboratory, Savoy.

8. Banich, M., Stokes, A.F., and Elledge, V. (1989), 'Neuropsychological screening of aviators', *Aviation, Space, and Environmental Medicine*, vol. 60, pp. 361-6.

9. Barnes, V.E., and Monan, W.P. (1990), 'Cockpit distractions: precursors to emergencies', *Proceedings of the Human Factors Society 34th Annual Meeting*, Human Factors Society, Santa Monica, CA.

10. Barthol, R.P., and Ku, N.D. (1959), 'Regression under stress to first learned behavior', *Journal of Abnormal and Social Psychology*, vol. 59, pp. 134-6.

11. Bergstrom, B. (1970), 'Tracking performance under threat-induced stress', *Scandinavian Journal of Psychology*, vol. 11, pp. 109-14.

12. Blake, M.J.F. (1967), 'Time of day effects on performance in a range of tasks', *Psychon. Science*, vol. 9, pp. 349-50.

13. Bowers, K.S. (1968), 'Pain, anxiety, and perceived control', *Journal of Consulting and Clinical Psychology*, vol. 32, pp. 596-602.

14. Braune, R., and Wickens, C.D. (1986), *A Componential Approach to the Investigation of Individual Differences in Time-Sharing*, University of Illinois Aviation Research Laboratory, Savoy.

15. Broadbent, D.E. (1971), *Decision and Stress*, Academic Press, New York.

16. Broadbent, D.E. (1978), 'The current state of noise research: a reply to Poulton', *Pychological Bulletin*, vol. 85, pp. 1052-67.

17. Broadbent, D., and Broadbent, M. (1988), 'Anxiety and attentional bias: state and trait', *Cognition and Emotion*, vol. 2, pp. 165-83.

18. Broadbent D.E., and Gregory, M. (1965), 'Effects of noise and signal rate upon vigilance organized by means of decision theory', *Human Factors*, vol. 7, pp. 155-62.

19. Buch, G., and Diehl, A. (1984), 'An investigation of the effectiveness of pilot judgment training', *Human Factors*, vol. 26, pp. 557-64.

20. Champion, R.A. (1950), 'Studies of experimentally induced disturbance', *Australian Journal of Psychology*, vol. 2, pp. 596-602.

21. Cohen, S. (1980), 'Environmental Load and the Allocation of Attention', in Baum, A., Singer, J.E., and Vallins, S. (eds.), *Advances in Environmental Psychology*, Erlbaum, Hillsdale, NJ, pp. 1-29.

22. Cohen, S., and Spacapan, S. (1978), 'The aftereffects of stress: an attentional interpretation', *Environmental Psychology and Nonverbal Behavior*, vol. 3, pp. 43-57.

23. Coleman, J.C. (1976), *Abnormal Psychology and Modern Life,* Scott, Foresman, Glenview, Illinois.

24. Colquhoun, W.P. (1971), 'Circadian Variations in Mental Efficiency', in Colquhoun, W.P. (ed.), *Biological Rhythms and Human Performance,* Academic Press, London, pp. 39-107.

25. Connolly, T.J., Blackwell, B.B., and Lester, L.F. (1987), 'A simulator-based approach to training in aeronautical decision making', *Proceedings of the Fourth International Symposium on Aviation Psychology,* Ohio State University, Columbus.

26. Daneman, M., and Carpenter, P. (1980), 'Individual differences in working memory and reading', *Journal of Verbal Learning and Verbal Behaviour,* vol. 19, pp. 450-6.

27. Darke, S. (1988), 'Anxiety and Working Memory Capacity', *Cognition and Emotion,* vol. 2, pp. 145-54.

28. Davies, D.R., and Parasuraman, R. (1982), *The Psychology of Vigilance,* Academic Press, London.

29. Davies, D.R., and Tune, S. (1970), *Human Vigilance Performance,* Staples Press, London.

30. Duffy, E. (1962), *Activation and Behavior,* McGraw-Hill, New York.

31. Easterbrook, J.A. (1959), 'The effect of emotion on cue utilization and the organization of behavior', *Psychological Review,* vol. 66, pp. 183-201.

32. Entin, E.E., and Serfaty, D. (1990), *Information Gathering and Decisionmaking under Stress* (TR-454), Alphatec, Burlington, Massachussetts.

33. Eysenck, M.W. (1979), 'Anxiety, learning, and memory: a reconceptualization', *Journal of Research in Personality,* vol. 13, pp. 363-85.

34. Eysenck, M.W. (1982), *Attention and Arousal. Cognition and Performance*. Springer, Berlin.

35. Firetto, A., and Davey, H. (1971), 'Subjectively reported anxiety as a discriminator of digit span performance', *Psychological Reports*, vol. 28, p. 98.

36. Fox, E. (1993), 'Allocation of visual attention and anxiety', *Cognition and Emotion*, vol. 7, pp. 207-15.

37. Fox, E., O'Boyle, C.A., Lennon, J., and Keeling, P.W.N. (1989), 'Trait-anxiety and coping style as predictors of preoperative anxiety', *British Journal of Clinical Psychology*, vol. 28, pp. 89-90.

38. Frankenhaueser, M., Nordheden, B., Myrsten, A., and Post, B. (1971), 'Psychophysiological reactions to understimulation and over-stimulation', *Acta Psychologica*, vol. 35, pp. 298-308.

39. Frazier, J.W., Repperger, D.W., Thoth, D.N., and Skowronski, V.D. (1982), 'Human tracking performance changes during combined -Gz and +Gy stress', *Aviation, Space, and Environmental Medicine*, vol. 53, pp. 435-9.

40. Friedland, N., and Keinan, G. (1992), 'Training effective performance in stressful situations: three approaches and implications for combat training', *Military Psychology*, vol. 4, pp. 157-74.

41. Galinsky, T.L., Rosa, R.R., Warm, J.S., and Dember, W.N. (1993), 'Psychophysical determinants of stress in sustained attention', *Human Factors*, vol. 35, pp. 603-14.

42. Garvey, W.D. (1957), *The Effects of Task Induced Stress on Man-Machine System Performance*, NRL report no. 5015, Washington DC, ASTIA no. AD 143 347.

43. Giffen, W.C., and Rockwell, T.H. (1987), 'A methodology for research on VFR flight into IMC', *Proceedings of the Fourth International Symposium on Aviation Psychology*, Ohio State University, Columbus.

44. Gliner, J.A., Horvath, S.M., and Mihevic, P.M. (1983), 'Carbon monoxide and human performance in a single and dual task methodology', *Aviation, Space, and Environmental Medicine*, vol. 54, pp. 714-7.

45. Haggard, E.A. (1949), 'Psychological Causes and Results of Stress', in Committee on Undersea Warfare (ed.), *Human Factors in Undersea Warfare*, National Research Council, Washington, DC.

46. Hamilton, V. (1982), 'Cognition and Stress: An Information Processing Model', in Goldberger, L. and Breznitz, S. (eds.), *Handbook of Stress: Theoretical and Clinical Aspects*, Free Press, New York, pp. 105-20.

47. Hammerton, M., and Tickner, A.H. (1969), 'An investigation of the effect of skill upon stressed performance', *Ergonomics*, vol. 12, pp. 851-5.

48. Hancock, P.A. (1982), 'Task categorization and the limits of human performance in extreme heat', *Aviation, Space, and Environmental Medicine*, vol. 53, pp. 778-84.

49. Hancock, P.A., and Warm, J.S. (1989), 'A dynamic model of stress and sustained attention', *Human Factors*, vol. 31, pp. 519-37.

50. Hockey, G.R.J. (1970), 'Effects of loud noise on attentional selectivity', *Quarterly Journal of Experimental Psychology*, vol. 22, pp. 28-36.

51. Hockey, G.R.J. (1978), 'Effects of Noise on Human Work Efficiency', in May, D. (ed.), *Handbook of Noise Assessment*, Van Nostrand-Reinhold, New York.

52. Hockey, G.R.J. (1979), 'Stress and the Cognitive Components of Skilled Performance', in Hamilton, V. and Warburton, D.M. (eds.), *Human Stress and Cognition*, John Wiley & Sons, New York.

53. Hockey, G.R.J. (1986), 'Changes in Operator Efficiency as a Function of Environmental Stress, Fatigue, and Circadian Rhythms', in

Boff, K.R., Kaufman, L., and Thomas, J.P. (eds.), *Handbook of Perception and Human Performance* (vol. 2), John Wiley & Sons, New York.

54. Houston, B.K. (1969), 'Noise, task difficulty, and Stroop color-word performance', *Journal of Experimental Psychology,* vol. 82, pp. 403-4.

55. Hovanitz, C.A., Chin, K., and Warm, J.S. (1989), 'Complexities in life stress-dysfunction relationships: a case in point -- tension headache', *Journal of Behavioral Medicine,* vol. 12, pp. 55-75.

56. Hudgens, G.A., Torre, J.P, Chatterton, R.T., Wansack, S., Fatkin, L., and DeLeon-Jones, F. (1986), 'Problems in modeling combat stress: a program to meet the challenge', *Proceedings of the Tenth Symposium on Psychology in the Department of Defense,* United States Air Force Academy, Colorado Springs.

57. Idzikowski, C., and Baddeley, A.D. (1983), 'Fear and Dangerous Environments', in Hockey, R. (ed.), *Stress, Fatigue, and Human Performance,* John Wiley & Sons, Chichester, pp. 123-144.

58. Janis, I.L. (1971), *Stress and Frustration,* Harcourt Brace Jovanovich, New York.

59. Janis, I., Defares, P., and Grossman, P. (1983), 'Hypervigilant Reactions to Threat', in Selye, H. (ed.), *Selye's Guide to Stress Research* (vol. 3), Van Nostrand Reinhold, New York, pp. 1-42.

60. Jensen, R.S. (1982), 'Pilot judgment: training and evaluation', *Human Factors,* vol. 24, pp. 61-73.

61. Jensen, R.S., and Benel, R.A. (1977), *Judgment Evaluation and Instruction in Civil Pilot Training,* Final report FAA-RD-78-24, National Technical Information Service, Springfield, Virginia.

62. Jorna, P., and Visser, R. (1991), 'Selection by Flight Simulation: Effects of Anxiety on Performance', in Farmer, E. (ed.), *Human Resource Management in Aviation,* Avebury Technical, Aldershot.

63. Keinan, G., and Friedland, N. (1984), 'Dilemmas concerning the training of individuals for task performance under stress', *Journal of Human Stress*, vol. 10, pp. 185-90.

64. Keinan, G., Friedland, N., and Arad, L. (1991), 'Chunking and integration: effects of stress on the structuring of information', *Cognition and Emotion*, vol. 5, pp. 133-45.

65. Kern, R.P. (1966), *A Conceptual Model of Behavior under Stress with Implications for Combat Training*, HumRRO Technical Report No. 66-12, The George Washington University, Washington, DC.

66. Kleitman, N. (1963), *Sleep and Wakefulness*, University of Chicago Press, Chicago.

67. Kornovich, W. (1992), 'Cockpit stress', *Flying Safety*, August, pp. 20-23.

68. Kragh, U. (1960), 'The Defense Mechanism Test: a new method for diagnosis and personnel selection', *Journal of Applied Psychology*, vol. 44, pp. 303-9.

69. Kragh, U. (1962), 'The prediction of success of Danish attack divers by the Defense Mechanism Test (DMT)', *Perceptual and Motor Skills*, vol. 15, pp. 103-6.

70. Lezak, M.D. (1983), *Neuropsychological Assessment*, Oxford University Press, New York.

71. Mackworth, N.H. (1950), 'Research in the Measurement of Human Performance' (MRC Special Report Series No. 268), H.M. Stationery Office, London, reprinted in Sinako, W. (ed.), *Selected Papers on Human Factors in the Design and Use of Control Systems*, Dover, New York, 1961.

72. Meichenbaum, D., and Cameron, R. (1983), 'Stress Inoculation Training: Toward a General Paradigm for Training Coping Skills', in Meichenbaum, D. and Jaremko, M. (eds.), *Stress Reduction and Prevention*, Plenum Press, New York.

73. Meichenbaum, D., and Novaco, R. (1977), 'Stress Inoculation: A Preventive Approach', in Spielberger, C., and Sarason, I. (eds.), *Stress and anxiety* (vol. 5), Halstead Press, New York.

74. Miller, S.M. (1979), 'Controllability and human stress: method, evidence and theory', *Behavioral Research and Therapy,* vol. 17, pp. 287-304.

75. Munday, R., cited in Middlebrook, M. (1990), *The Berlin Raids,* Viking, New York.

76. Novaco, R., Cook, T., and Sarason, I. (1983), 'Military Recruit Training: An Arena for Stress-Coping Skills', in Meichenbaum, D. and Jaremko, M. (eds.), *Stress Reduction and Prevention,* Plenum Press, New York.

77. Pamperin, K.L., and Wickens, C.D. (1987), 'The effects of modality and stress across task type on human performance', *Human Factors Society 31st Annual Meeting,* Human Factors Society, Santa Monica, California.

78. Pepler, R.D. (1953), 'The effect of climatic factors on the performance of skilled tasks by young European men living in the tropics: IV. A task of prolonged visual vigilance', *Medical Research Council, Applied Psychology Reports,* vol. 156.

79. Poulton, E.C. (1970), *Environment and Human Efficiency,* C.C. Thomas, Springfield, Illinois.

80. Raby, M., and Wickens, C.D. (1990), 'Planning and scheduling in flight workload management', *Human Factors Society 34th Annual Meeting,* Human Factors Society, Santa Monica, California.

81. Sperandio, J.-C. (1978), 'The regulation of working methods as a function of work-load among air traffic controllers', *Ergonomics,* pp. 193-202.

82. Stokes, A.F., Belger, A., Banich, M.T., and Bernadine, E. (1994), 'The effects of alcohol and chronic aspartame ingestion upon per-

formance in aviation relevant cognitive tasks', *Aviation, Space, and Environmental Medicine,* vol. 65, pp. 7-15.

83. Stokes, A.F., Belger, A., and Zhang, K. (1990), *Investigation of Factors Comprising a Model of Pilot Decision Making, Part II: Anxiety and Cognitive Strategies in Expert and Novice Aviators,* University of Illinois Aviation Research Laboratory, Savoy.

84. Stokes, A.F., Kemper, K.L., and Marsh, R. (1992), *Time-Stressed Flight Decision Making: A Study of Expert and Novice Aviators,* University of Illinois Aviation Research Laboratory, Savoy.

85. Stone, R.B., Babcock, C.L., and Edmunds, M.S. (1985), 'Pilot judgment: an operational viewpoint', *Aviation, Space, and Environmental Medicine,* vol. 56, pp. 149-52.

86. Stroop, J.R. (1935), 'Studies of interference in serial verbal reactions', *Journal of Experimental Psychology,* vol. 18, pp. 643-62.

87. Swenson, R.M., and Vogel, W.H. (1983), 'Plasma catecholamine and corticosterone as well as brain changes during coping in rats exposed to stressful footshock', *Pharmacology, Biochemistry, and Behavior,* vol. 18, pp. 689-93.

88. Taylor, R.M. (1989), 'Crew Systems Design: Some Defence, Psychology Futures', in Jensen, R.S. (ed.), *Aviation Psychology,* Gower Technical, Aldershot, Hants., pp. 38-49.

89. Telfer, R. (1987), 'Pilot judgment training: the Australian study', *Proceedings of the Fourth International Symposium on Aviation Psychology,* Ohio State University, Columbus.

90. Tonner, M. (1990), 'The Controller in Human Engineering', in Wise, J.A., Hopkin, V.D., and Smith, M.L. (eds.), *Automation and Systems Issues in Air Traffic Control,* Springer, Berlin.

91. Wachtel, P.L. (1967), 'Conceptions of broad and narrow attention', *Psychological Bulletin,* vol. 68, pp. 417-29.

92. Wachtel, P.L. (1968), 'Anxiety, attention, and coping with threat', *Journal of Abnormal Psychology,* vol. 73, pp. 137-43.

93. Walker, R., Sannito, T., and Firetto, A. (1970), 'The effects of subjectively reported anxiety on intelligence test performance', *Psychology in the Schools,* vol. 3, pp. 241-3.

94. Walker, R., and Spence, J. (1964), 'Relationship between digit span and anxiety', *Journal of Consulting Psychology,* vol. 28, pp. 220-3.

95. Warm, J.S., Dember, W.N., and Parasumraman, R. (1991), 'Effects of olfactory stimulation on performance and stress in a visual sustained attention task', *Journal of the Society of Cosmetic Chemists,* vol. 42, pp. 199-210.

96. West, L.J. (1958), 'Psychiatric aspects of training for honorable survival as prisoners of war', *American Journal of Psychiatry,* vol. 15, pp. 329-36.

97. Wickens, C.D. (1992), *Engineering Psychology and Human Performance* (2nd ed.), HarperCollins, New York.

98. Wickens, C.D., Stokes, A.F., Barnett, B., and Hyman, F. (1991), 'The Effects of Stress on Pilot Judgment in a MIDIS Simulator', in Svenson, O., and Maule, J. (eds.), *Time Pressure and Stress in Human Judgment and Decision Making',* Cambridge University Press, Cambridge, England.

99. Wilkinson, R.T. (1959), 'Rest pauses in a track affected by lack of sleep', *Ergonomics,* vol. 2, pp. 373-80.

100. Williams, H.L., Lubin, A., and Goodnow, J.J. (1959), 'Impaired performance with acute sleep loss', *Psychological Monographs: General and Applied,* vol. 138, pp. 685-6.

101. Williams, J.M., Tonymon, P., and Anderson, M.B. (1990) 'Effects of life-event stress on anxiety and peripheral narrowing', *Behavioral Medicine,* pp. 174-84.

102. Williams, J., Watts, F., MacLeod, C., and Mathews, A. (1988), *Cognitive Psychology and Emotional Disorders*, John Wiley & Sons, Chichester.

103. Yates J.F., Klatzky, R.L., and Young, C.A. (1992), 'Cognitive Performance under Stress', in Committee on Human Factors, *Research Needs Report*, National Research Council, Washington, DC.

104. Zajonc, R.B. (1965), 'Social facilitation', *Science*, vol. 149, pp. 269-74.

105. Zhang, K. (1989), *Effects of Noise and Workload on Performance with Object Displays versus Separated Displays*, unpublished doctoral dissertation, University of Illinois.

4 Decision making and communication

For a split second a wave of uncontrollable panic surged through me.
On reflection I do not honestly think this was due to the knowledge of the
possible consequences, so much as the fatal decision I was forced to
make.
> -- Alex Henshaw, *Sigh for a Merlin: Testing the Spitfire*

As well as those problems which are inherent in any communication
system, the human decision-maker is the victim of another hazard --
namely that attention, perception, memory and thinking are all liable to
distortion or bias by emotion and motivation.
> -- Norman F. Dixon, *On the Psychology of Military Incompetence*

Chapter 3 reviewed a number of general cognitive abilities important in flight and ATC operations, and the ways in which these abilities can be affected by stress. An additional skill that was mentioned, but not discussed at any length, was that of judgement or decision making. As we noted previously, faulty decision making has been implicated in a large proportion of pilot error accidents.[18,28,29,60] Once thought to be an intangible aspect of airmanship or 'The Right Stuff' (see Chapter 6), aeronautical decision making has increasingly been recognized as a cognitive function amenable to analysis and responsive to formal training. Decision making has developed into an important research field both within psychology generally and in specific applied areas such as aviation.

Within the field of decision research stress effects have become an important topic. This chapter is, therefore, primarily concerned with the effects of stress upon pilot judgement and decision making. We begin with a general review of the types of thought processes in which humans engage when deciding upon a course of action, and proceed to an examination of individual flight decision making and the effects of state and trait anxiety. The second half of the chapter examines group or crew decision making, beginning with a consideration of stress and communication in general. We then move up the hierarchy of stress effects, from acoustic, phonetic and lexical changes, to syntactic and semantic effects, to broader issues of group understanding, shared mental models, and social behaviour.

Models of decision making

Analytical decision making: weighing the options

Traditional conceptions of decision making describe a cognitive sequence that is heavily inferential and analytical. The process runs as follows: the individual faced with a decision to be made assesses the situation, considers all available alternatives (calculating the costs and benefits of each), and ultimately arrives at the best solution to the problem.[27] In this view, the goal is to select the best alternative (what is sometimes referred to as 'maximizing utility'), and good decision makers invest whatever resources are required (time, energy, etc.) in order to do so.

This type of strategy is thought to yield the most positive outcome -- if it is fully implemented (that is, if situational factors are comprehensively weighed and viable alternatives fully considered). Conversely, it is assumed that if all steps in the process are not completed, defective decision making will result. It is not difficult to imagine such a process being short circuited under conditions of high workload and psychological distress. Analytical decision making makes heavy demands on working memory resources*, for example, and working memory capacity can, as we discussed in Chapter 3, degrade very significantly under stress.

Psychologist Giora Keinan of Tel Aviv University has made an extensive study of the effects of stress on the selection of alternatives, and suggests three mechanisms by which decision quality might degrade under stress.[30,31,32] The first of these, *premature closure,* refers to the forming of a decision before all possible options have been evaluated. It is possible that this results from the cognitive tunnelling referred to in Chapter 3, in which the decision maker, under pressure, concentrates exclusively on a small subset of the information available and ignores everything else.[51,72,73] This, of course, leaves fewer options from which to choose. But premature closure also brings to mind the personality trait of impulsiveness, which, as we discuss in Chapter 6, has been put forth as one of several 'hazardous thought patterns' in pilots.

---

*Consider, for example, trying to analyze the costs and benefits of three competing life insurance policies.

Nonsystematic scanning, the second threat to decision quality, occurs when the reviewing of options becomes frantic and disorganized rather than logical and orderly. The individual may even appear to switch back and forth between the same alternatives in a random manner.[26] This is a symptom of 'hypervigilance', a stress condition described in Chapter 3.

Finally, in what Keinan calls *temporal narrowing*, all decision options may be considered, but insufficient time is allocated to each option such that it cannot be adequately assessed. Studies by Keinan and colleagues requiring subjects to solve a series of logical analogy tests under threat of electric shock have demonstrated the presence both of premature closure and of nonsystematic scanning, but (arguably for methodological reasons) have failed to demonstrate temporal narrowing. Interestingly, however, studies by Stokes show that experienced pilots invest more time in decision making and make better decisions than inexperienced flyers. These results diverge from the common expectation that proficiency is necessarily marked by rapid, as well as accurate decision performance.[57,58] It is also important to note that Keinan's studies, unlike some others, have excluded time pressure as a stressor (potentially a confounding variable). This allows the conclusion to be drawn that "psychological stress, in and of itself, has a significant effect on the manner in which the decision makers scan the alternatives available to them" (Keinan,[31] p. 642).

While analytical decision making strategies are probably used from time to time by pilots, there is some doubt as to whether most pilots, most of the time really go about decision making in the 'traditional' analytical way. If this is true, the stress effects described by Keinan, while real, may not be as commonplace in operational flying as might otherwise be the case. Next, therefore, we consider some of the drawbacks of the analytical approach as a model of aeronautical decision making, and then go on to discuss an alternative approach which suggests that good decision making may stem less from exhaustive analysis than from applying the lessons of experience.

The best versus good enough: problems with the analytical model. The analytical model of decision making may be a reasonable approximation of what corporate traders and foreign policy makers do or try to do. However, it does not seem to be entirely representative of the kind of decision making most often encountered in flying, or, for that matter, emergency room medicine, firefighting, or other dynamic, risk filled occupations. The combination of critical time pressure and raw emotion that sometimes

Suddenly, without a spit or cough the engine stopped and I was in an awful ominous silence, other than the noise of the slipstream which slowly died away as the machine went into a normal glide. I looked below in desperation but all I could see in that depressing black country-side was steelworks, electric pylons, terraced houses and the odd highly banked canal. For a split second a wave of uncontrollable panic surged through me. On reflection I do not honestly think this was due to the knowledge of the possible consequences, so much as the fatal decision I was forced to make. It was Russian Roulette with a double-barrelled gun, but both barrels were loaded. I could bail out, but would I make it? I could try to put the machine down -- but where -- and would I survive? I didn't want to make the final decision but in the seconds I had to spare I was compelled to act and to do it instantly. Once I had decid-ed on my course of action I became calm but I felt in my heart that this was my last flight.

-- Alex Henshaw, *Sigh for a Merlin: Testing the Spitfire*

characterizes flight decision making under stress is illustrated by the epi-graph at the head of the chapter. This is taken from Alex Henshaw's account of a skewgear failure in a Spitfire, a fuller account of which may be found in the sidebar above. Henshaw eloquently expresses the cognitive turmoil, the oscillation of attention between task and threat (see Chapter 3), that makes the analytic model seem quaint and implausible, either as a description of, or prescription for, decision making under stress in fast moving contexts.

In evaluating the analytical model it is not necessary, however, to invoke situational extremes. Consider a relatively commonplace situation: a pilot encountering deteriorating weather conditions. Among other things, she may elect to climb, to descend, or to maintain altitude; to slow down, to speed up, or to maintain airspeed; to divert, to continue, or to turn back; or some combination of these. There are twenty-seven combinations or action alternatives in this simple scenario alone; allowing only a minute or so for analyzing the short and long term implications of each one and comparing it with all the others for optimality, the very safest and most efficient course of action can probably be determined -- in about half an hour, weather permitting! It comes as no surprise, then, to learn that analytical strategies have been shown experimentally to be ineffective in situations where time limits constrain the amount of cognitive processing that can be done, and so prevent a fully comprehensive analysis of the situation.[24,46,74]

There is also reason to doubt that pilots, especially experienced pilots, are really trying to whittle down all possible alternatives to some single very best option. Indeed, Shanteau[50] has suggested that

> Although expert decision makers may make small errors, they generally avoid large mistakes. They seem to have discovered that for many decisions coming close is often good enough: the key is not to worry about being exactly right, but to avoid making really bad decisions. (p. 208)

For example, protocols obtained from fireground commanders have shown shown that these expert firefighters do not spend precious time weighing alternative options or evaluating probabilities.[35] Rather, they report seeking 'workable', 'timely', and 'cost effective' courses of action. Similarly, expert aviators may, instead of investing substantial mental resources in identifying an optimal solution, invest the minimum resources consistent with arriving at a strategy that is workable and adequate for the extant problem, even if it is not necessarily the most elegant one. This decision strategy is sometimes referred to using the (admittedly unlovely) neologism 'satisficing'.[52] An alternative model of decision making that is more consistent with this view, therefore, focusses on the experienced pilot's ability to use long term memory to invoke a decision response without major recourse to deliberations in (highly stress vulnerable) working memory.

Flying and chess: pattern recognition models

Experiments conducted within the slow moving, fustian world of chess playing might not, at first blush, appear to be an ideal place to begin an analysis of flight decision making. In fact, however, these studies throw considerable light on what experienced pilots probably do and don't do when deciding on their 'next move'. Several researchers have used chess to investigate the nature of expertise because chess is a very formalized domain with well recognized skill levels.[8,12,37] One study showed, for example, that chess masters (an advanced skill classification) were far more capable than novices of accurately replacing chess pieces removed from a board *if those pieces had formerly been arranged in a coherent game position*. The conditional statement is key here: when the pieces were randomly placed, masters were no better than novices at recalling the configurations. Another interesting finding was that the two groups performed quite differently in the presence of time pressure: masters were not affected by it, but the quality of the moves made by novices was significantly worse.[7]

These findings provide little support for the common notion that expert chess players must have inherently better basic cognitive skills (prodigious memories, superior logical reasoning, etc). Rather, they are more consistent with the view that expertise in chess is a function of the size and quality of the repertoire of game states (i.e., the pattern of board positions) internalized over years of playing.

Within this model, chess masters match the board layouts that they see with 'mental layouts', that is, patterns or templates based on games played in the past and stored in long term memory. Thus, they are able to reconstruct board positions without overloading working memory with individual piece positions. Time pressure has very little effect upon this efficient pattern matching strategy, since the slow computational processes in working memory are largely bypassed. In other words, the experimental data suggest that the decision performance of experts is characterized by a 'top down' knowledge representational model rather than by a 'bottom up' information processing model.

For purposes of the present discussion, an important feature of the chess masters' performance is that the moment a board position is recognized and categorized, he or she appears to entertain only a few potential high value moves, each of which is analyzed no more than perhaps two or three moves into the future. This contrasts with the supposition that chess masters need to be able to analyze large numbers of pieces and mentally play out future moves in considerable depth.

The cognitive capabilities of experienced pilots may be analyzed in a fashion analogous to those of expert chess players. On the one hand, it could be that pilots -- highly selected personnel, after all -- have superior cognitive capacities which help them to exhaustively analyze situations and review all alternatives before selecting the best course of action (the analytical model). Alternatively, in parallel with chess masters and novices, proficient high time flyers may differ little from low time pilots in basic information processing skills. Rather, the seasoned fliers could be seen as accessing a large repertoire of well organized situational schemata -- aerial game states, as it were, which, once recognized and categorized, confine the consideration of action alternatives to a very few high value 'moves'.

(By high value we mean, of course, options in which the probability of success is high).

This kind of 'it worked before' strategy has been called 'pattern matching', 'pattern recognition', and (by one researcher) 'recognition primed decision making'.[34,35] It is based less on finding the 'best' solution to a given decision problem than merely a workable and timely one. Indeed, recent research indicates that both skilled pilots and chess players generate adequate options as the very first courses of action they consider. Often, the first *satisfactory* solution that presents itself is adopted as the most efficient course of action.[37,58]

An integrated model of pilot decision making under stress

Stokes has argued that experienced pilots (and for that matter, air traffic controllers) routinely function by using the pattern recognition strategy in flight management decisions.[56] Figure 4.1 presents a diagrammatic model of pilot decision making under stress, in which the large upper box represents the pilot's long term store of domain specific information: flight situations experienced, procedural 'scripts', and mental models (of aerodynamics, systems, the airspace, and so forth). The large lower box represents processes within working memory, non-domain specific, analytical processes such as logical inference, mental arithmetic, and the like. Other processes include the 'metacognitive' processes of appraisal (such as the evaluation of situational demands and personal coping resources) that, as we discussed in Chapter 1, are associated with the level of stress actually felt or experienced. High stress levels are assumed to significantly reduce working memory capacity, not least by using capacity for 'worry work', that is, for non-task related self referential thoughts. (For more on this, see the discussion of stress induced inaction in Chapter 7).

The decision making process is represented by the bold outline boxes. Going from left to right, the pilot 'samples' the world, registering instrument readings, ATC calls, the external scene, and so on. The 'picture' of the situation (equivalent to the chess master's board layout) is then matched to a situational 'schema' or template in long term memory. Most of the time an adequate match is found. With it comes at least one workable option (or, at least, one that has worked before), as well as the procedures to implement it. Part of the decision making process involves setting priorities; thus, the pilot slots the chosen procedures into an appropriate place in his flight management sequence and executes the decision.

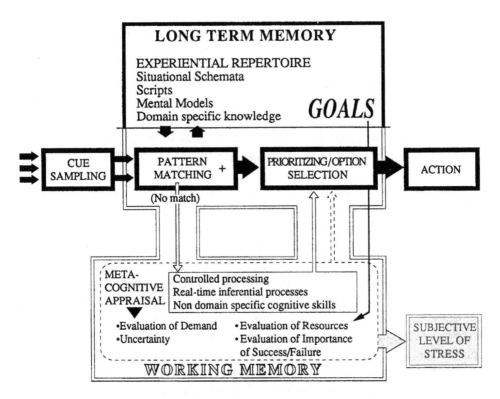

Figure 4.1 A model of decision making under stress *(from Stokes[56])*

Note that in this conception, the long term memory (LTM) strategy (in Stokes' terminology), or the recognition primed decision making (RPDM) strategy (in Klein's more precise terminology) forms the normal, pre-ferred, or 'default' strategy. The analytical approach -- that is, the time intensive computational and inferential use of working memory,* is resort-ed to only when the 'pattern matching' strategy cannot be utilized. This, in turn, occurs only when an appropriate schema is not evoked by the envi-ronmental cues -- as, for example, in unusual or abnormal flying condi-tions. (Of course, if the pilot is inexperienced this is likely to occur even in fairly routine circumstances.)

It is easy to see how failure to 'pattern match' may be due to the inexpe-rience of the pilot. Novice aviators, like novice chess players, simply have a smaller stock of situational schemata to operate with, and are therefore more often forced to 'drop down' into slow, inefficient analytical process-ing. An example may be seen in flight students' actions prior to the descent as they approach a terminal area. Even when the environmental cues appear (to their instructors) to be almost shouting "initiate the descent now!" (that is, when the cues closely reproduce a pattern in the instructor's long term memory), students are still sometimes heavily engaged in trying to calculate the descent point from some rule of thumb.[*] Students often find this computationally intensive process to be difficult to complete while actually flying the aircraft, talking to ATC, and so forth; by the time the calculation is complete, it is often too late for it to have much operational value.

Even where the pilot is very experienced, an appropriate schema may not be invoked by the environmental cues because of the unique features of the circumstances. For example, in 1979 the crew of an American Airlines DC-10 departing from O'Hare International Airport in Chicago was faced with the loss of an engine -- unbeknownst to them, the physical loss of the whole engine and nacelle, which had rolled up and over the left wing. This had, in turn, ripped out the hydraulics to a leading edge high lift device, causing it to retract. Nothing in the crew's experience -- certainly, no simulated engine failure emergencies -- had prepared the crew for such an eventuality. They followed normal engine out procedures (the DC-10 has plenty of power left even without an engine). When the aircraft began to roll left uncontrollably on climbout, the crew were taken by surprise. With sufficient time any crew could probably have 'figured out' what had to have happened. Unhappily, the length of time that it takes to run analytical diagnostics in working memory was less than the time it took for the aircraft to sustain the power loss, stall the left wing, and hit the ground.

In evaluating the circumstances in which pilots might 'drop into' a slow analytic decision making process, one element is striking, whether the discussion is of novices 'out of their depth' in ordinary circumstances, or experienced fliers faced with extraordinary circumstances. That is, the conditions are often just those calculated to maximize the mismatch between perceived demand and perceived resources to cope, where failure matters and uncertainty is high: in short, conditions of stress. It is an irony that the circumstances that may force a switch to intensive analytical

---

[*]One such rule is to multiply a range (in miles from the runway) by 3, convert it to hundreds of feet, and add the field elevation to give a height appropriate for a three degree glide slope at that range. Subtract this from the current height and factor in groundspeed in miles per minute to give a rate of descent in feet per minute that will put the aircraft at the correct glideslope height at the selected distance from the runway.

processes in working memory are also those that reduce the capacity of working memory and the efficiency of processes in it. In stress, then, an inefficient decision mechanism is rendered yet more inefficient.*

Empirical studies of pilot decision making

Analytical versus recognition primed decision making

Psychological research has a way of coming up with neat and tempting formulations that do not bear really close scrutiny -- the engineering analogy for human stress discussed in Chapter 1, for example, or the inverted U curve relationship between stress and performance discussed in Chapter 2. If the model of pilot decision making under stress outlined above is at all neat or tempting, it behooves us to give it close scrutiny. Fortunately a number of studies have been conducted which throw light on the claims made by the model.

A research team at the University of Illinois conducted a series of studies on aeronautical decision making for the US Air Force. The first of these studies, which proceeded from an analytical model of decision making, attempted to contrast the decision making of experienced and inexperienced aviators by exploring the extent to which decision quality was a function of information processing skills and flying knowledge -- the putative components of the decision making process.[67]

In the study, thirty-eight instrument rated pilots were identified as either experts or novices on the basis of their flight hours, and administered a set of domain independent cognitive tests. These were selected with a view to assessing the information processing skills traditionally believed to comprise decision making ability. They included, for example, tests of working memory capacity, logical reasoning skills, spatial ability, and visual cue sampling skill. The pilots subsequently 'flew' a simulated instrument flight in which they were presented with a series of decision scenarios with multiple choice responses. The answers they provided were used to assess the quality of their decision making.

The results showed that in low time pilots, very few of the information processing tests bore any relationship to the quality of decisions made. Those that did -- mainly the tests of working memory capacity and spatial

---

*For a discussion of this in an organizational context see pp. 336-337.

ability -- were only weakly or moderately predictive. Declarative knowledge (of flight rules, regulations, and other nonsituational 'ground school' topics) was no better a predictor of decision quality. And in high time or 'expert' pilots, information processing measures were hardly predictive of decision making ability at all. The authors concluded that these results provided little support for the idea that pilots normally use the working memory intensive 'analytical' decision strategy.

It will be noted, of course, that this study only provides negative evidence. While it suggests that pilots do not rely heavily on analytical decision making, it does not provide direct support for the alternative contention, that pilots utilize an LTM (or RPDM) strategy, much less that such a strategy is in any sense 'stress resistant. The question of pilots' preferred strategy was investigated in a 1989 experiment by the same University of Illinois team.[2] As in the previous study, expert and novice IFR pilots completed a battery of generalized information processing tests; this time, however, subjects also attempted three domain specific tasks designed to index representations of situational knowledge in long term memory.

The first, called the Air Traffic Control (ATC) Recall Task, involved reconstructing both randomized and coherent radio call sequences from memory; it was hypothesized that by controlling out memory effects (using recall of the *jumbled* transmissions), the quality of reconstruction would be primarily influenced by the availability of appropriate situational 'scripts' in the pilot's repertoire. A second task, called the ATC Recognition Task, involved building a mental 'picture' of a situation from ATC calls and selecting appropriate diagrams of the scenario. The third task, the Dynamic Diagnosis Task, involved recognition of failures or flight problems (e.g., wind shear, suction pump failure, pitot icing), solely by reference to instrument panel indications. Finally, as before, subjects completed a simulated instrument flight with multiple choice problem scenarios.

The results showed that for the novice pilots, the risk assessment and logical reasoning tests were significant predictors of decision performance. For experts the tests of working memory, visual scanning, and logical reasoning were predictive of decision quality, but the aviation specific knowledge representation tasks were much more so. These findings provide positive support for the model shown in Figure 4.1. However, they do not demonstrate that 'top down' strategies (i.e., the use of direct retrieval of situational schemas from LTM) are particularly robust in the presence of task related stress, or that 'fragile' computational and integrative processes in working memory are more readily disrupted by stress.

Stress and decision performance

The preceding hypothesis was examined in two additional studies. The first was a between-subjects design,[68] in which twenty novice instrument pilots were pair matched by flight hours and test battery results. Each pilot flew a single simulated flight: ten in a nonstressed condition, and ten while being subjected to several (putative) stress manipulations. These included the following:

1. *Time pressure:* pilots were instructed to finish the flight in one hour (the mean time taken by the nonstressed group).

2. *Additional workload:* pilots were required to perform a secondary task, which involved responding to visually presented letters on the instrument panel which were stimuli for a Sternberg memory search task.

3. *Financial risk:* pilots were told that their earnings (as paid subjects) would be depleted for every minute in excess of one hour; secondary task errors were linked to further financial decrement.

4. *Irritating noise:* failure to perform the secondary task rapidly and accu rately produced an annoying tone of moderate volume (72 dBa). Even with successful completion of the task, the tone was periodically (and randomly) presented in order to create uncertainty and doubt over per- formance.

It is important to note that the experiment was not attempting to separate the effects of these manipulations, but rather to impose conditions that would affect the pilots' appraisal of demand, their ability to cope, and the importance of success. Pilots emerged from the test sweating and shaking their heads about their performance, but no formal pre- and post-test evaluation of stress was reported -- an unfortunate omission.

In fact, the stress manipulations did seem to provoke significantly poorer flight decision making. Interestingly, however, this deterioration was not found for all problem types. Decisions depending heavily on retrieval of textbook knowledge from long term memory, although not (in these nov- ices) very good to begin with, were no worse in the stress condition. However, decisions requiring spatial skills were highly disrupted by stress. This suggests that problems with a high demand for spatial operations in working memory may be particularly sensitive to the degrading influence of stress, again as predicted by the model.

Whether this result was, in fact, caused by a stress induced reduction in working memory capacity, however, is questionable in the light of a third set of results. These appeared to indicate that decision performance was essentially unaffected by the demand for verbal working memory, and this insensitivity was observed equally for stressed and control subjects alike. Working memory is where the clearest stress related decrements might have been expected.[23] This result, therefore, is not consistent with the model presented earlier; however, it may be an artifact of methodological limitations inherent in that particular study.

First, stress effects were inferred from decision performance on problems rated subjectively (albeit by pooled expert ratings). While it is relatively easy to rate a problem as being high or low in demand for spatial skills or declarative knowledge, it is much harder to rate the working memory demand of a problem scenario. Thus, these ratings may simply have been inaccurate. Alternatively, the decrement in decision performance observed for spatial problems may have been partially due to the visual/verbal (screen displayed) nature of the workload increasing Sternberg task. Since most of the spatial problems involved instrument scanning, it is possible that these were disrupted more by the need to visually time share with the Sternberg display than by a reduction in working memory capacity. On the other hand, a further study demonstrated that very similar stress manipulations can give rise to significant decrements in performance on working memory and spatial tasks as tested in an aviation relevant test battery.[59] Moreover, in this latter study, declarative knowledge scores were not significantly different in the stress and nonstress conditions, consistent with the findings of the simulation experiment.

A second stress study was accordingly designed which, in addition to replicating the first, included a number of modifications intended to permit a clearer test of the hypothesis that the source of stress resistance in expert aviators is indeed 'recognition primed decision making'.[57] For example, the earlier work had only *inferred* stress effects upon putative components of decision making (such as working memory and spatial ability) from decision making performance on specific problem types (memory problems, spatial problems, etc.). This placed a great burden upon the accurate content analysis of the problems.

In the follow-up experiment, however, stress effects were measured directly and outside the criterion task. This was done by utilizing the same stress manipulations used in the flight simulation during administration of the cognitive test battery. In fact, stress effects on the performance of knowledge representation tasks were also measured separately. Second, the study used a within-subjects design and two different simulated flights (stressed and nonstressed, in a counterbalanced design). This eliminated the difficult task of trying to match pairs of pilots by skill and flight hours in order to run stressed and unstressed groups on a single criterion flight. Third, the stress manipulations used in this study are believed to adhere more closely to a cognitive appraisal model of stress, and involved a closer replication of noise stress conditions that have been found to simulate anxiety in their effects upon performance.[23] Last, the study contrasted novice and expert IFR pilots, as in the initial experiment in the series, rather than observing a relatively homogeneous set of low time pilots. It was anticipated that these changes in the research design would permit the experimenters to observe the extent to which stress gave rise to (domain independent) cognitive performance decrements in experts and novices, as well as the extent to which these effects were either reproduced or resisted by experts and novices in the simulated operational setting.

In the experiment, thirty instrument pilots flew two simulated IFR cross-country flights (one stressed and one unstressed). The battery of automated tests was also administered under stress and control conditions, providing data on the effects of the stress manipulation upon the putative cognitive components of decision making, independent of the criterion task. The results were dramatic. They clearly showed significant decrements in performance under stress for both experienced and inexperienced pilots in non-aviation specific information processing tasks. These decrements were of the same magnitude for experts and novices, and involved the same tasks. However, as hypothesized, this was *not* associated with any performance decrement in simulated flight decision making by experienced pilots. Although decision quality was about equal for the two groups in the control condition, only the novice pilots made significantly poorer decisions under stress, and only on "dynamic" scenarios (problems involving attention to moving display indicators). This not only comports with earlier results showing the vulnerability of spatial processes to stress, but is consistent with the view that novice pilot performance is more dependent than expert performance upon an analytic decision making strategy that is particularly susceptible to disruption by stress.

Perhaps more significant than this, it was found that high *trait* anxiety was associated with markedly worsened decision performance only in novice aviators exposed to acute stress. No impairment of flight decision performance was observed in experts exposed to acute stress. This is an all the more interesting result insofar as the trait anxious group within the experts actually exhibited higher trait anxiety scores than the trait anxious group within the novices. Domain specific knowledge, the researchers concluded, may not only provide a 'stress inoculation', but may be a more important variable in resistance to acute stress than personality -- at least insofar as trait anxiousness is concerned. Put another way, the hypothesis (discussed in Chapter 1) that trait anxiety predisposes individuals to respond to stressful circumstances with more marked state anxiety was found to be true for the low time aviators in the study, but untrue for the high time aviators.

The final study in this series investigated the relationship of cue recognition and hypothesis generation to proficient aeronautical decision making in the presence of one particular stressor, time pressure.[58] As in the preceeding studies, low and high time pilots were administered tests both of general (domain independent) information processing ability and of experience related (domain specific) cognitive schemata. The flight simulation portion of the study differed, however, in that the problem scenarios permitted open ended (as opposed to multiple choice) responses. In addition, subjects were required to identify the cues underpinning their decisions and to list all viable decision alternatives. Time limits were also imposed.

Results showed that under time pressure, the experienced pilots detected significantly more *relevant* cues than did their junior colleagues. They also chose to execute their first option alternatives significantly more often, suggesting that their decision making was also more efficient. Pilot's certification level was easily the most powerful predictor of decision performance. (Total flight hours, in contrast, had no predictive value.) Among the psychometric variables, the best predictors of decision making proficienc included spatial memory skills and the knowledge representation test measures.

Further support for this model of analytical versus experience based decision making comes from Cohen,[10] who conducted a study of decision strategies adopted by a group of airline pilots. The experiment was a paper and pencil exercise involving a series of inflight problem scenarios. In each scenario a flight was defined, followed by the announcement of unexpected weather problems requiring a diversion/no diversion decision to be made. The weather problem consisted of a fog bank that might obscure both destination and alternative, one but not the other, or neither.

As an additional variable, dispatch recommended continuation in half the cases and diversion in the other half.

Examination of the strategies adopted by the pilots revealed three groups: risk takers, less experienced non-risk takers, and experienced non-risk takers ('experience' being defined as having twenty years of experience or more). Only the latter pilots took the dispatch advice seriously. While not following it slavishly, they did tend to begin their decision making from the dispatch recommendation -- utilizing a 'provisional acceptance' and attempted rebuttal approach.

Cohen notes that the decision process observed in these pilots was at variance with the analytical model in several respects. First, the options were evaluated sequentially, rather than being compared concurrently. Second, pilots analyzed potential outcomes selectively, not exhaustively, concentrating on the worst case and the expected case. Third, potential courses of action were evaluated using an 'accept and critique' strategy, instead of by reference to quantitative weightings, as attached to decision alternatives in the analytical model.

Cohen makes the important observation that while the decision making strategies of experienced and inexperienced pilots may indeed be qualitatively different, this is not merely the result of the repertoire of situational experiences ("specialized recognitional templates" -- p. 247) that experience brings. Rather, experience in a particular domain (for example, aviation) also brings with it characteristic strategies for using that information. These could be described as metacognitive skills which only evolve over extended periods of time.

Crew decision making

This chapter has thus far focussed primarily upon the strategies and processes adopted by pilots acting as individual decision makers. Another dimension is added, however, when decision problems are addressed collectively by teams -- as is, of course, the case in multicrew aircraft. Faulty crew coordination has been implicated in a very large number of aviation mishaps; more than one study, in fact, has attributed the *majority* of flight crew errors or accidents not to failures of individual members but to breakdowns in group process.[47] Thus, the study of group decision making processes among pilots has important implications for flight safety, and is likely to receive increasing attention in the future.

Of course, group decision making can 'go wrong' in a number of ways. Most obviously, perhaps, there may be communication problems between team members. Existing research on group decision making (and, also, cockpit resource management) has devoted considerable attention to the social aspects of communication in groups, and to the ways in which this can be affected by stress or other factors. We will return to this subjevct later in the chapter; however, another area of potential interest concerns the effects of stress on speech itself. This is, unfortunately, a somewhat neglected topic; however, because of its clear importance to the study of group decision making, it seems fitting to review here such findings as do exist.

Stress effects on communication

Speech production under stress. Speech communication undergoes various changes under stress: some acoustical and phonetic, and some lexical, syntactic, and semantic. These changes can be important indicators of stress and, in addition, potential sources of communication degradation, misunderstanding, and error. In examining these changes we will move up the hierarchy of effects from the purely acoustical (of most relevance, perhaps, in *detecting* stress), through phonetic changes, to semantic effects.

Acoustical changes in speech. It has been known for well over a century that emotional state has specific and quantifiable effects on speech production.[20] A number of investigators, most notably in Russia and Japan, have applied this knowledge to the study of aircrew speech, generally in the context of accident investigation: the idea is to analyze radio communications to determine the pilot's emotional state in the period leading up to the accident (particularly when the pilot has not survived to render an account). These studies report consistent changes in pilots' speech quality in times of stress, presumably resulting in part from an increase in muscle tension around the larynx and vocal cords. The changes include increases in pitch[33,45,53,70] and vibration,[41,42] as well as frequency, amplitude and speech rate.[6,38,61,71]

These studies have tended to involve extreme levels of stress, with the individuals involved being in mortal peril. However, the same types of changes have been shown to occur in conditions of increased workload or task difficulty,[5,19] which, while suggesting a common psychophysiological mechanism, may also represent a methodological difficulty in discriminating high workload from actual distress. Some of the observed changes (e.g., increased speech rate) clearly represent a possible source of communication degradation; however, the extent to which the overall set of changes influences transfer of information in realistic settings is not clear.

Phonetic changes. Phonetic changes represent another stress related speech alteration which has clear implications for overall intelligibility, in particular, the articulation of vowel sounds. Both depressed[20] and affectively aroused[62] individuals tend to blur the distinction between different vowels in favor of a neutral 'schwa' sound (that is, the sound of the 'e' in the word 'the').[63] Although this finding has, to date, received little attention from aviation psychology, it may have significant implications for flight deck operations. Vowel sounds are, of course, important and sometimes crucial in distinguishing one word from another, and the accurate identification of such sounds is likely to be especially important where nonnative English speakers (on the flight deck or in ATC) are attempting to comprehend a message that may already be degraded by other effects.

Lexis, syntax, and semantics. While changes in the acoustic and phonetic characteristics of speech production represent an interesting (if not fully explored) topic, potentially more important stress effects exist at the level of sentence structure, grammar, and word choice. In a 1990 review of research in voice analysis in workload and stress research, a French team noted that lexical choice had not been the subject of any special study.[48] They also noted that there had been little systematic research in lexico-grammatical and semantic changes with stress and workload. This is a surprising omission, for these may be areas of great potential.

For example, in conditions of high excitement or time pressure, speech appears to become simplified and telegraphic. An interesting (if nonaviation) example is found in the excited and cliche ridden 'patter' of highly aroused sports commentators. Wanta and Leggett have shown that the rate at which commentators resort to cliches is predicted by the importance of the game (as indexed by the ranking of the teams and the degree of 'upset' in the games).[65] Indeed, the British satirical magazine *Private Eye* carries a column entitled 'Colemanballs' which routinely exploits the entertaining infelicities of speech uttered by overexcited, time pressured sports commentators. Under pressure there appears to be a tendency to revert to easy and familiar ways of communicating, 'down home' dialects, the use of cliches and other 'ready made', often imprecise, abbreviated, or cryptic shorthand expressions. Attempts to express more complex ideas may break down, as the sports commentators' splendidly mixed metaphors attest. The

LaGuardia Airport, September, 1989: USAir Flight 5050, a Boeing 737-400, was departing on runway 31 for Charlotte, North Carolina. As the first officer began the takeoff he felt the aircraft drift left (later found to have been caused by a mistrimmed rudder). The captain noticed the left drift also, and used the nosewheel tiller to help the first officer steer. As the takeoff run progressed, the aircrew heard a 'bang' and a continuous loud rumbling noise. The first officer maintained force on the right rudder pedal and later testified that the aircraft once more began to track true. However, the captain had some anxiety over the unidentified bang (later identified as probably the left nosewheel tire coming off the rim as a result of the tiller input). The Cockpit Voice Recorder shows that the captain then said "Got the steering". Later the captain reported this to investigators as "You got the steering". The first officer, however, reported it as "I got the steering", and, on the understanding that directional control was now being exercised by the captain, released pressure on the right rudder pedal. As the takeoff progressed, the rumbling (caused by the extreme nosewheel angle) continued, and less than three seconds after the captain's remark "got the steering", the (now directionally pilotless) aircraft swerved left. These symptoms prompted the captain to abort the takeoff late in the sequence. The aircraft ran off the end of the runway into Bowery Bay, killing two passengers.

-- condensed from NTSB Accident Report AAR-90/03

reversion to less elaborated speech is probably both a time pressure effect and a manifestation of the often cited phenomenon of stress related regression to first learned responses (see Chapter 3, pp. 65-6).[1,3]

One of the effects of this may be overpronominalization, said to be a feature of childhood speech, especially in lower socioeconomic strata.[4] Stressful circumstances are sometimes characterized by exchanges like this: "Oh no, it's on fire!" "What is?" "There, right there!" "Where?" These exchanges are only humourous after the incident, and if no harm has been done. British investigators point to the captain's command "throttle *it* back", in an aviation emergency in which the wrong engine was shut down, leading to the loss of the aircraft (discussed later). Weick[66] describes the role of reversion and communication degradation in his account of the 1977 Tenerife air disaster, the runway collision between a KLM Boeing 747 and a Pan Am 747 which resulted in 583 deaths:

The Pan Am captain wanted to hold short of the active runway, but he was asked to proceed down the active runway by a ground controller who spoke with a heavy accent and who did not seem to comprehend fully what Pan Am was requesting. Rather than attempt a potentially more complex negotiation to get permission to hold short, the Pan Am captain chose the more overlearned option of compliance with the controller's directive. Controller communiques also became more cryptic and harder to understand as controllers tried to cope with too many aircraft that were too big. These pressures may have made their use of English, a language which they used less frequently, more tenuous and increased the likelihood that more familiar Spanish instructions would be substituted. (p. 123)

Despite evidence from accounts such as this,* research on speech degradation in terms of its acoustical, phonetic, lexical and syntactic/semantic changes under stress still has a long way to go. This is even more true for fatigue. Other than at the acoustic-phonetic end of the scale, these are almost virgin research areas in the aviation domain. While the research that has been done in acoustics and phonetics is often very sophisticated technically, even at this level many serious problems remain. Laboratory workload manipulations are idiosyncratic and difficult to generalize, and it is not known how well they represent operational workloads. Significant results tend only to be associated with extremes of stress and workload, making it difficult to calibrate these variables on a continuum.[48] Finally, variations in emotional response and in workload have not been well discriminated, either conceptually or experimentally.

Reception of information under stress. The negative effects of stress upon transmission of information may also be compounded by decreased ability to receive and interpret messages. Chapter 3 discussed a number of stress effects on information processing, many of which can combine in subtle ways. A simple but classic example from flight training runs as follows. The student has reduced power from a 'level approach' power setting and is descending toward a short runway. However, she remains too high on the approach: she has not reduced power enough. Every additional second at the selected power setting is making a successful landing less likely. Various hints do not alert the student (who does not seem to hear -- she is tense and 'whiteknuckling' the controls; her attention appears to be tunnelled on salient visuospatial stimuli, and she is not processing peripheral

---

*For another example of an accident in which communications and language difficulties (also English/Spanish) played a pivotal role, see the sidebar on p. 367.

auditory stimuli). Finally the instructor commands (very loudly and saliently), "Throttle back!" The technical register of the command is part of a newly learned repertoire for the student, and she responds on the basis of her nonaviation language experience and automatic compliance with the authority figure. She promptly puts the throttle 'back' -- that is, back to its previous position, level approach power -- ruining any chance of landing but providing insufficient power to 'go around', i.e., to climb away. The instructor hurriedly intervenes, wiser or with another anecdote about 'foolish' students.

Obviously, not all interpretation errors can be attributed to stress. However, time pressure and psychological distress may make such errors much more likely to occur, and often compound the confusion. One reason for this is that in stressful circumstances team members may not be 'listening up' as efficiently as usual: attentional tunnelling and working memory restrictions may cause individuals to miss advice, information, or instructions from ATC or flight deck colleagues. Indeed, entire crews have been known to miss warning horns when anxious and distracted.[69] Crew members under stress may miss more subtle cues, as well -- for example the confusion or hesitation in a first officer's voice (see the sidebar on the Kegworth crash), or the *absence* of a comment where one might have been expected. The same is true for nonverbal information -- for example, failure to notice the hand that hesitates over the fuel switches and then moves away without switching tanks.

Where crews are concerned, however, there may also be broader interpersonal dynamics at work. Information exchange, even information connected solely with the task at hand, does not take place in a social vacuum. We now consider some of the social aspects of communication within teams.

Are two (or more) heads better than one?

In theory, at least, decision making by teams should be more efficient and effective than decision making by individuals. After all, as Orasanu[43] has pointed out, a group can collectively take in and process more information than any one member could manage unaided:

> Multiple eyes, ears, hands, and minds increase cognitive capacity, increasing the potential for better decisions. Crews can consider a larger picture, contribute more viewpoints, offer multiple options, use more information, share workload, critique proposals, and avoid traps." (p. 13)

Kegworth, Leicestershire, 8 January, 1989: A Boeing 737 twin engined airliner departed Heathrow for Belfast. Climbing through 28,300 feet the No. 1 engine (on the left of the aircraft) suffered a blade failure, causing airframe shuddering, smoke within the aircraft, and fluctuations in No. 1 engine instrument readings on the flight deck. The crew diverted to East Midlands Airport. The presence of smoke led the captain to suspect the No. 2 (right) engine, on the basis of his conception of the air conditioning system in the 737. The captain asked the first officer which engine was causing the trouble. The latter replied, "It's the le... It's the right one." The captain said, "OK. Throttle it back". Shortly thereafter engine instruments stabilized and the smoke cleared. The captain went on to order the shutdown of the right engine. In order to calm panicky passengers, he announced that problems with the right engine had caused the smoke but that it was now shut down. The busy cabin attendants did not hear the announcement. Passengers who could see the left engine on fire were puzzled but did not communicate the discrepancy to the cabin attendants. The aircraft continued its descent and approach to East Midlands Airport until, at 900 feet and just over two miles short of the runway, the No. 1 engine suddenly lost power. Attempts to restart the No. 2 engine failed, and the aircraft crashed onto the M1 motorway. Forty-seven passengers died, and seventy-four suffered serious injury.

-- Adapted from an Air Accidents Investigation Branch Report cited in *Flight Deck*, Winter, 1991, pp. 3-9.

Whether teams really do make better decisions than individuals, however, is partly a matter of context. Mullen and Goethals have observed that individuals tend to function well in situations where there exist both a clear 'best' answer and a well defined procedure for arriving at it: in these instances, the presence of more than one person may not necessarily result in better decision making.[40] However, tasks which require the integration of information from many sources (as is true of aviation) are often accomplished more efficiently by groups or teams -- at least, potentially.

Sometimes, however, decision making by groups can actually be *less* efficient than when only a single individual is involved. This has been demonstrated, for example, in controlled studies in which identical problem situations are presented both to individuals and to teams.[44] Aviation specific evidence along these lines is reported by Clothier, who found that in airline operations, two person crews exhibited superior performance to three person crews, whether the criterion was actual line performance or performance in simulator based Line Oriented Flight Training (LOFT).[9] Clothier ascribed this decrement to inefficiencies introduced via the third communication node.

In such instances, instead of saying that "two heads are better than one", a more applicable cliche might be "too many cooks spoil the broth". While teams of decision makers may have superior powers of information gathering and integration, they are also subject to certain vulnerabilities over and above those that apply to individuals, as we shall see.

The concept of the 'team mind'. What exactly is a team or a crew, if not merely the sum of its parts? One decision theorist, Klein, has conceptualized the team almost in terms of a supernumary individual, an emergent entity -- the 'fourth man' in a flightdeck crew of three, for example.[36] In this view the crew has a 'team mind' distinct from the individual minds that contribute to it. This type of thinking can quickly degenerate into mysticism, of course; however, the concept does not in fact depend upon numinous notions of belonging or identity. Rather, the idea of the team mind derives from the notion of shared information and pooled knowledge. Each of the three individual flightdeck crew members are monitoring a wide range of phenomena, but each draws the other's attention to but a few items (by speech, but also by pointing, control movements, and body language).[49] In other words, the team mind only has access to that which is publicly shared. The team's 'subconscious' mind consists of the knowledge that is not yet, but is potentially available to the team, data that some individual crew member may be fully aware of but has not communicated to the others. One example of the failure of a team mind can be seen in the KLM crew involved in the Tenerife disaster, which has been described as functioning less like a coordinated team than like three individuals working in parallel.[66]

Special problems of team decision making

Group understanding. One rather obvious area in which crews can experience difficulties is in the establishment and maintenance of communal understanding. Misunderstandings can occur, for example, about the nature of the task, the proper procedure for executing it, or the wishes and intentions of the group leader. Also, there may be a lack of consensus as to where individual responsibilities lie and precisely who should be doing what; this may stem from actual disagreements or from nothing more than a failure to question assumptions. Whatever their causes, such communication breakdowns can lead to duplicated (and possibly conflicting) efforts, or, more seriously, to neglect of individual responsibilities (on the assumption that "someone else will take care of it").

Mental modelling. Related to the issue of communication in groups is what we might term the 'convoy' problem, after the well-known requirement for convoys to steam at the speed of the slowest ship. In a rapidly developing situation, the 'mental model' or 'picture' of the situation needs to be updated regularly to keep abreast of events. If each individual provides part of that picture, then the complete model is available to the team mind only when the last element of information has been supplied. That is, there will be a tendency for a team's appreciation of a dynamic situation to lag behind the real rate of change. Through various mechanisms already discussed, stress is likely to exacerbate this feature of team performance. Given these difficulties, the 'team mind' may be left with a simplified, partial, distorted, and out-of-date representation of the true state of affairs. Indeed, this is seen all the time in accounts of military command (and is part of what Clausewitz called the 'fog of war').

Social aspects of crew interactions. Group decision making can also be compromised by certain kinds of social dynamics among team members. Personal animosities can obviously impede cooperation; two notable examples of this relating to sexism and union/nonunion confrontations on the flight deck are discussed in Chapter 11). Other effects may occur simply because there is more than one person present.

For example, one kind of social factor that can come into play in team decision making is the feeling that there is 'safety in numbers'. As social animals, humans tend to be more confident in their opinions when these are shared by other group members; thus, an error in judgement made by one individual may, instead of being identified and corrected, receive social reinforcement and propagate through the system. By the same token, people are typically *less* confident about perceptions that appear to contradict the majority opinion: thus, a crew member who correctly identifies a developing problem may nevertheless fail to take appropriate action if she believes that her assessment is not shared by the rest of the team. Related to this, perhaps, is the observation that people are often more willing to take risks when they are in groups, possibly because it is easier to avoid individual culpability.[11]

There may also exist certain dynamics relating to rank or status differences between teammates. Several researchers have noted, for example, that people who feel themselves to be under threat often tend to be more obedient, to look more to authority figures. (As Norman Dixon[13] has put it, "in times of stress even the poorest leaders, like drunken fathers and rabbits' feet, are clung to with pathetic, if misplaced, dependency" -- p. 237). Such behaviour has been observed in (for example) disaster victims,[25] but it can also occur in cockpit crews.[21] Certainly there are many cases on record of junior crew members becoming so passive and deferential that they fail to supply the captain with vital information.[15,16] Similar behaviour can be noted in the passengers in the Kegworth crash (see sidebar on p. 117), who were loth to question the captain's judgement despite the evidence of their own eyes.

In explanation, some researchers have turned to the discipline of organizational psychology, noting that when organizations come under threat, responsibility for decisions tends to become increasingly centralized and to devolve upon the highest levels of authority.[22,56,57] This phenomenon is well established at the organizational level (see Chapter 11), but there is somewhat less consensus about its applicability to smaller groups such as cockpit crews. One implication of the model is that not only may subordinates become more acquiescent in times of stress, but leaders may be less open to input from below.[14] In the cockpit, such a dynamic might well create a kind of vicious circle, with captains refusing to accept input from copilots, and copilots becoming more unwilling than ever to volunteer information. Chapter 6 describes several incidents of this sort (see in particular the discussion of ego defence mechanisms), although it should be noted that it is not clear in those cases whether stress was an exacerbating factor, or whether this was simply normal behaviour for the pilots in question.

However, some investigators have placed a different interpretation on the behaviour of teams under stress. There have been a number of studies in which the dominant reaction to perceived threat has been for *all* group members, irrespective of their status, to become more cooperative with one another.[14,39,64] Within this paradigm, subordinates in the group are still more obedient to authority under stress; however, the leaders, far from rejecting others' opinions, become more receptive and information seeking. Obviously, both of these hypotheses cannot be exclusively correct; most likely, both apply at different times. One variable in determining the type of organizational stress response that is activated is likely to be the type of command structure already in place, and, in particular, the rigidity of the hierarchy. In the flight environment there is typically a well-defined hierarchy: it might extend from captain to first officer to cabin staff to passengers, or from flight instructor to student, for example. This has important implications for the operation of the team: as Weick[66] puts it, "communication dominated by hierarchy activates a different mindset regarding what is and is not communicated and different dynamics regarding who initiates on whom" (p. 128).

Hierarchical communication is also subject to particular types of distortion.[17] For example, information that might displease a superior may be summarized, simplified, subtly recast with a different emphasis, not so subtly altered in its nature, or even withheld outright. Interestingly, it has been observed that these kinds of distortions are not unlike some that occur in the presence of heavy workload,[55] which may make them all the more difficult to eliminate. In Weick's words, "the mutually reinforcing 'solutions' to two distinct problems of crises -- overload and centralization -- should exert continuing pressure on communication in the direction of distortion and away from accuracy" (p. 128).

Conclusion

While much of the published literature on individual pilot decision making under stress is anecdotal or the result of post hoc incident analysis, there is, as we have discussed, a growing body of research which connects the operational world of flying to the literature of cognitive psychology. A number of these studies have been quantitative, experimental, and have addressed the issue of individual differences in information processing strategies. At the same time, a rather separate body of research has tackled the question of crew (as opposed to individual) decision making under a variety of operational conditions. This research has been influenced more by social and personnel psychology, focussing upon group dynamics and the efficient management of small teams (cockpit resource management -- CRM). Both traditions of research have provided insights into decision making under stress, although CRM studies have had more influence on operational practices. Both need to keep the workload/distress distinction more clear and explicit than has often been the case.

A strong argument could be made for research which more closely integrates these two lines of inquiry. For example, more studies could be designed which examine cockpit resource management from the perspective of cognitive psychology and, especially, individual differences. Individual aircrew or controllers may, for example, have distinctive personal predilections or tendencies in the way in which they formulate or interpret language communications under psychological stress -- tendencies which may be significant influences upon (and, perhaps, predictors of) the performance of teams under duress.

Another area of potential research integration relates to individual decision 'biases' or heuristic preferences. Cognitive psychology has provided some insights into the effects of these biasses (a number of papers contain reviews from an aviation perspective;[57,67,68] see also Chapter 3, p. 69). This work, while occasionally referred to in after-the-fact critiques of individual pilot decisions, is barely exploited at all in the analysis of superior and inferior *team* performance, least of all in predictive modelling. Some issues to be explored include whether particular biasses in the decision making process are enduring characteristics of individuals; whether any of these biasses change systematically and differentially under stress and workload;* and whether certain combinations of individuals (and their respective biasses) exacerbate or, alternatively, tend to 'cancel out' individual crew members' decision making idiosyncracies.

Issues can also be raised with respect to team selection. Individuals wishing to fly or control air traffic are, of course, subjected to intensive scrutiny: computerized testing, interviews, checkrides, medical examinations, and so forth. However, decision making teams, both in the military and in civilian contexts, are often assembled (some would say randomly thrown together) on no principled basis whatsoever, and with very little consideration of the psychology involved. The decision making proficiency and stress resistance of the group *as a team* or crew is, therefore, largely left to chance, just as individual judgement and decision making prowess was once considered to be an intangible element of proficiency donated or withheld by Fortune. One of the challenges facing us, therefore, is to make team communication and decision making under stress matters that can be modelled and predicted using *all* of the available data, including probable group dynamics and the cognitive 'profiles' of the potential team members.

*Preliminary evidence suggests that some may.[57]

References

1. Allnut, M. (1982), 'Human Factors: Basic Principles', in Hurst, R. and Hurst, L.R. (eds.), *Pilot Error* (2nd ed.), Jason Aronson, New York, pp. 1-22.

2. Barnett, B. (1989), 'Information Processing Components and Knowledge Representations: An Individual Differences Approach to Modeling Pilot Judgment', *Proceedings of the 33rd Annual Meeting of the Human Factors Society,* Human Factors Society, Santa Monica, California, pp. 878-82.

3. Barthol, R.P., and Ku, N.D. (1959), 'Regression under stress to first learned behavior', *Journal of Abnormal and Social Psychology,* vol. 59, pp. 134-6.

4. Bernstein, B. (1959). 'A public language: some sociological implications of a linguistic form. *British Journal of Sociology,* vol. 10, pp. 311-26.

5. Brenner, M., and Shipp, T. (1987), 'Voice Stress Analysis', NASA Conference Publication 2504, National Aeronautics and Space Administration, Scientific and Technical Information Division.

6. Brenner, M., Shipp, T., Doherty, E.T., and Morrissey, P. (1985), 'Voice Measures of Psychological Stress: Laboratory and Field Data', in Titze, I.R. and Scherer, R.C. (eds.), *Vocal Fold Physiology, Biomechanics, Acoustics, and Phontory Control,* Denver Center for the Performing Arts, Colorado.

7. Calderwood, R., Klein, G.A., and Crandall, B.W. (1988), 'Time pressure, skill and move quality in chess', *American Journal of Psychology,* vol. 101, pp. 481-93.

8. Chase, W., and Simon, H. (1973), 'Perception in chess', *Cognitive Psychology,* vol. 4, pp. 55-81.

9. Clothier, C. (1991), 'Behavioral differences in advanced technology and standard aircraft: results of systematic observations of line opera-

tions and simulations', *Proceedings of the Sixth International Symposium on Aviation Psychology*, Ohio State University, Columbus.

10. Cohen, M.S. (1993), 'Taking risks and taking advice: the role of experience in airline pilot diversion decisions', *Proceedings of the Seventh International Symposium on Aviation Psychology*, Ohio State University, Columbus.

11. Davis, J.H., and Stasson, M.F. (1988), 'Small group performance: past and present research trends', *Advances in Group Processes,* vol. 5, pp. 245-77.

12. De Groot, A. (1965), *Thought and Choice in Chess,* Mouton, The Hague.

13. Dixon, N.F. (1976), *On the Psychology of Military Incompetence,* Futura Publications, London.

14. Driskell, J.E., and Salas, E. (1991), 'Group decision making under stress', *Journal of Applied Psychology,* vol. 76, pp. 473-8.

15. Foushee, H.C. (1984), 'Dyads and triads at 35,000 feet: factors affecting group process and aircrew performance', *American Psychologist,* vol. 39, pp. 885-93.

16. Foushee, H.C., and Helmreich, R.L. (1988), 'Group Interaction and Flight Crew Performance', in Wiener, E.L., and Nagel, D.C. (eds.), *Human Factors in Aviation,* Academic Press, San Diego, California.

17. Fulk, J., and Mani, S. (1985), 'Distortion of Communication in Hierarchical Relationships', in McLaughlin, M. (ed.), *Communication Yearbook* (vol. 9), Sage Publications, Beverly Hills, California, pp. 483-510.

18. Giffen, W.C., and Rockwell, T.H. (1987), 'A methodology for research on VFR flight into IMC', *Proceedings of the Fourth International Symposium on Aviation Psychology,* Ohio State University, Columbus.

19. Griffin, G.R., and Williams, C.E. (1987), 'The effects of different levels of task complexity on three vocal measures', *Aviation, Space, and Environmental Medicine,* vol. 58, December.

20. Helmholtz, H.V. (1954), *On the Sensation of Tone,* Dover, New York (Original work published in German in 1864).

21. Helmreich, R.L. (1979), *Social Psychology on the Flight Deck,* paper presented at the NASA Workshop on Resource Management Training for Airline Flight Crews, San Francisco.

22. Hermann, C.F. (1963), 'Some consequences of crisis which limit the viability of organizations', *Administrative Science Quarterly,* vol. 8, pp. 61-82.

23. Hockey, G.R.J. (1986), 'Changes in Operator Efficiency as a Function of Environmental Stress, Fatigue, and Circadian Rhythms', in Boff, K.R., Kaufman, L., and Thomas, J.P. (eds.), *Handbook of Perception and Human Performance* (vol. 2), Wiley, New York.

24. Howell, G.E. (1984), Task influence in the analytic intuitive approach to decision making. Final Report. (Office of Naval Research contract N00014-82 C-001 Work Unit (NR197-074)), Rice University, Houston, Texas.

25. Janis, I.L. (1954), 'Problems of theory in the analysis of stress behavior', *Journal of Social Issues,* vol. 10, pp. 12-25.

26. Janis, I.L. (1982), 'Decision-Making under Stress', in Goldberger, L. and Breznitz, S. (eds.), *Handbook of Stress: Theoretical and Clinical Aspects,* Free Press, New York, pp. 69-80.

27. Janis, I.L., and Mann, L. (1977), *Decisionmaking: A Psychological Analysis of Conflict, Choice, and Committment,* Free Press, New York.

28. Jensen, R.S. (1982), 'Pilot judgment: training and evaluation', *Human Factors,* vol. 24, pp. 61-73.

29. Jensen, R.S., and Benel, R.A. (1977), *Judgment Evaluation and Instruction in Civil Pilot Training'* (Final Report FAA-RD-78-24), National Technical Information Service, Springfield, Virginia.

30. Keinan, G. (1986), 'Confidence Expectancy as a Predictor of Military Performance under Stress', in Milgram, N.A. (ed.), *Stress and Coping in Time of War: Generalizations from the Israeli Experience*, Brunner/Mazel, New York.

31. Keinan, G. (1987), 'Decision making under stress: scanning of alternatives under controllable and uncontrollable threats', *Journal of Personality and Social Psychology,* vol. 52, pp. 639-44.

32. Keinan, G., Friedland, N., and Ben-Porath, Y. (1986), 'Decision making under stress: scanning of alternatives under physical threat', *Acta Psychologica,* vol. 64, pp. 219-28.

33. Khachatur'yants, L., and Grimak, L. (1972), *Cosmonaut's Emotional Stress in Space Flight,* NASA TT F-14, 654.

34. Klein, G.A. (1989), 'Recognition-Primed Decisions', in Rouse, W. (ed.), *Advances in Man-Machine Systems Research,* vol. 5, JAI Press, Inc., Greenwich, Connecticut, pp. 47-92.

35. Klein, G.A., Calderwood, R., and Clinton-Cirocco, A. (1986), 'Rapid Decision Making on the Fire Ground', *Human Factors Society 30th Annual Meeting,* Human Factors Society, Santa Monica, CA.

36. Klein, G.A., and Thordsen, M.L. (1990), *Cognitive Processes of the Team Mind,* Yellow Springs, Ohio, Klein Associates, Inc.

37. Klein, G., Wolf, S., Militello, L., and Zsambok, C. (in press), 'Characteristics of Skilled Option Generation in Chess', in *Organizational Behavior and Human Decision Processes.*

38. Kuroda, I., Fujiwara, O., Okamura, N., and Utsuki, N. (1976), 'Method for determining pilot stress through analysis of voice communication', *Aviation, Space, and Environmental Medicine,* vol. 47, pp. 528-33.

39. Lanzetta, J.T. (1955), 'Group behavior under stress', *Human Relations*, vol. 8, pp. 29-52.

40. Mullen, B., and Goethals, G.R. (1987), *Theories of Group Behavior*, Springer-Verlag, New York.

41. Niwa, S. (1970), 'Changes of voice characteristics in urgent situation (1)', *Report of the JASDF Aeromedical Laboratory*, vol. 11, pp. 51-8.

42. Niwa, S. (1971), 'Changes of voice characteristics in urgent situation (2)', *Report of the JASDF Aeromedical Laboratory*, vol. 11, pp. 246-51.

43. Orasanu, J. (1992), 'Decision Making in the Cockpit', in Wiener, E., Kanki, B., and Helmreich, R. (eds.), *Cockpit Resource Management*, Academic Press, New York.

44. Orasanu, J., and Salas, E. (in press), 'Team Decision Making on Complex Environments', in Klein, G., Calderwood, R., and Zsambok, C. (eds.), *Decision Making in Action: Models and Methods*, Ablex, Norwood, New Jersey.

45. Popov, V.A., Simonov, P.V., Frolov, M.V., and Khachatur'yants, L.S. (1971), *'The Articulatory Frequency Spectrum as an Indicator of the Degree and Nature of Emotional Stress in Man*, NASA TT F-13, 772.

46. Rouse, W.B. (1978), 'Human problem solving performance in a fault diagnosis task', *IEEE Transactions on Systems, Man and Cybernetics*, vol. 4, SMC-8, pp. 258-71.

47. Ruffel Smith, H.P. (1979), *A Simulator Study of the Interaction of Pilot Workload with Errors, Vigilance, and Decisions*, (NASA Technical Memorandum No. 78482), NASA-Ames Research Laboratory, Moffett Field, California.

48. Ruiz, R., Legros, C., and Guell, A. (1990), 'Voice analysis to predict the psychological or physical state of a speaker', *Aviation, Space, and Environmental Medicine*, vol. 61, pp. 266-71.

49. Segal, L.D. (1989), 'Differences in cockpit communication', *Proceedings of the Fifth International Symposium on Aviation Psychology*, Ohio State University, Columbus, pp. 576-81.

50. Shanteau, J. (1988), 'Psychological characteristics and strategies of expert decision makers', *Acta Psychologica,* vol. 68, pp. 203-15.

51. Sieber, J.E. (1974), 'Effects of decision importance on ability to generate warranted subjective uncertainty', *Journal of Personality and Social Psychology,* vol. 5, pp. 688-94.

52. Simon, H.A. (1955), 'A behavioral model of rational choice', *Quarterly Journal of Economics,* vol. 69, pp. 99-118.

53. Simonov, P.V., and Frolov, M.V. (1973), 'Utilization of human voice for estimation of man's emotional stress and state of attention', *Aerospace Medicine,* vol. 44, pp. 256-8.

54. Staw, B.M., Sandelands, L.E., and Dutton, J.E. (1981), 'Threat-rigidity effects in organizational behavior: a multilevel analysis', *Adminstrative Science Quarterly,* vol. 26, pp. 501-24.

55. Stohl, C., and Redding, W.C. (1987), 'Messages and Message Exchange Processes', in Jablin, F., Putnam, L., Roberts, K., and Porter, L. (eds), *Handbook of Organizational Communication,* Sage Publications, Newbury Park, California, pp. 451-502.

56. Stokes, A.F. (1991), 'Flight Management Training and Research using a Microcomputer Flight Decision Simulator', In Sadlowe, R. (ed.), *PC based Instrument Flight Simulation: A First Collection of Papers,* American Society of Mechanical Engineers, New York, pp. 25-32.

57. Stokes, A.F., Belger, A., and Zhang, K. (1990),*Investigation of Factors Comprising a Model of Pilot Decision Making: Part II. Anxiety and Cognitive Strategies in Expert and Novice Aviators,* University of Illinois Aviation Research Laboratory, Savoy.

58. Stokes, A.F., Kemper, K.L., and Marsh, R. (1992), *Time-Stressed Flight Ddecision Making: A Study of Expert and Novice Aviators*, University of Illinois Aviation Research Laboratory, Savoy.

59. Stokes, A.F., and Raby, M. (1989), 'Stress and cognitive performance in trainee pilots', *Proceedings of the Human Factors Society 33rd Annual Meeting*, pp. 883-7.

60. Stone, R.B., Babcock, C.L., and Edmunds, M.S. (1985), 'Pilot judgment: an operational viewpoint', *Aviation, Space, and Environmental Medicine*, vol. 56, pp. 149-52.

61. Sulc, J. (1977), 'To the problem of emotional changes in human voice', *Activ. Nerv. Sup. (Praha)*, vol. 19, no. 3.

62. Tolkmitt, F., Helfrich, H., Standke, R., and Scherer, K.R. (1982), 'Vocal indicators of psychiatric treatment effects in depressives and schizophrenics', *Journal of Communication Disorders*, vol. 15, pp. 209-22.

63. Tolkmitt, F.J., and Scherer, K.R. (1986), 'Effect of experimentally induced stress on vocal parameters', *Journal of Experimental Psychology*, vol. vol. 12, pp. 302-13.

64. Torrance, E.P. (1967), 'A Theory of Leadership and Interpersonal Behavior under Stress', in Petrullo, L. and Bass, B.M. (eds.), *Leadership and Interpersonal Behavior*, Holt, New York, pp. 100-17.

65. Wanta, W., and Leggett, D. (1988), 'Hitting pay dirt: capacity theory and sports announcers' use of cliches', *Journal of Communications*, vol. 38, p. 82.

66. Weick, K.E. (1991), 'The Vulnerable System: An Analysis of the Tenerife Air Disaster', in Frost, P.J., Moore, L.F., Louis, M.R., Lundberg, C.C., and Martin, J. (eds.), *Reframing Organizational Culture*, Sage Publications, Newbury Park, California, pp. 117-30.

67. Wickens, C.D., Stokes, A., Barnett, B., and Davis, T., Jr. (1987), *A Componential Analysis of Pilot Decision Making,* University of Illinois Aviation Research Laboratory, Savoy.

68. Wickens, C.D., Stokes, A.F., Barnett, B., and Hyman, F. (1988), *The Effects of Stress on Pilot Judgment in a MIDIS Simulator,* University of Illinois Aviation Research Laboratory, Savoy.

69. Wiener, E.L. (1977), 'Controlled flight into terrain accidents: system induced errors', *Human Factors,* vol. 19, p. 171.

70. Williams, C.E., and Stevens, K.N. (1969), 'On determining the emotional state of pilots during flight: an exploratory study', *Aerospace Medicine,* vol. 40, pp. 1369-72.

71. Williams, C.E., and Stevens, K.N. (1981), 'Vocal Correlates of Emotional States', in Darby, J. (ed.), *Speech Evaluation in Psychiatry,* Grune & Stratton, New York, pp. 221-40.

72. Wright, P. (1974), 'The harassed decision maker: time pressures, distractions, and the use of evidence', *Journal of Applied Psychology,* vol. 59, pp. 555-61.

73. Wright, P., and Weitz, B. (1977), 'Time horizon effects on product evaluation strategies', *Journal of Marketing Research,* vol. 14, pp. 429-43.

74. Zakay, D., and Wooler, S. (1984), 'Time pressure, training and decision effectiveness', *Ergonomics,* vol. 27, pp. 273-84.

5 Life stress

Unresolved environmental demand requiring adaptive behaviors in the form of social readjustments

-- Rabi Bhagat and Stephen Allie[5]

The bread of adversity and the water of affliction

-- Isaiah 30:20

It has been suggested that aircrew performance can be affected by three types of stress: acute reactive stress, environmental stress, and what is called life stress (that is, events such as divorce, bereavement, and so forth).[9] These may differ in subjective intensity, and also qualitatively: for example the patterns of arousal likely to be associated with many 'life events' can, as discussed in Chapter 2, be very different from those associated with acute reactive stress. Nevertheless, the tripartite classification has, to date, been less a psychological claim that there are three qualitatively different sorts of stress than a way of focussing attention upon *sources* of stress thought to be important in aviation. Certainly each of these category labels refers to a set of phenomena that may potentially influence performance on the operational task of interest, be that controlling the aircraft, navigating, or operating weapons systems. It might be more accurate, therefore, to say that the three classes of stress differ in their breadth of inclusiveness and remoteness from the task at hand -- the difference between acute test anxiety, say, and chronic unhappiness. Their relevance or legitimacy as putative causes of particular mishaps or episodes of poor performance depends partly upon the 'causal field' invoked.[*]

Acute reactive stress is generally seen as a short term effect closely linked to the execution of operational duties. It is not just an 'on the job'

[*]"For want of a nail the horseshoe was lost ... for want of a battle the kingdom was lost." Whether the loss of the realm was caused by equipment failure, poor military judgement (too few reserves), or the divorce of the royal blacksmith depends upon the causal field the analyst is prepared to consider (a topic discussed further in Chapter 11, 'Organizations, Stress, and Accidents').

phenomenon; it is, as it were, a 'because of the job' phenomenon. Acute reactive stress can be defined as a response to a threatening event or circumstance -- for example, a sudden emergency or the clash of combat. It is in its nature an aversive experience, a 'power' stressor in McClelland's terminology (see Chapter 2, p. 41), probably associated with elevated adrenalin and noradrenalin levels.[15]

The category of environmental stress is much more vague. In aviation, the term is generally used to refer to a rather narrow set of ambient physical conditions, including noise, temperature, and vibration. There is no doubt that such conditions may interfere with cognitive performance, judgement, control, or communication, especially at unusual or unaccustomed levels. However, as noted in our discussion of stimulus based definitions of stress (Chapter 1), the mere presence of these factors need not be taken as evidence of psychological distress in the crew member, even if performance is, indeed, influenced in some way. That is, environmental 'stressors' are not necessarily associated with psychological 'distress'.

It could be argued, of course, that in real terms all stress is in some sense environmental, since our experience as humans is inevitably tied in with our surroundings. For example, the appearance of smoke on the flight deck (an 'environmental' phenomenon, strictly speaking) could obviously lead to acute reactive stress. Likewise, an unpleasant social atmosphere might generate stress among the crew that could lead to poor cockpit resource management. (An example of this would be a domineering captain imposing a very hierarchical authority structure and ignoring or rejecting input from other crew members[7] -- see Chapters 4, 6, and 11.)

The concept of life stress

Life stress is not, it might be thought, a concept that is easily separated from the notion of suffering. However, in its conventional technical useage, the phrase has few emotional overtones and refers merely to life *changes*. Life stress, it is often said, may result from such unhappy circumstances as the death of a family member or favoured pet, difficulty with employers, medical problems, or any of the other "slings and arrows of outrageous fortune" that make up the human condition; however, it can equally result from positive events such as winning the lottery or being promoted to captain. (At least, this is the standard view of life stress -- more on this model later). A key element is that the stress inducing events

or circumstances are relatively remote from the operational task of immediate concern. To this extent we are concerned, then, with chronic effects,
and, frequently, with the phenomenon of 'affiliative stress'[15] discussed in
Chapter 2. As noted there, such stress may not, in biochemical terms, be
strongly associated with the adrenergic arousal patterns of acute reactive
stress, but rather with elevated dopamine levels, and, perhaps, other (as
yet inadequately researched) long term changes that could influence performance and sense of well-being.

Within this framework, the kinds of events most often thought responsible for the majority of 'life stress' (and, therefore, the events most frequently studied) are, understandably, major life changes, turning points,
and crises. However, some investigators maintain that it is the smaller
worries and frustrations of life, the everyday hassles or 'microstressors'
(e.g., traffic jams, 'phone tag', losing of keys) that create the most psychological distress[13] (see sidebar below). There is recent research evidence that such microstressors do indeed account for more daily worry and
trait anxiety than larger 'life events', and that daily 'hassles' are significantly related to measures of both trait anxiety and worry.[22]

Others suggest that it may not be life stress itself which presents the
primary danger to aircrew; rather, they argue, it is the interaction of life
stress with acute stress in nonroutine events that produces significant
changes in performance.[26] This model of events is not dissimilar from that
embodied in Spielberger's state/trait hypothesis,[27] sharing with it the notion

---

*Boston, Maryland, April, 1990: The spot 3 helicopter pilot walked his
blades 90 degrees to the cockpit prior to entering the helicopter. As the
spot 2 helicopter flew to his spot for shutdown, his rotor downwash may
have caused the spot 3 helicopter's blade to go off the 90-degree start
position. The helicopter on spot 3 began its start cycle while the spot 2
(landing) helicopter was still at flight idle for its two-minute cool down.
As rotor speed increased on the spot 3 helicopter, blade contact was
made and damage resulted. The rules of the road -- not to have two
adjacent helicopters running simultaneously -- were not followed. The
spot 3 pilot appeared to be having the proverbial 'bad day' with other
distractions and aggravations, which clouded his decision making.*

-- NASA Aviation Safety Reporting System (Accession No. 143383)

of a 'background' anxiety state upon which task related stress states are superimposed.

Nevertheless, while many post hoc accident reconstructions and reports implicate life events in the aetiology of accidents and incidents, and many of these mishaps involve emergencies or other unusual events, it is notoriously difficult to prove causality after the fact (a problem that dogs many of the studies reviewed in this chapter). Moreover, studies that attempt to predict accidents before the fact are very difficult to conduct; problems include difficulties in the measurement of life stress, individual differences in response to events, and the exigencies of providence -- that is, chance.[21] In general, there is a paucity of hard evidence on the matter.

Measuring life stress

Questionnaires and 'normative biography'

In many incident and accident investigations, significant life events relating to the mishap become known purely through the relevant information being volunteered by a pilot ("my mind kept going back to my wife's hospitalization and I forgot to lower my undercarriage"). Sometimes pertinent life events are 'stumbled upon' by investigators during the course of interviews with pilots or pilots' colleagues or relatives. In major accidents, formal background checks are conducted on all personnel connected with the accident, including aircrew, controllers, and maintenance personnel.

The evidence from all these sources, while occasionally compelling, nonetheless remains largely anecdotal and difficult to quantify. In order to investigate the relationship between life events and performance in any kind of systematic way, test instruments have been developed that attempt to define and formalize precisely which life events count as 'stressful', and to quantify their cumulative impact on the individual.

The evaluation of life events in the context of medical diagnosis can be traced at least as far back as 1934.[16,30] However, the names most associated with initial attempts to develop a standardized, quantitative approach in this area are Holmes and Rahe of the US Navy. These investigators were initially most concerned with the relationship of life events or crises to physical and psychiatric illness. In the late 1960s they conducted a number of scaling studies intended to provide some idea of the importance of various events in terms of their effects upon individuals' lives, and on the social and psychological adjustments that had to be made. Social readjustment was defined solely in terms of the amount and duration of change an event imposed, "regardless of the desirability of this event" (Holmes and Rahe,[11] p. 213). This nonspecificity is a biographical analogue of the biological nonspecificity assumed by Hans Selye (see Chapter 1). Selye, too, regarded the eliciting conditions of stress as unimportant, and maintained that the stress response involves a nonspecific adjustment -- a general 'one response fits all stressors' adaptation.[25]

The event chosen to anchor the scale was marriage, which was simply declared to be 'worth' 500 points. Subjects then rated all other events by reference to this value. A questionnaire was devised called the SRE, or Schedule of Recent Experiences, which contained forty-two questions concerning changes in finances, employment, health status, domestic life, and related matters. Each 'event' was given a weighting based upon the scaling studies. The weightings were simply the event ratings divided by 10, thus marriage was 'worth' 50 'Life Change Units' (LCUs). The events in the SRE ranged in importance from 11 LCUs (a minor infraction of the law) to 100 (death of a spouse). In this way a total combined 'life change score' could be tallied for any year.[20]

It was demonstrated that health and LCU score were inversely correlated. For example, in one study approximately four out of five individuals with scores over 300 reported illnesses and injuries, as compared to only a little over one in three of those with scores between 150 and 199.[10] Health changes tended to lag behind the reported life crises by about one year. A similar study using 2,500 shipboard personnel gave similar results and showed that it was the total sum of LCUs that predicted overall susceptibility to illness, rather than any single identifiable life event or crisis.[18]

One difficulty with this approach is that it assumes that a given event has the same meaning for everyone. This is oversimplistic, as events can differ markedly in their significance for different individuals. A modified version of the SRE, the Recent Life Change Questionnaire (RLCQ), therefore permits the test subject to subjectively rate the personal impact of the events. Total scores are given not only for LCUs, but also for Subjective Life Change Units (SLCUs), and allows investigators to compare the two. A high value for LCUs combined with a low value for SLCUs is assumed to indicate efficient coping.[19] This test meets objections to the normative approach, although it does retain the notion of nonspecificity.

The Life Events Questionnaire (LEQ), developed by Sarason and colleagues, is an attempt to improve upon these methods. This instrument is made up of 110 questions divided into a number of categories, such as legal/financial, family, medical, work, relationships, and so forth. Some of the test items are occupation specific and permit the forms to be 'customized' to particular groups -- students, for example, or general aviation pilots. However, perhaps the most significant innovation in the design of the questionnaire is its consideration of the recency of events and of individual differences in coping with these events. Subjects not only specify whether an event has occurred to them, but also when (i.e., in the preceding week, month or year), and this provides some basis for differentiating between acute and chronic stress. In addition, the putative stress inducing events are rated by the subject on a three point scale to indicate the extent to which the event has been troubling and a cause for concern.[23]

Difficulties with life event questionnaires

Typically, life event questionnaires have contained questions about both positive and negative events. Even a brief 20-item questionnaire is long enough to list both positive and negative occurrences while remaining easy to administer and score. The logic of combining both positive and negative event scores has been questioned, however, and it is not clear what evidence exists to justify the assumption that major life changes are stressful irrespective of their desirability.[23] There is evidence that negative events are predictive of, among other things, anxiety and depression, while positive life events are not[29] -- which would certainly seem to accord with common sense. Also, not all events can even be classified as universally positive or negative: such circumstances as pregnancy or a cross country move may be viewed as desirable by some and undesirable by others.

Another issue is that of questionnaire length and complexity. Short, simple questionnaires offer certain advantages. First, they are more likely to be completed and returned to the investigator, and a high return rate enhances the validity of the study. Simplicity and brevity also enable easy and rapid data analysis. However, short questionnaires by definition omit many events, and may therefore make the subject's life appear less stressful than it actually has been (i.e., they encourage a bias toward false negatives). Moreover, it is generally only recent events that are taken into account, effectively denying the potential impact of chronic factors (e.g., long term grief, sequelae of medical events, and so forth). Finally, in many brief questionnaires events are weighted equally, despite the fact that certain events may have far more impact than others.

Texas, January, 1991: After shooting the last approach at Greeneville Airport we were flying VFR back to Addison Airport at 2500 feet. I began briefing my student on Addison weather. We saw and missed a light aircraft by no more than ten feet under us. It happened so fast that no reaction was possible. As the instructor I should have insisted that we requested radar service en route to Addison. I should have also waited until we were in radar contact receiving flight advisories from Regional Approach before I stuck the card in the other pilot's face to brief him on the weather. Furthermore, I believe I was distracted by personal problems due to the fact that I had recently had a death in my family.

-- NASA Aviation Safety Reporting System (Accession No. 200527)

Longer questionnaires have their own advantages and disadvantages. They can contain a larger number of items, and thus may be less subject to false negatives. In addition, items can be weighted according to how stressful the researcher considers the event or experience to be. This added complexity may create problems, however, as the weightings may be of dubious validity, and individual differences may be disregarded. Also, the problem of recent versus chronic experiences is obviously not solved merely by comprehensiveness. Finally, other things being equal, lengthy questionnaires also suffer from a lower return rate. The bias and false negatives eliminated by expanding the questionnaire may be reintroduced as poorly motivated, overworked, harassed, or otherwise preoccupied subjects effectively exclude themselves from the study.

Finally, although this is not a function of questionnaire design itself, it should be noted that the entire methodology rests heavily upon correlation, and as a statistical precept correlation has some significant limitations. It is a common logical error to assume that correlation implies causality, and, moreover, causality in a particular direction. An individual may, for example, suffer from malaise and depression, and also be involved in an high number of accidents or incidents. It may therefore be said that the depression and the accident rate correlate with one another. However, this correlation provides no basis for assuming that the accidents are caused by the depression: it is also quite possible that the depression is caused by the accidents, or, alternatively, that there is no causal relationship at all between the two phenomena. Another possibility is that both the depression and the accidents result from some third, unidentified factor.

It is particularly tempting to read causality into the data when the chronological sequence of putative stressors and incidents is clear (although in the operational world it is often unclear). While there may indeed be some causal links, to assume them based on the sequence of events is to commit the fallacy known to logicians as *post hoc ergo propter hoc*. This may be irreverently and somewhat loosely translated as "if it follows breakfast it was caused by breakfast".

In summary, studies based on conventional life events questionnaire techniques have a number of potential methodological difficulties and limitations. These should be borne in mind when evaluating the research studies reviewed subsequently in this chapter.

Life stress, performance, and accidents

In 1977 Dr. Robert Alkov, a US Navy psychologist, suggested that life changes assumed to affect the health of naval aviators could also conceivably result in aircraft accidents. He and his colleagues initiated a number of questionnaire studies which attempted to relate life events to accidents.[1,2] The investigators, working at the Naval Safety Center in Norfolk, Virginia, developed a 50-item questionnaire drawing on the work of Holmes and Rahe discussed previously. The questionnaire favoured recent life events. In the first study 129 questionnaires were returned; this represented an excellent return rate of 83 percent.[1] In the second study a 22-item questionnaire was developed from the original one, and 248 of these were returned (an 82 percent return rate).[2] It should be noted that the individuals involved in accidents did not complete the questionnaires themselves. Rather, they were completed by squadron flight surgeons on the basis of information obtained from the accident victim or from his relatives (if he did not survive). In each study a distinction was made between subjects who in some degree contributed to the accidents, and those who were merely involved in accidents without playing a causal role. The investigators found nine questions whose answers indicated a difference between these two groups. However, the criterion for significance was set at $p < 0.10$, which is not a very stringent test of the relationships in the data.

Four of the questions judged to discriminate between the two groups concerned personality characteristics: maturity and stability, professionalism, sense of humour, and quick-wittedness in difficult situations. However, the interpretation of these data presents certain difficulties. As the researchers point out, the flight surgeons who rated the subjects on these qualities are likely to have been influenced by the knowledge that the pilots had or had not made errors which were responsible for the mishap. The remaining five questions, which concerned life events, are at least relatively objective. The five life events cited as significant markers for the 'at fault' accident group included, in order of statistical significance,

(1) recent major decision about the future
(2) recent trouble with superiors, peers, or subordinates
(3) recent death of a family member or close friend
(4) difficulty with interpersonal relationships
(5) recent marriage engagement.

The first of these, 'recent major decision', appears to be statistically strong ($p=0.0002$), while the second, 'trouble with superiors, peers, or subordinates', is moderately so ($p=0.03$). The remainder are rather weak, ranging between $p=0.06$ and $p=0.07$. Closer inspection illustrates some of the difficulties that can arise in attempting to interpret correlational data. For example, a not uncommon 'major decision' was the decision to leave the service. While this event might be assumed to be a 'stressor' that led to the accident, it is entirely possible that the reverse is true -- that aircrew who had made this decision then relaxed their vigilance, became less motivated, or had already determined that military flying was not their strength and vocation. Alternatively, the decision to leave the service and the accident may both be sequelae of other factors, such as an individual's tendency to get into 'scrapes' or his ill-suitedness for military flying.

In 1983 Alkov's team reported a further study of life events in American naval aviators, this time focussing on stress coping and accidents.[3] The investigators were interested in the relationship between errors in performance and inadequate stress coping, which, they maintained, was signalled by the aggressive 'acting out' of frustrations (as indicated in points (2) and (4) above), 'trouble with associates', and 'difficulty with interpersonal relationships'.

The subjects of the study were pilots and other aircrew members who had been involved in serious aircraft mishaps and who had roles that could have influenced events (pilots, copilots, navigators, and so forth). Flight surgeons on aircraft mishap boards completed the 22-item questionnaire on

Pennsylvania, 1988: On November 2 the crew of a Federal Aviation Administration aircraft, a Rockwell Jet Commander, was slated to complete an inspection of the Instrument Landing System at Latrobe airport in Pennsylvania. Weather conditions were marginal, but the captain decided to proceed with the inspection flight. At around 10:00 a.m. the aircraft flew into an area of forecasted icing conditions. When the wing de-icing system was activated, ice broke away and was ingested by both engines, which then flamed out. The crew was geographically disoriented and did not know where nearby Latrobe airport was. The pilots made no 'Mayday' emergency call and ATC was unable to give timely vectors for Latrobe (only two miles away). The crew initially requested vectors for Johnstown airport, sixteen miles distant. Engine restart procedures during the emergency descent were unsuccessful and the aircraft crashed in Oak Grove. All three crew members were killed.

Both pilots had been seen drinking beer the night before the crash, but postmortem examination suggests that alcohol was probably not a factor in the accident. However, the captain, a 17,000 hour veteran, had made the decision to retire that day and the copilot had recently had his driving licence revoked. The NTSB concluded that both pilots had personal stresses which may have preoccupied their thoughts and influenced performance. Inattention and the psychological condition of the pilots were found to be contributory factors in the accident.

-- Condensed from NTSB accident report no. MIA-89-MA-023

each individual in the study. This time about 500 questionnaires were returned (an 86 percent return rate). As in the earlier studies the investigators built in an ingenious control condition: half of the aircrew surveyed had been found to be at fault in the mishaps in which they were involved, while the other half were not at fault. The data were analyzed using the Fisher-Irwin Exact Test to discriminate between the two groups on the basis of the 22 questionnaire items. It was found that at-fault aviators could be distinguished from controls in several respects. The aviators who had made errors appeared more likely to have had marital problems, recent trouble with superiors and peers, and difficulties with personal relationships. They also appeared to be less mature and stable. Significant life events for this group included marriage engagement and the making of a recent major decision concerning the future.

This study has to be interpreted in several lights, not least of which is the fact that naval aviators are a very highly selected group that is not representative of the pilot population as a whole. Among the traits selected for in officer training are low levels of self doubt and general anxiety, high self reliance, and good stress coping skills. It could be argued, therefore, that the detection of significant relationships between life events and accidents is doubly important since a study using such subjects provides such a stringent test of the hypothesis.

There are, however, certain drawbacks inherent in using military personnel in a study organized around the concept of life event related accident proneness. The military in general and naval aviation in particular are efficient organizational systems for weeding out the truly accident prone. First, in these closely monitored social settings, individuals thought to be liable to mishaps are identified early and moved out of harm's way. Second, aviation is an unforgiving environment, rather sparing with second and third chances, and this is certainly no less true of naval aviation. Thus there may be little opportunity to become prone to accidents since death or serious injury are likely to intervene and prevent the accumulation of any extensive accident record.

Interesting comparisons with the US Navy's data are provided by Royal Air Force and Canadian Armed Forces studies of life stress in military pilots. One British study, which scrutinized 149 military flying accidents, included the observations of a number of psychologists who were permitted to conduct their own investigations alongside the boards of inquiry responsible for determining the circumstances surrounding the accidents.[6] Of all the cases in the study, only seventeen were identified as having even potential life stress involvement; most of these featured domestic/marital or work problems. In only two cases was a direct link established between a stressful 'life event' and behaviour in the accident flight. In one case the pilot had recently experienced being under fire and reacted to a tactical situation in a manner that might have been appropriate under fire; in the other, the pilot involved was suffering from a terminated marriage engagement.

These results are not strongly supportive of Alkov's US Navy studies. However, the RAF survey was never intended to serve as a formal experiment in life stress and error, and consequently was not as methodologically sophisticated as the American studies, lacking, for example, any control groups or fault/no-fault distinctions. A further consideration, if Rahe's original findings are valid, is the possibility that it is the accumulation of stressful life events that compromises well-being. If so, it may be naive to hope to associate single life events with specific operational errors.

The Canadian study was somewhat more formal, and was part of an initiative whose purpose was to develop a method for screening accident prone aviators. In the study, Holmes and Rahe's Recent Life Change Questionnaire (RLCQ) was administered to 158 Canadian Forces aviators and two control groups.[14] The aviators were drawn from ten operational squadrons in Canada and Europe and had a broad range of duties, including transport, training, maritime patrol, and fighter interception. The larger of the control groups consisted of 127 aircraft maintenance personnel, matched with the pilots for both age and location. The other control group consisted of 46 additional personnel matched for rank. No significant differences in life event scores were found between the aviators and either of the control groups, although all had scores that, the authors claimed, would give rise to health changes in half the general population. As no accident data were examined, the safety implications of these findings cannot be determined. In general, then, these studies are rather inconclusive, leaving the impression that the jury is still out on the issue of life stress in military aircrew.

It is helpful, in this context, to consider the evidence from studies of civilian pilots. In 1987 Platenius and Wilde reported the results of an extensive and detailed survey of Canadian civilian pilots.[17] The questionnaire, which contained over three hundred items, attempted to assess both accident involvement and life events, although it also covered a range of personality and 'lifestyle' variables. Some fourteen work and family related matters were included as life event items; in this respect the questionnaire resembled those developed by Rahe and colleagues.[18-21] Events were not differentiated as to recency, but were limited to those which had occurred within the previous twelve months. Reactions to the events were coded on a tripartite scale similar to that used in the LEQ. Respondents were divided into four groups (private, commercial, helicopter and airline transport pilots), and the data for each group were analyzed separately.

The picture that emerged of the overall relationship between life events and accidents was not particularly clear. Some two-thirds of the life event items "served as accident markers in at least one pilot group" (p. 740), although no single item did so across all groups. In general, business and divorce worries appear to have been the most frequently cited concerns associated with accident involvement. The study did make a number of intriguing and surprising findings concerning personality variables, including an apparent relationship between involvement in aircraft accidents and a lack of 'humour appreciation'. Persons who engaged in sedentary forms of recreation such as reading and gardening were also associated with a higher rate of accidents than those who favoured more active pastimes such as skydiving and motorcycling.

This study does have a number of important limitations. First, although nearly nine thousand individuals returned questionnaires, this represented less than twenty percent of the total surveyed population. Second, accident involvement was not independently determined, but was reported by the respondents themselves; it is possible that safety conscious individuals may have been more inclined to complete the questionnaire than those suffering from feelings of guilt. Third, the questionnaire was an extremely lengthy one and, as noted previously, this can have the effect of discouraging the more overworked or harassed individuals from replying.

A further important limitation of the study, as its authors note, is the uncertainty about cause and effect. It is not obvious whether having an accident prompted, set a context for, or exacerbated worry over other life events, or whether, alternatively, the life events themselves played a determining part in bringing about the accidents. As Alkov and his colleagues point out, quarrels with a spouse or troubles at work could just as easily be symptoms of stress as causes of stress.[3] Even the most self confident skydiver or motorcyclist, for example, might take up reading or gardening after the sobering experience of an aircraft accident. Certainly there is a considerable body of literature devoted to the emotional problems that result from aircraft accidents.[4,8,12]

Research on the role of life stress in human error is not limited to retrospective studies of accidents; life events questionnaires can also be used in conjuction with more precise performance measures. Simmel's Life Events Questionnaire (LEQ) has been used to investigate the relationship of life stress to performance on a simulated air traffic control task.[26] Of 220 subjects screened with the LEQ, and those with the sixteen highest and lowest scores participated in a computer presented approach control task. Subjects gave verbal altitude and airspeed instructions to an experimenter who controlled the screen based simulation, and were instructed to preserve aircraft separation (i.e., to avoid collisions or near misses on final approach). At various points, proceedings were halted and the subject was required to declare the developing situation to be routine, urgent, or critical. It was anticipated that those subjects with high life events scores would make more errors in assessing the situation.

However, this proved not to be the case: many over- and underassessments were made by both groups, and the results of the experiment failed to demonstrate any relationship between these misassessments and measured 'life stress'. There are several reasons why this might have been so. First, the subjects were psychology students in a university rather than professional air traffic controllers. While this is in keeping with a long tradition in American psychological research, it means that results cannot easily be generalized to populations whose daily performance has the most profound implications for public safety and private careers. Moreover, the obvious artificiality of the task and the tripartite simplicity of the responses required may have reduced the resolution of the experiment to the point where false negatives were more likely than not. However, perhaps the most important limitation of the experimental procedure, given the hypothesis that it is the interaction of life stress with acute reactive stress that matters, is that the ATC exercise contained no task related stressors (e.g., sudden increases in workload, emergencies, or noise).

Nevertheless, not all the results of this experiment were negative. A potentially important finding was that in the 'high stress' group, scores for chronic stress were significantly higher than scores for acute stress (i.e., stress related to recent events). In the 'low stress' group, however, the two scores were about the same. As the authors point out, if this finding has general validity, accident investigators and researchers may need to broaden their attention to include not only recent events and proximate causes, but long term stresses as well.

Theoretical problems with life events research

Biographical events as environmental stimuli

The idea of life events as 'stressors' which influence flight deck performance is, at first sight, a very attractive and intuitively reasonable one. Nevertheless, there are serious problems with the life stress construct.

In one sense, life events research is firmly in the tradition of stimulus based stress models, in which stress is, in Sir Charles Symonds' phrase (quoted in Chapter 1) "a set of causes".[28] The causes here are non-task-related events, such as marriage and divorce. As is the case with almost all stimulus based approaches to stress, life stress research has not traditionally taken into account individual differences in response to (putative) stressors. Methodologies which attempt to do this are an important step forward, but to date remain crude.

A General Adaptation (to life events) Syndrome?

In another sense, life stress research follows in the tradition of response-based approaches to stress, especially the approach most closely associated with Hans Selye. As discussed in Chapter 1, Selye saw stress in terms of the organism's nonspecific response to events or circumstances. That is, irrespective of the nature of the eliciting condition, the response is supposedly the same: the General Adaptation Syndrome. Similarly, life stress research asserts that *change* evokes a stress response, and it does not matter much whether those life changes are for better or for worse, since all that matters is a general social and nonspecific adaptation to change.

If the life stress idea sounds appealing and intuitively correct at first, the nonspecificity of response to events and a normative approach to biography does *not* accord well with our intuitions.* Perhaps getting divorced *is* very stressful for Captain Smith, as it would be, perhaps, for most of his colleagues, but it may be a great relief from worry for Captain Brown. Moreover, no amount of averaging across pilots will tell us about Captain Brown's response. Apart from the theoretical inadequacy of 'normative biography' (and life events research has been broadly criticized for its lack of theory[30]), such an approach has rather limited policy usefulness (precisely because it has little predictive power). We cannot ground Captain Brown for a month just because she recently divorced, or First Officer Smith because he has been promoted to captain!

Additive and synergistic effects

One convenient result of the nonspecificity assumption for life event questionnaire designers is that life events are additive in terms of their stress producing potential. Thus, marriages and deaths, promotions and prosecutions, can all be summed into one overall life stress score. On top of this is the attractive and compelling hypothesis that life stress and acute reactive stress are also additive or synergistic. However, hard evidence for this is

---

*The 'Life Experiences Survey' (LES) devised by Sarason, Johnson, and Siegel[24] abandons both the normative and nonspecificity assumptions of other life events approaches, and focusses upon negative events within a full-blown cognitive appraisal model of stress. We know of no aviation studies using this approach, however.

as difficult to come by as anecdotal evidence is plentiful. An intriguing paper from sports psychology has demonstrated one potential mechanism by which life events could interact with task related 'stress' (in fact, high workload); in this study, student athletes with high life event scores (as determined using Sarason's sophisticated LES methodology) were found to exhibit the classical narrowing of peripheral visual attention in a laboratory dual task situation.[31] Evidence from the biochemical research referred to in Chapter 2, however, suggests that very different adaptive responses may be associated with acute reactive stress and life events: an 'adrenalin rush' in the former, and in the latter a 'sedating' increase in dopamine and opioid secretions. The very mischievous might suggest that a really numbing level of life stress ought to be the best preparation for terrifying inflight emergencies, since the combined biochemical responses should put average arousal in the middle of the Yerkes-Dodson inverted U curve -- right at optimum performance! The serious point, of course, is that we do not understand the complexities of endocrine and cognitive responses to multiple stressors, or how alternative mechanisms of psychological defence and coping will be invoked by individuals with varying personalities and life event backgrounds. Differentiating among these variables can be difficult.

It may be made more so by the characteristics of pilots themselves. Flying, as Chapter 6 describes, selects for outgoing, assertive, confident, and self reliant individuals. It is possible that pilots' lives are in general happier, or a least less eventful (in the life event sense) than those of nonpilots, although no studies have shown this (cf. the Canadian military study). Perhaps it is in the psychological 'makeup' of pilots to feel the stress of life's crises less than others, although this doesn't seem probable. Perhaps, as control oriented individuals, aviators merely cope better with life stress. On the other hand, it is equally likely that it is denial rather than real coping which leads to the downplaying of life stress by pilots whose self image and peer respect may depend upon the projection of a positive 'can do' attitude. Certainly the workplace can be very unforgiving of pilots perceived as 'bringing their domestic problems to work'.

Conclusion

There is little doubt that life's 'slings and arrows' can and do influence individuals' sense of well-being in many occupational walks of life. Moreover, life events research in aviation has performed the important function of raising our awareness of the potential influence of life stress on pilot performance. Other than this, however, it has not brought us much more insight than accident investigators have provided on the basis of case studies. We believe that to date much of the life events research work has been underpinned by too much that is speculative, intuitive, and nontheoretical. The best work on life events in flight performance remains to be done, and will feature, among other things, hypothetical mechanisms for performance change as a result of multiple stressors and workload variables. It will employ an enlightened and updated methodology for testing these hypotheses, one that, we trust, will abjure normative biography and nonspecificity, and not shrink from the (complicating but necessary) recognition of individual differences in the cognitive appraisal of events. In the meantime, questions remain whether pilots and flight activities are more or less vulnerable to life stress than individuals in other occupational activities; whether life 'events' can be related to flight performance in systematic, predictive and operationally useful ways; and, indeed, whether we should be focussing attention upon 'large' negative events or upon the cumulative effect of 'microstressors'.

References

1. Alkov, R.A. (1977), 'The Life Change as a Possible Predictor of Accident Behavior', paper presented at the 43rd Annual Scientific Meeting of the Aerospace Medical Association, Miami Beach.

2. Alkov, R.A., and Borowsky, M.S. (1980), 'A questionnaire study of psychological background factors in U.S. Naval aircraft accidents', *Aviation, Space, and Environmental Medicine,* vol. 51, pp. 860-3.

3. Alkov, R.A., Borowsky, M.S., and Gaynor, J.A. (1983), 'Pilot error as a symptom of inadequate stress coping', *Proceedings of the Second International Symposium on Aviation Psychology,* Ohio State University, Columbus, pp. 401-5.

4. Barnes, I., and Lurie, O.E. (1989), 'The descent from Olympus: the effect of accidents on aircrew survivors', *AGARD Conference Proceedings No. 458: Human Behaviour in High Stress Situations in Aerospace Operations,* NATO, Neuilly-sur-Seine, France.

5. Bhagat, R.S., and Allie, S.M. (1989), 'Organizational stress, personal life stress, and symptoms of life strains: an examination of the moderating role of sense of competence', *Journal of Vocational Behavior,* vol. 35, pp. 231-53.

6. Chappelow, J.W. (1989), 'Causes of aircrew error in the Royal Air Force', *AGARD Conference Proceedings No. 458: Human Behaviour in High Stress Situations in Aerospace Operations,* NATO, Neuilly-sur-Seine, France.

7. Day, W.R. (1984), 'Resource management', *Air Safety,* May, pp. 18-21.

8. Fowlie, D.G., and Aveline, M.D. (1985), 'The emotional consequences of ejection, rescue, and rehabilitation in Royal Air Force aircrew', *British Journal of Psychiatry,* vol. 146, pp. 609-13.

9. Green, R.G. (1985), 'Stress and accidents', *Aviation, Space, and Environmental Medicine,* vol. 56, pp. 638-41.

10. Holmes, T.H., and Masuda, M. (1972), 'Psychosomatic syndrome', *Psychology Today,* April, pp. 71-2, 106.

11. Holmes, T.H., and Rahe, R.H. (1967), 'The social readjustment rating scale', *Journal of Psychosomatic Research,* vol. 11, pp. 213-18.

12. Jones, D.R. (1982), 'Emotional reactions to military aircraft accidents', *Aviation, Space, and Environmental Medicine,* vol. 53, pp. 595-8.

13. Lazarus, R.S., and DeLongis, A. (1983), 'Psychological stress and coping in aging', *American Psychologist,* vol. 38, pp. 245-54.

14. McCarron, P.M., and Haakonson, N.H. (1982), 'Recent life change measurement in Canadian forces pilots', *Aviation, Space, and Environmental Medicine,* vol. 53, pp. 6-13.

15. McClelland, D.C., Patel, V., Stier, D., and Brown, D. (1987), 'The relationship of affiliative arousal to dopamine release', *Motivation and Emotion,* vol. 11, pp. 51-66.

16. Meyer, A. (1934), 'The Psychobiological Point of View', in Bentley, M. and Cowdrey, E.V. (eds.), *The Problem of Mental Disorder,* McGraw-Hill, New York, pp. 51-70.

17. Platenius, P., and Wilde, G. (1987), 'Personal characteristics related to accident histories of Canadian pilots', *Fourth International Symposium on Aviation Psychology,* Ohio State University, Columbus.

18. Rahe, R.H. (1967), *Life Crisis and Health Change,* Report No. 67-4, Navy Medical Neuropsychiatric Research Unit, San Diego.

19. Rahe, R.H. (1975), 'Epidemiological studies of life change and illness', *International Journal of Psychiatric Medicine,* vol. 6, pp. 133-46.

20. Rahe, R.H. (1978), 'Editorial: life change measurement clarification', *Psychosomatic Medicine,* vol. 40, pp. 95-8.

21. Rahe, R.H., Mahan, J.L., Arthur, R.J., and Gunderson, E.K. (1970), 'The epidemiology of illness of naval environment. I. Illness types, distribution, severities and relationship to life change', *Military Medicine,* no. 135, pp. 443-52.

22. Russell, M., and Davey, G.C.L. (1993), 'The relationship between life event measures and anxiety and its cognitive correlates', *Personality and Individual Differences,* vol. 14, pp. 317-22.

23. Sarason, I.G., De Monchaux, C., and Hunt, T. (1975), 'Methodological Issues in the Measurement of Life Stress' in Levi, L. (ed.), *Emotions: Their Parameters and Measurement,* Rover Press, New York.

24. Sarason, I.G., Johnson, J.H., and Siegel, J.M. (1978), 'Assessing the impact of life changes: development of the Life Experiences Survey', *Journal of Consulting and Clinical Psychology,* vol. 46, pp. 932-46.

25. Selye, H. (1956), *The Stress of Life*, McGraw-Hill, New York.

26. Simmel, E.C., Cerkovnik, M., and McCarthy, J.E. (1987), 'Sources of stress affecting pilot judgment', *Proceedings of the Fourth International Symposium on Aviation Psychology*, Ohio State University, Columbus, pp. 190-4.

27. Spielberger, C.D. (1966), 'Theory and Research on Anxiety', in Spielberger, C.D. (ed.), *Anxiety and Behavior*, Academic Press, New York.

28. Symonds, C., cited in Cox, T. (1978), *Stress*, Macmillan, London.

29. Vinokur, A., and Selzer, M.L. (1975), 'Desirable versus undesirable life events: their relationship to stress and mental distress', *Journal of Personality and Social Psychology*, vol. 32, pp. 329-37.

30. Vossel, G. (1987), 'Stress conceptions in life event research: towards a person-centred perspective', *European Journal of Personality*, vol. 1, pp. 123-40.

31. Williams, J.M., Tonymon, P., and Anderson, M.B. (1990), 'Effects of life-event stress on anxiety and peripheral narrowing', *Behavioral Medicine*, pp. 174-81.

6 Stress and pilot personality

Character generates the mysterious force that often holds things together when aviation's grand design comes apart at the seams.

-- Editorial, *Business Aviation Safety*

Don't expect to find a typical pilot. They come in all shapes and sizes and not one of them looks like Paul Newman.

-- Ken Beere, *Bluff Your Way on the Flight Deck*

Within the model discussed in Chapter 1, stress, or the extent to which things are perceived to be 'coming apart at the seams', is a matter of cognitive appraisal. Likewise, it should be obvious that an important variable in this process is the 'character' or personality of the individual making the appraisal. It is fair to say, however, that the notion of the 'pilot personality' has often been surrounded by a considerable degree of mystique. In the public mind, especially, aviators are sometimes seen as a breed apart, a rare class of individuals endowed with nearly superhuman courage and discipline -- the 'Right Stuff', as Tom Wolfe called it in his famous account of test pilots' derring-do. (Indeed, a passing mention of this work seems to be more or less obligatory in discussions of the subject, and even the term itself has made its way into the research literature -- although with a variety of meanings, as we shall see.)

Some of the more picturesque traits associated with the Hollywood stereotype are detailed in the sidebar on the following page; in more positive terms, one of the most salient aspects of the popular image seems to be the idea that the best pilots are unusually cool-headed and impervious to stress. We will consider this hypothesis later in the light of more general research on personality traits, cognitive appraisal patterns, and attitudes associated with stress resistance; first, however, we will review actual research on the psychology of aviators and the personality traits they commonly display.

> *The conventional misconception is that all pilots and especially military fighter pilots are notorious for exhibiting some form of the following set of behavioral and personality characteristics:*
>
>   *1. Devil-may-care value systems.*
>   *2. Live-for-the-moment attitudes.*
>   *3. Womanizing sexual ethics.*
>   *4. Rebellion against authority and cultural conventions.*
>   *5. Low level of professional commitment.*
>   *6. So individualistic that they make poor team players.*
>   *7. Inconsiderate, self-centered and self-serving.*
>   *8. Macho, egomaniacs who cannot tolerate criticism.*
>   *9. Deficient in self-analysis.*
>   *10. Power and status hungry authoritarians.*
>   *11. Superstitious beliefs in magical solutions.*
>
>   *-- Robert Besco,[15] p. 687*

The study of pilot personality

Historical background

The study of aircrew personality characteristics originated largely within a military context, as a device for screening candidates for flight training programs. A primary reason for this, obviously, is that would-be aviators who enter such programs and subsequently fail or drop out incur substantial expense to the taxpayer; one American report published in 1987 reported an average cost of over $800,000 per pilot.[23] Thus, one important goal of applicant selection processes within the military has been to minimize this costly attrition. Similar procedures have also sometimes been adopted by commercial airlines, particularly by those who train their own aircrew; however, the vast majority of research on pilot selection continues to be conducted by and for the armed forces. A second effect of this research focus, as we shall see, is that success as a pilot has often been measured largely in terms of the ability to complete a training programme, rather than by performance over the course of an individual's entire flying career.

Actually, prior to the Second World War such programmes had few entry requirements other than basic medical fitness. However, as the scope of military flight operations expanded, the practical and financial costs of attrition also increased, and recruiters began to impose more selective criteria.[91] This development was also stimulated by advances in the field of personnel psychology and applicant testing: where previously trainee attrition had been regarded as largely beyond human prediction, there was a growing perception that the power of science could be brought to bear on the problem. (It may be noted that while our discussion here is concerned with personality measures, this was of course by no means the only, or even primary, dimension of interest to recruiters. Other screening criteria have included general intelligence, psychomotor skills, and aviation relevant knowledge.)

Over the decades, a number of different approaches have been adopted in research on pilots' personalities. One has been simply to administer conventional personality tests to groups of pilots and observe to what extent (if any) their scores differ from population norms. Often these tests have been used to compare the traits of 'superior' and 'inferior' pilots, the criterion often being success or failure in flight training. These were the prevailing methodologies before the 1970s, at which point traditional paper-and-pencil inventories began to be supplemented by performance based assessments of qualities thought likely to be of direct relevance to flying performance (for example, risk taking propensity or decision making style). More recently still, the criteria used to identify 'superior' pilots have expanded to encompass not only their performance at the training stage but also such operationally relevant measures as long term safety records.[23] In the area of personality, one current topic of inquiry concerns the pilot's underlying attitudes toward safety procedures, authority figures, their own level of competence, and so forth, and the relationship of these to flying performance.

Personality measures and training outcomes

Early efforts to apply personality measures to the process of pilot selection were not greatly encouraging. As a rule the tests employed were traditional ones already in use with the general population, such as the Rorschach Test and the Thematic Apperception Test.[47] Of course, many of these had been designed to identify psychiatric abnormalities, not to discriminate among groups of healthy individuals or to predict performance,[4,27] and pilots' scores on such tests tended to show little correlation with success or failure in flight training.[47,140] Even more recent measures, some of them specifically designed for use in occupational testing, have often yielded frustratingly inconclusive results, as the following example will illustrate.

A case study. A 1987 study by Paul Retzlaff and Michael Gibertini (entitled "Hard Data on the 'Right Stuff'") sought to determine the relationship between personality traits and training success in a group of US Air Force cadets.[111] With the aid of two inventories, the Personality Research Form[59] and the Millon Clinical Multiaxial Inventory,[95] they identified three distinct 'types' within their subject pool. The pilots in the largest cluster were described as achievement oriented, dominant, and outgoing, as well as stable and level headed, with a structured, matter-of-fact approach to problem solving. As they comprised 58 percent of the sample, they were labelled 'typical' pilots. The second group, which comprised 21 percent of the total sample, was, like the first, outgoing and achievement oriented, but also unusually aggressive, socially dominant, exhibitionistic, and self aggrandizing. Because these pilots resembled the macho aviators of popular myth they were described (perhaps inevitably) as the 'right stuff' group. The final 21 percent were described as being neither outgoing nor achievement oriented, but instead as "cautious, compulsive, and socially retiring". As it was hypothesized that they might be less effective or successful in the cockpit, this group was referred to as having the 'wrong stuff' -- at least with respect to aviation.

These personality groupings were empirically derived via cluster analysis. The hypothesized performance correlations had a substantive basis in the research literature (as we shall see), and were, it may be said, suggestive and interesting in their implications for aircrew selection and training. What they were not, however, was operationally significant, at least as far as this particular study was concerned.

That is, the investigators were unable to find any correlations at all between the personality profiles they identified and the pilots' success in flight training.[14] The cautious and retiring 'wrong stuff' pilots fared no worse than the other two groups, and the level-headed 'typical' pilots, who were assumed to possess an optimal personality profile, fared no better. Neither did personality have any bearing on the type of aircraft to which the student was ultimately assigned, despite predictions that the individualistic 'right stuff' pilots might function better in single seater aircraft than as members of larger cockpit crews. Similar results, incidentally, were found in a separate study of experienced US Army pilots: while the investigator, James Picano, was able to identify personality types analogous to those found in Retzlaff's and Gibertini's Air Force trainees, no relationship was evident between the types of missions flown, years of service, or number of flight hours.[108]

Of course, conventional personality tests have not universally failed to predict flying performance; those which appear to have at least some value in this respect are discussed as follows, along with the traits that they have identified as characteristic of successful pilots.

Minnesota Multiphasic Personality Inventory. The Minnesota Multiphasic Personality Inventory (MMPI) is a very widely used personality instrument originally developed for clinical diagnostic purposes. The dimensions it measures include hypochondriasis, depression, hysteria, psychopathic personality, masculinity-femininity, paranoia, psychasthenia, schizophrenia, hypomania, and social introversion. In general, studies using the MMPI have found pilots to be relatively high in sociability, aggression, self confidence, and intellectual striving and low in hypochondriasis, anxiety, and schizoid tendencies.[22,33,39] A 1954 study[93] found, interestingly, that a cluster of high scores in hysteria, masculinity-femininity, and mania predicted successful completion of flight training in a US Navy sample, while low scores in these traits were predictive of failure. However, another study from the 1950s[38] found no such discrimination, a finding consistent with more general reviews of its validity as a tool for personnel selection.[50]

Eysenck Personality Inventory. The Eysenck Personality Inventory[31] assesses two separate dimensions of personality, extraversion/introversion and neuroticism/stability. Research using this test indicates that military pilots, at least, are significantly less neurotic than the general population.[12] A study of RAF trainees in the early 1970s found that 60 percent of those who failed to complete flight training belonged belonged in the category of neurotic introverts, whereas those individuals who successfully completed their training were typically classified as stable introverts.[60] Other evidence suggests that stability alone may have been the relevant factor: a study of naval aviation trainees that utilized only the introversion/extraversion component of the inventory was unable to predict training outcome on this basis alone.[43]

Edwards Personal Preference Schedule. The Edwards Personal Preference Schedule (EPPS)[26] is a personality inventory that assesses fifteen different personality 'needs'. Based on the idea that different occupations fulfill different kinds of personal and emotional needs,[75] the EPPS has proven to be effective in identifying traits typical for given occupational groups, and also in differentiating (at a statistical level) between successful and unsuccessful members of particular occupations.

Several studies have employed the EPPS to obtain normative data on the personality characteristics of different groups of pilots.[1,6,37,101,102] The results have been fairly consistent across the groups: in four separate studies pilots have been found to exceed the general population in their need for what the EPPS calls 'achievement' (striving, attainment), 'dominance' (control or leadership of others), and 'change' (variety, doing different things), but to be lower than average in 'deference' (following instructions) and 'order' (planning, neatness). In addition, in most of the studies pilots have obtained higher than average scores in 'aggression' (the tendency to criticize, to become angry, to attack the views of others), and lower scores in 'abasement' (timidity, feelings of inferiority), 'nurturance' (kindness, helpfulness), and 'succorance' (the tendency to seek help and understanding from others).

Personality Research Form. A relatively new general assessment tool is the Personality Research Form,[58] developed in the 1970s. A 1980 study of trainee pilots in the Canadian armed forces[61] found that the trait of aggressiveness correlated positively with successful completion of training, but only in individuals who were also assessed as having strong leadership or interpersonal abilities. Conversely, the combination of aggressiveness and poor leadership or interpersonal skills was associated with failure to complete training.

Behaviourally based tests. With the advent of applicable computer technologies, the paper-and-pencil inventories traditionally used in aviation selection are increasingly being supplemented by a variety of automated test batteries. While these are primarily used to assess psychomotor and perceptual skills (e.g., reaction time, spatial orientation), they may also include behavioural components that can be used to assess certain personality traits and attitudes.

One example is the Basic Attributes Tests (BAT) battery developed by the United States Air Force.[62] Among its fifteen subtasks are several that are concerned with personality characteristics, including compulsiveness versus decisiveness, field dependence, confidence in decision making, and risk taking. However, only the confidence task has proved to have even marginal statistical signficance in predicting training success. This item, the Self-Crediting Word Knowledge Test, consists of a series of multiple choice vocabulary matching trials; before each set subjects are informed that the difficulty level will increase and are invited to wager points based upon how well they believe they will perform. In one study conducted by the US Air Force, successful completion of flight training was observed most often in subjects who spent a long time on each trial and wagered relatively few points; these behaviours are believed to indicate a cautious decision making style.[128]

The BAT also contains a measure of risk taking propensity which, although of uncertain predictive validity, appears to be worthy of further investigation and development. In this test, subjects are presented with a row of ten boxes and invited to 'select' as many as they wish. All but one contain points in varying amounts which are awarded cumulatively; the tenth is a 'penalty' box which, if selected, erases all points accumulated for that trial. Thus, with each additional selection, the subject gambles all of his existing points on the chance of gaining yet more; the number of boxes chosen in each trial is taken as an indication of willingness to take risks.

In the Air Force study this test was not found to be predictive of success in flight training.[128] However, significant results were obtained by a Navy study which used a variation of the test. In the latter group, risk takers (i.e., those who selected a large number of boxes) were more likely to complete their training; interestingly, however, within the subset of those who graduated, it was the low risk takers who tended to receive better grades from their flight instructors.[127]

General comments. To summarize, then, the research described above suggests an individual who is aggressive (MMPI, EPPS, Personality Research Form); dominant or competitive (EPPS); achievement oriented (MMPI, EPPS); self confident (MMPI, EPPS); unanxious (MMPI, Eysenck); and socially outgoing (MMPI, Personality Research Form), although not to the extent of *needing* to be liked (EPPS). The profile generated by the EPPS further suggests a person who is somewhat insensitive emotionally and not by nature introspective. This picture is often echoed in the literature, as in the following description by a Norwegian researcher[96] of 'the typical fighter pilot':

He is capable, competitive, individualistic, [and] scores high on achievement and exhibition.

His values are capitalistic rather than radical.

He is intelligent, athletic, and blessed with good health.

He lives an active life, has many acquaintances but few close friends.

He is well adapted and independent, prefers physical activity to intellectual [pursuits].

He has limited contact with his own feelings and is not prone to introspection.

Safety based criteria

Another way of exploring the relationship between pilot personality and performance has been via the study of accident rates. In the mid-1970s, Michael Sanders and Mark Hoffman[117] of the US Army Aeromedical Research Laboratory in Fort Rucker, Alabama, examined the accident files of fifty-one Army aviators and also administered standard personality measures, including the Sixteen Personality Factor Questionnaire (16PF)[18] to the same individuals. Three of the factors on this scale correlated highly with accident history: using only these three scores, the investigators were able to determine with 86 percent accuracy whether a given subject had previously been involved in an accident where pilot error had been implicated.

The first of these factors concerned the dimension of self sufficiency versus group dependence. In general, persons who score highly on this scale can be described as being independent and resourceful, while low scorers have a higher need for social approval and often prefer to consult others before making decisions. Those pilots who had previously been in accidents had average scores (relative to the general population); those who had not had high scores, indicating that they were unusually self reliant.

The second factor concerned the dimension of practicality versus imaginativeness. Persons scoring high on this part of the questionnaire tend to be imaginative, unconventional, and sometimes absent-minded, while low scorers are more practical-minded and rooted in the present. Interestingly, the accident-free pilots had high scores on this dimension, while the scores of the accident group were average or slightly lower. Sanders and Hoffman considered this finding to be counterintuitive: certainly qualities such as absent-mindedness are not normally considered to be conducive to flight safety. It should be borne in mind, however, that the pilots in the study were not specifically found to be absent-minded; rather, these qualities are merely common among high scorers in the population at large. It could well be argued, in fact, that imaginativeness itself is a desirable quality for a pilot, if by this we mean the ability to visualize the far-reaching implications of present situations, and to anticipate trouble before it arrives.

The third personality dimension found to correlate with accident history was that of forthrightness versus shrewdness. Low scores on this scale are associated with spontaneity and lack of pretension; a high score suggests a more polished or sophisticated individual. Those pilots who had been in accidents had average scores on this measure. Those who had not were slightly below average, that is, more forthright than the average person. The reason for this effect was unclear.

These results might appear to suggest that it is possible to identify not only a typical 'pilot personality', but also an ideal one (at least as far as safety is concerned). However, a cross-validation study carried out the following year on another group of pilots failed to replicate the first study's results.[118] This time, no correlations were found between any personality variables and accident history. This inconsistency was attributed in part to the vagueness of the term 'pilot error'; one recommendation for future research was that errors be more closely analyzed by type.

Attitudes and thought patterns

Another area of research that touches on the interaction between pilot personality and accident risk has been the notion of 'hazardous thought patterns'. This concept grew out of an investigation conducted by the Federal Aviation Administration and Embry-Riddle Aeronautical University in the early 1980s.[14] The purpose of the research was isolate specific 'attitudes' or 'thought patterns' that might serve as precursors to faulty pilot judgement. Five thought patterns identified as hazardous in an aviation context included resistance to authority, impulsivity, invulnerability, macho attitudes, and external control or resignation (see sidebar overleaf).

While the selection of these particular five traits was determined intuitively and anecdotally rather than through any empirical process, there has been something of a tendency in subsequent literature to refer to them in all-inclusive terms, as *the* five hazardous thoughts. Actually, only three of the five have been found to occur with significant frequency among aviators; studies of civilian pilots have thus far identified the invulnerability pattern as the most prevalent, followed by impulsivity and macho. The

---

Hazardous 'Thought Patterns' [A Speculative List]

Anti-Authority: "Don't tell me!" This thought is found in people who do not like anyone telling them what to do. They think, "Don't tell me!" In a sense, they are saying "No one can tell me what to do." The person who thinks, "Don't tell me," may either be resentful of having someone tell him or her what to do or may just regard rules, regulations, and procedures as silly or unnecessary.

Impulsivity: "Do something -- quickly!" This is the thought pattern of people who frequently feel the need to do something, anything, immediately. They do not stop to think about what they are about to do -- they do the first thing that comes to mind.

Invulnerability: "It won't happen to me." Many people feel that accidents happen to others but never to them. They know accidents can happen, and they know that anyone can be affected; but they never really feel or believe that *they* will be involved. Pilots who think this way are more likely to take chances and run unwise risks, thinking all the time, *"It won't happen to me!"*

Macho: "I can do it." People who are always trying to prove they are better than anyone else think, *"I can do it!"* They 'prove' themselves by taking risks and by trying to impress others. While this pattern is thought to be a male characteristic, women are equally susceptible.

Resignation: "What's the use?" People who think, *"What's the use?"* do not see themselves as making a great deal of difference in what happens to them. When things go well, they think, *"That's good luck"*. When things go badly, they attribute it to bad luck or feel that someone is *'out to get them'*. They leave the action to others: for better or worse.

-- cited in Lester and Bombaci,[85] p. 568

---

anti-authority pattern appears to be fairly uncommon, and the pattern of resignation, extremely so.[85,86]

Opinion has also been divided as to whether pilots can be taught to recognize and correct these thought patterns, or whether they represent enduring personality traits that are relatively resistant to change. In support of the first view it may be noted that the hazardous thought patterns

Denver, Colorado, October, 1990: After a delay vector en route we were asked to descend to Flight Level 310 from Flight Level 350. The captain was flying and upset at the descent clearance. He got on the microphone and requested Flight Level 350 again after traffic descent. Center said he would be on request. Captain then began a slower than normal descent. Next came anther vector off course and another terse exchange between him and center. The captain kept the nonstandard descent going. About five minutes later we got another descent clearance to a lower altitude and another vector off course, followed by another terse conversation between the two. At this point I became a passenger and told the captain he was in a no win situation. It didn't help. I don't know if he realized he caused most of his own problems by a slow rate of descent or not. When I said the same he chose to ignore me. It was war. I'm aware that this could come back to haunt me as a crew member by FAA action, even though he took it upon himself to win a no win situation. My reaction is to say to ATC to cross certain areas in such and such a time or within a specified fix or DME so as not to put other crew members in the middle of this childish behavior.

-- NASA Aviation Safety Reporting System (Accession No. 159440)

concept has been used with favourable results as a teaching aid in pilot judgement training programmes.[14,17,87] On the other hand, correlations have been identified between the same thought patterns and certain well-established personality dimensions. For example, Lester and Bombaci[85] found that general aviation pilots exhibiting the macho thought pattern also obtained high scores on the Rotter Locus of Control Scale[115] (discussed later), and the integration/self concept control scale of the Cattell 16PF,[18] while pilots characterized by the impulsive and invulnerable thought patterns were both less internally controlled and less well-integrated.[85] This finding was replicated in a later study by Lester and Connolly,[86] who also found that pilots displaying the invulnerable pattern were somewhat less conscientious than those with impulsive or macho attitudes. It remains to be determined what other personality dimensions might map onto the hazardous thought pattern construct; one promising area for future research might be the relationship between hazardous thought patterns and psychological defence mechanisms (a subject addressed later in this chapter).

Personality issues in crew coordination

Historically, personality research in aviation has been directed nearly exclusively at the psychological traits of individual pilots. However, this focus may be overly narrow in the modern era of multicrew aircraft. Foushee and Helmreich[35] point out the while the macho, risk taking maverick qualities popularly associated with pilots may have been desirable or even necessary in the early, 'barnstorming' days of aviation, they are increasingly less so now -- and not only because flying has progressed from being the most dangerous mode of transportation to being the safest and most highly regulated one:

> It has been suggested that those characteristics associated with the right stuff are 'the wrong stuff' as far as effective group function is concerned, and therein lies the paradox. Since so much value has been placed upon personality characteristics such as self-sufficiency, machismo, and bravery, we may be selecting individuals who tend to keep themselves to themselves, communicate less than the average person, and are not very good at sharing responsibility with others -- not exactly the characteristics one would look for when trying to put together a group that well. (p. 193)

At the University of Texas at Austin, Robert Helmreich and other researchers studying the psychology of aircrew interactions have focussed on two personality dimensions in particular, instrumentality and expressivity. The former includes orientation toward work, achievement, and task mastery; the latter incorporates the qualities of interpersonal sensitivity and communicativeness. Both of these qualities can assume negative as well as positive forms (for example, an undesirable form of expressivity would be verbal aggressiveness; negative instrumentality might take the form of excessive competitiveness). These qualities have been assessed with the use of a test battery called the Personal Characteristics Inventory (a composite of several other scales, including the Work and Family Orientation Questionnaire[53] and the Extended Personal Attributes Questionnaire.[132]

Based on various combinations of these traits, a 1989 study[45] identified three different clusters within a sample of military pilots enrolled in a recurrent training seminar on cockpit resource management. The first exhibited a strong orientation toward work, achievement, and mastery, combined with high levels of positive expressivity and low levels of competitiveness and verbal aggression. Other research suggests that this

Milwaukee, December, 1991: After receiving clearance and instructions to taxi to runway 1L via the inner on terminal taxiway captain and copilot completed checklists and powered up. In blizzard conditions with visibility near zero in blowing snow we made our way slowly through 10-14 inches of fresh drifting snow. Progress was impaired often by deep snowdrifts and stuck aircraft that we had to make our way around. As our taxi continued outside visibility was impaired further by snow on the side windows allowing us to only see forward. Snow was also sticking to taxiway signs making them unreadable. From the inner taxiway we transitioned to what we thought was the romeo taxiway and crossed runway 7R. After the crossing we discovered that we were not on romeo but on mike taxiway and had crossed 1L, the active runway. We notified ground control of our predicament and were cleared back across the active runway and on our way with no further problems. In retrospect I cannot attribute this incident to fatigue as we were both fresh after a full weekend rest. However, there was a certain amount of frustration involved with the fact that the airport would be closing shortly making it a sort of race to get out of there.

The captain compromised safety with his 'must go' attitude. This particular captain is very hard to work with because of his huge ego. In order to work in peace with the man I have to be overly submissive to his authority as captain. He seems to feel that the flight officer is not really needed and resents it when I point out his mistakes. It does not matter how big or small, or how nicely it is pointed out to him, he just can't deal with it and gets angry. I am still on probation with this company and this captain is well liked by the management. This Catch-22 situation causes me to have to choose between doing my job and keeping peace with this captain. I feel that I would have noticed and prevented the runway incursion if I had not been so worried about stepping on this man's very sensitive toes.

-- NASA Aviation Safety Reporting System (Accession No. 195859)

profile is the optimal one for work in multicrew cockpits,[131] and this group did indeed enjoy the highest military promotion rate. It was, accordingly, labelled the 'right stuff' group. Pilots who were equally high in achievement motivation but also competitive and verbally aggressive were identified as having the 'wrong stuff' (in contradiction to the stereotype). A third group, which displayed relatively low levels both of instrumentality and expressiveness (either positive or negative), was assigned the label 'no stuff'. (These labels should not be equated with those in the Retzlaff and Gibertini[111] study cited earlier; in fact, the macho and aggressive 'right stuff' pilots in that study probably have more in common with the 'wrong stuff' pilots in the one discussed here.)

Before undergoing the crew coordination training for which they were enrolled, all three groups completed a test called the Cockpit Management Attitudes Questionnaire (CMAQ).[51,54] This instrument assesses three attitudes relevant to cockpit resource management.[44] The first, 'communication and coordination', or the degree of willingness to communicate and work with others, was found to be highest in the 'right stuff' group, and lowest in the 'no stuff' group. The second attitude dimension, 'command responsibility', concerns the issue of whether responsibility for the flight is believed to rest with the crew as a whole or with the captain only; the latter, more authoritarian belief system is regarded as undesirable. Within this particular sample of pilots, beliefs about command responsibility initially showed no relationship to the personality profile identified; following training, however, 'right stuff' pilots improved markedly in this respect, 'wrong stuff' pilots evinced little attitude change, and 'no stuff' pilots actually showed a decreased in their appreciation of collective responsibility.

The third attitude measured by the CMAQ is referred to as 'recognition of stressor effects', or the willingness to acknowledge and compensate for diminished capacities brought about by stress. In some respects this would seem to be related (in an opposite sense) to the 'macho' thought pattern described by Berlin and colleagues.[14] The relationship that emerged between this attitude dimension and the instrumentality/expressivity personality cluster was a highly interesting one. Initially, the so-called 'right stuff' pilots were the *least* disposed to recognize and work around their own limitations or those of others (perhaps because of their high achievement motivation); however, upon completing the cockpit resource management course they exhibited the *highest* scores in 'recognition of stressor effects', indicating a dramatic attitude change in response to training. (The other two groups, the 'wrong stuff' and 'no stuff' pilots, displayed only modest attitude changes in this area).

Actually, of course, this mature attitude toward stress is likely to be important in both single crew and multicrew operations. Skilled leaders, in particular, can elicit the best performance from themselves and from their crews by setting high standards without losing sight of the fact that teams are comprised of fallible human beings. To acknowledge one's limitations is not to 'make excuses' or to settle for mediocre performance: in the study just described, the pilots most receptive to stress education were, after all, the highly motivated 'right stuff' group. We are reminded of the following words, which appeared in a popular aviation magazine some years ago: "Good pilots will go to the limit, but that is because they know what the limit is."[105]

Methodological issues

Problems with conventional personality tests. It has been observed that question and answer personality inventories of the type described above often have considerable potential for response bias. It is well established, for example, that personality characteristics that are perceived as negative may be deliberately concealed in order to secure employment or acceptance into a training program,[4] and pilots, being fairly intelligent, tend to be well equipped to manipulate their scores in this way.[46] It has also been suggested that the responses they give may be influenced by their own stereotyped notions of what pilots are 'supposed' to be like.[100]

Training based evaluation: a sufficient criterion? There have also been difficulties with the other side of the equation, the evaluation of pilots' performance. As noted, one important impetus for research on pilot personalities has been to provide selection guidelines for the military, and perhaps for this reason the primary criterion of 'success' used has often been completion of flight training. Another measure of flying performance has sometimes been the grade assigned by the student's instructor. However, it has never been easy to ensure objectivity and consistency across instructors.[24,126]

One specific problem is that of the 'halo effect', in which a student's past performance influences the instructor's perception of current performance, or when positive or negative performance in one area influences the evaluation of performance in another.[92] Also of interest here is the 'honeymoon effect',[52] wherein high levels of motivation during training or in the initial stages of employment have an improving effect on behaviour, which is, however, only temporary.

Until relatively recently researchers did not, in general, address the issue of what personality factors might influence a pilot's later flying career. For example, one early review noted that while prediction of actual operational effectiveness was also a worthwhile goal, there was an unfortunate lack of empirical data capable of shedding light on the subject.[47] (Russian research has reportedly had greater success with pilot personality tests in part because, under the former Soviet system, state flying school students could be tracked right through early training and well into their careers with Aeroflot.[135]) Finally, successful completion of training is in some respects not the most relevant of criteria, insofar as *all* active pilots have, by definition, completed training. (An analogy could be made with, for example, schoolteachers: since all teachers are required to have graduated from an approved training course, this is not a useful yardstick with which to rate one against another.)

Occupational categories. As noted previously, much of the research on pilot personality has been conducted within a military context. The subjects in these studies therefore comprise a fairly homogenous group of individuals. First, of course, they belong to a narrow age range and until quite recently were all males; in addition, they can be assumed to possess motivations and personality traits compatible with life in the armed forces. As such they may well share certain personality traits for these reasons alone, reasons that do not bear directly on their operational effectiveness in the cockpit. The same is presumably true of airline pilots, who in addition to possessing a specific set of vocational inclinations are preselected for their ability to fit in with a particular sort of lifestyle and corporate culture.

Of interest here are two studies from the 1970s by Novello and Youssef, which examined the personalities of male and female general aviation pilots, respectively.[101,102] The male pilots were found to have the same suite of traits as that already noted to be typical in the military, although to a less marked degree. So, indeed, did the female pilots: in fact, on some dimensions of the MMPI their scores were closer to the norms for male pilots and for men in general than to female population norms. Nevertheless, the point remains valid that caution should be exercised in attempting to generalize research findings from one group of aviators to another.

Operational relevance: does descriptive equal prescriptive? Eric Farmer of the Royal Air Force Institute of Aviation Medicine has pointed out that while traditional personality tests may well tell us what pilots are like, the question of which traits are actually desirable for aviation is a separate issue.[32] There are obvious logical pitfalls inherent in applying data of the kind described above in a prescriptive manner. The following *reductio* argument will help to illustrate this point. If a study indicates that the majority of pilots are (say) white, male, and politically conservative (as per the Norwegian description noted earlier[96]), does it follow that these qualities specifically lead to safe and efficient flying? Should nonwhite female liberals be excluded from flight training programs or denied jobs in airlines on the grounds that they represent a poor risk? While the use of personality tests to predict occupational success does have some empirical support, the correlation occurs at the statistical rather than individual level, and the importance of identifying actual causative mechanisms should never be overlooked.

General comments

Thomas Chidester of NASA-Ames Research Center in California has stated that "personality research in aviation has mostly been a bust".[21] By this he apparently means that the dimensions of personality that psychologists have typically sought to measure do not seem to correlate very reliably with operational effectiveness in the cockpit. Robert Besco,[15] a researcher with extensive flying experience himself, describes the situation in the following terms (with specific reference to fighter pilots):

> This writer has observed "Top Guns" who are shy and retiring. Some are domineering and authoritative. Some are intellectual and bookish. Some are religious and spiritual. Some are loud and boisterous. Some are comical. Some are somber. Some are athletically gifted. Some cannot walk and chew gum at the same time. I have even observed some who fit the macho-fighter-pilot-type personality stereotype. The point is that all of these characteristics can be observed in the same proportions in all categories and performance levels of pilots from "top guns," to "average pilots" and even in the "tail end Charlies." What does distinguish the good pilots from the mediocre pilots is the performance they achieve at work. (p. 688)

While we agree that personality research in aviation needs to be grounded in operational relevance, it would be overstating the case to conclude that 'personality' is an entity that functions completely independently of 'performance'. As far as empirical research is concerned, the problem has partly been one of definition: which traits should be measured and how, and which aspects of performance should be evaluated and how. Over the years, personality research has become increasingly sophisticated in both of these respects. However, there is a more fundamental difficulty inherent in the search for 'causes' and 'effects'. A pilot's personality traits do not necessarily *cause* mishaps or failures, but they may *enable* them -- that is, they may contribute to the establishment of conditions which, in combination with other factors, make failures more probable. In other words, certain personality characteristics could be described as 'gateways' to error. As such they will have concrete effects only some of the time -- in some cases, perhaps, not very often at all. This variability simply underscores the importance of analyzing specific causal mechanisms as well as statistical correlations.

Stress resistance

Pilot training manuals, not to mention books and articles on flight safety, abound with descriptions of the 'good' or 'ideal' aviator. Needless to say, these prescriptions for success place little if any emphasis on superhuman levels of 'right stuff', much less on MMPI scores and the like. One such description, again from Robert Besco,[15] is excerpted below. While the qualities described here are not empirically derived, they have a strong commonsense appeal, and it is interesting to note that a recurring theme is the quality of not becoming flustered or stressed when problems develop:

> Good pilots detect mistakes immediately after they are made. First their own errors, then their fellow crew members and then the errors of others.
>
> Good pilots cope, correct and compensate for these errors gracefully and uneventfully.
>
> Good pilots communicate their assessment of these errors immediately to their fellow crew members and to supporting personnel.
>
> Good pilots accept that errors will occur and know that they can compensate for them.
>
> Good pilots do not let the threat of past, current, or future errors increase their own error rates or their ability to cope.
>
> Good pilots develop and maintain an attitude of wariness and anticipation of errors.
>
> Good pilots have the character strength to say N-O to marginal conditions and to resist the organizational pressures to "Press on".
>
> Good pilots exert a stabilizing influence on others when the system is degenerating and goal conflicts are developing.
>
> Good pilots adapt quickly to changes in the demands and environmental conditions of their profession. (pp. 688-9)

While stress resistance should not, of course, be viewed as a single, discrete 'trait' (any more than stress itself is a unidimensional phenomenon), psychologists have in recent years been exploring (fairly independently from one another) a number of different personality variables that appear to affect the level of stress that an individual experiences. This would appear to be a promising area for applied research in aviation, and, as we shall see, some of the specific traits thought to decrease vulnerability to stress effects have in fact been included in recent aviation selection batteries.

The subject of individual differences in stress tolerance received little attention before the 1970s and 1980s. The reasons for this neglect are rooted in the ideas about the overall nature of stress which prevailed up to that time. Certainly stimulus based models, which regard 'stress' as inherent in situations rather than in persons, must by their nature ignore this dimension.[89] Response based models could, in theory, consider individual factors but in practice have rarely done so; such investigations as do exist have typically focussed on physiological functions,[76,77] a tendency that has doubtless been reinforced by the predominance of Selye's views on the nature of stress.[123,124] In general, both stimulus and response oriented theorists have tended to view individual differences merely as sources of random variation or error variance.[134]

Interest in the role of individual differences has increased, however, with the advent of transactional models of stress, which explore the interplay between the person and his or her environment. Some of the dimensions along which individuals may vary include prior experiences with given stressors, actual physical or intellectual coping abilities, and motivation levels. Perhaps the most intriguing dimension, however, is that of personality. Beginning with the work of Lazarus in the mid-1960s,[78,104] there is a growing body of research devoted to identifying specific character traits likely to increase or decrease vulnerability to stress. Indeed, the importance of personality variables in stress research is now widely acknowledged,[5,20,74,88,90,120] particularly by those theorists concerned with the role of cognitive appraisal. In fact, the study of personality could even be regarded as intrinsic to a cognitive appraisal view of stress:

> The process of appraisal which takes place in the individual is always a subjective one, and this means, among other things, that it runs differently in different people. If we take this understanding of stress as a point of departure, then the conclusion must be that the individual differences approach should be considered as one of the most important paradigms in the study of stress. (Strelau,[134] p. 156)

Psychological traits influencing cognitive appraisal

Cognitive appraisals are affected not only by an individual's specific perceptions of a situation, but also, inevitably, by certain general belief systems. These relate both to the surrounding environment -- i.e., whether it is fundamentally friendly or hostile -- as well as to the person's place in it -- i.e., whether he is basically a competent individual, or someone who is chronically 'out of his depth'.[8] These sorts of ideas, which tend to operate at an implicit level, can obviously influence whether a given situation is viewed as a negative threat or a positive challenge.[34] Thus, it is entirely possible that two individuals in the same environment and with seemingly equivalent abilities may form quite different perceptions, either of the nature and degree of threat present or of their capacity to respond appropriately. This is even more the case in unfamiliar and ambiguous situations, where concrete information necessarily contributes less to appraisal.[78] We will therefore examine some specific personality traits and belief systems likely to influence cognitive appraisals -- and, by extension, performance -- under stress.

Locus of control. One such dimension concerns the extent to which an individual regards control over events to be under his own influence. This variable is known as locus of control.[115] Viewed purely in situational terms, the perception of control has long been recognized as an important mediator of stress: there is voluminous evidence to the effect that people (and animals) object less to an aversive stimulus when they possess some type of control over its administration.[94] This is true even when control is objectively lacking but is *perceived* to be present.[16,19] The term 'locus of control', however, refers not to specific situational appraisals, but to a more basic attitude concerning the effects of one's own behaviour, as assessed by means of the Rotter Locus of Control Scale.[115]

Pilots with an internal locus of control generally feel that they have significant influence over the course of events: they have confidence that their actions lead to predictable results. They are likely to believe that 'you make your own luck'. Individuals with an external locus of control, on the other hand, are more likely to ascribe the outcome of any given situation to the workings of fate, chance, the weather, their flight instructor, air traffic controllers, or other factors external to themselves.[143] Possession of an external locus of control has frequently been associated with greater vulnerability to stress.[80,81,107] One mechanism for this, obviously, is the association with helplessness; persons with this particular personality trait tend to exhibit a general skepticism that their actions can really be depended upon to bring about the results desired. This is probably part of what lies behind the (so-called) hazardous thought pattern termed 'resignation'.

Interestingly, however, the locus of control variable has also been linked to differences in mental functioning and performance. Wichman and Oyasato[143] have described internally controlled individuals as being 'cognitively more active': in other words, they are apparently better both at acquiring new information[83,121,122] and at applying it effectively.[25,106] This effect seems to be especially pronounced in highly ambiguous situations.[82,109] There is also evidence that internal locus of control is associated with greater awareness of environmental cues (and, of course, persons who succeed in perceiving relevant information are also in a better position to act upon it).[25,83,107]

This correlation invites speculation concerning cause and effect: it is unclear whether internally controlled pilots monitor their environment more actively *because* they are internally controlled (and hence perceive this to be a profitable use of resources), or whether pilots who are in the habit of keeping track of external cues then develop an internal locus of control, thanks to a positive track record of accomplishments. Certainly, a series of studies by Wichman and Ball[142] demonstrated that pilots are significantly (or even, as they put it, "dramatically") more internally controlled than the average person (p. 509). This suggests that the Rotter Locus of Control Scale deserves additional attention as a predictor of pilot performance in general, and of performance under stress in particular.

Self efficacy. Another important coping variable (which will receive further attention in our discussion of combat stress in Chapter 7) is known by the term 'self efficacy'. Based upon the work of Bandura, perceived self efficacy refers to the extent to which an individual judges himself able to perform an imminent task, and as such may, like locus of control, also be related to the hazardous thought pattern labelled 'resignation'. Doubters are said to be more easily deterred, invest less effort, and exhibit less resolve. By the same token, individuals with perceptions of higher self efficacy are said to enter the task with more resolve, to persist longer, and to invest more resources in success.[10,11]

The concept of self efficacy is obviously related to that of locus of control, but refers less to a global conviction about the world in general than to beliefs about one's own level of control, often within particular contexts. These beliefs can, therefore, vary from one domain to another. Like locus of control, however, the perception of self efficacy (or its absence) is highly relevant to cognitive appraisal models of stress:

> It seems sensible to assume that persons who believe that they can master most demands and threats by doing what is needed or by discovering what to do and how to do it are less likely to be threatened or to feel helpless or hopeless in stressful transactions. The obverse of this is the chronically anxious person who can be thought of as someone who maintains a general belief both that the environment is hostile, and that he or she is incapable of mastery. Such persons are anxious even in situations in which the ordinary person does not experience threat because the very act of engaging the environment carries with it the implication of danger. (Folkman, Schaefer, and Lazarus,[34] p. 286)

The conceptual relationship between self efficacy and locus of control has been likened to Allen and Potkay's[2] broader state-trait distinction.[79] Whether generalized or specific, control expectancies are thought to assume the greatest importance in unfamiliar or ambiguous situations.[115,116] That is, when few concrete cues are available as to the probable outcome of a situation or the kinds of control inputs possible, personality factors are likely to play a relatively greater part in appraisal of the level of threat present. However, ambiguity and personality may also interact in another respect.

Tolerance of ambiguity. As mentioned in Chapter 1, one factor that has been shown to increase stress is uncertainty: the less clear the outcome of a situation, the more likely it is to be experienced as stressful. This has been amply demonstrated, for example, by Shalit, who subjected over 300 studies of performance under stress to multiple scalogram analysis and found that the more ambiguous the situation, the poorer the performance.[125] It has also been observed that more ambiguous a given situation is to the person evaluating it, the more appraisal is influenced by personality factors such as locus of control.[34]

For the most part, research on stress and uncertainty has focussed on situational variables, that is, on the degrees and types of ambiguity possible; these include, for example, the question of whether an event will happen, when it will happen, what actions are possible, and so forth.[34] However, a few investigators have also looked at the possible human variables and their effects, reasoning that there are likely to be individual differences in the extent to which uncertainty is found to be actually threatening.

The term 'tolerance of ambiguity' was originally coined by Frenkel-Brunswik,[36] who considered this personality dimension to be "one of the basic variables in both the emotional and cognitive orientation of the person toward life" (p. 113). It has been defined as "a willingness to consider multiple aspects of reality and a more flexible adaptation to varying circumstances and degrees of abstraction".[34] Frenkel-Brunswik regarded this adaptability as a coping resource, noting that intolerant (or 'closed minded'[114]) persons tended to resolve ambiguous situations by seeking premature 'closure', which, as described in the decision making section of Chapter 4, refers to the adoption of decisions or courses of action before all of the relevant facts are available. Premature closure probably relates to the hazardous thought pattern termed 'impulsivity'.

There is clear evidence that humans have an increased tendency to seek closure under stressful conditions.[64,130] However, even in the absence of unusual stress, individuals classified as neurotic have shown a significantly greater tendency to avoid ambiguous situations than have normals.[48,49] The relationship between tolerance of ambiguity and general resistance to stress remains a promising area for future research. Some specific issues yet to be clarified include situational factors conducive to increased or decreased tolerance, and the identification of other personality traits associated with tolerance or the lack of it.

Defence mechanisms. The concept of defence mechanisms has its origins in the psychoanalytic literature. Defence mechanisms can be defined as mental 'compromises' and other processes, usually unconscious, that allow the individual to make positive cognitive appraisals in situations that might otherwise be distressing. They exist in many forms, but for the purposes of the present discussion it should suffice to say that they typically involve the repression, denial, or rationalization of unpleasant and threatening information. A certain amount of this is healthy and indeed necessary: for example, the pilot engaged in a difficult instrument approach cannot afford to become preoccupied by the small but genuine possibility of failure and imminent death.[84] Similarly, military aircrew on combat missions will likely be unable to function emotionally if they truly acknowledge to themselves that they may well not survive.

On the other hand, the tendency to close one's mind to threatening information can also interfere with more substantive, action oriented coping strategies.[42,134] There is no doubt that self delusion can be dangerous (e.g., "this emergency isn't happening to me / this isn't a problem, therefore no action on my part is needed"). The sidebar on the Riyadh tragedy is from an account by David Beaty, a well respected commentator on the human factors of accidents, who puts this accident forward explicitly as an account of defensive denial at work.

Defence mechanisms can come into play not only with respect to external situational appraisals, but also with personal imperfections or weaknesses. The 'well-defended' individual has a powerful need to believe in his or her own competence and invulnerability, and may react quite aggressively to anything that challenges this belief. Qualities typically seen in such people include a lack of tolerance for personal failures or shortcomings, avoidance of introspection and denial of emotions, a reluctance to

---

Riyadh, Saudi Arabia, 19 August, 1980: A Lockheed TriStar departed Riyadh for Jidda, taking pilgrims to Mecca. It is believed that one of the pilgrims began to operate a portable gas stove within the passenger cabin of the aircraft. Shortly after takeoff the crew heard a smoke alert. The flight engineer went back into the passenger cabin to investigate. He returned to the flight deck to announce. "We've got a fire back there!" The captain turned back to Riyadh, while the flight engineer made a second visit to the cabin. This time he announced, "Just smoke in the aft." Then another smoke warning sounded. "What can I say?" asked the engineer." "OK", supplied the captain. "I think it's all right now," said the engineer. A third warning then sounded, and a stewardess arrived on the flight deck to say that there was, indeed, a fire in the cabin and that people were "fighting in the aisles". The engineer then said there was no smoke at the back, a comment which was followed by a fourth smoke warning. Five minutes before touchdown, a stewardess asked the captain if they should carry out an emergency evacuation after landing. Twice more the crew asked the captain the same question. It was not until half a minute before landing that the captain at last decided. "Tell them, tell them to not evacuate!" The TriStar landed. Emergency services waited for the crew to open the door. They saw fire at the back of the aircraft. A last message came from the TriStar: "We are trying to evacuate now!" But the crew did not open the doors. Attempts to open them from the outside were at first unsuccessful. It was twenty-three minutes after engine shutdown before door 2 on the right side was opened. It was too late. All 301 people on board had died.

-- Adapted from Beaty,[13] p. 23

rely on others, a rigid need for order and routine, and a tendency to attribute mistakes to external circumstances or persons rather than to one's own failings.[137]

Defensive personality traits may also make it more difficult for a pilot to work cooperatively with others.[42] The literature on aviation accidents contains many accounts of captains who refused to listen to attempts by their subordinates to point out critical errors or omissions -- often with tragic results. John Nance[97] relates several instances of this sort of behaviour. For example, the captain of Air Illinois Flight 710, which crashed in Pinckneyville in 1983, had a reputation for routinely doing precisely the opposite of whatever another crew member suggested, simply as a way of asserting his status as pilot in command; a copilot had even complained that this man had on one occasion deliberately flown the aircraft into extremely hazardous weather conditions after she had had the 'temerity' to point them out.

Another case recounted by Nance concerns a older captain (and airline vice president) who was well known for simply ignoring input from other crew members and generally behaving as though he were the only pilot on board. During a final approach he (apparently) became medically incapacitated, but the copilot, accustomed to the man's uncommunicativeness and intimidated by his high status and abrasive personality, elected not to query the aircraft's abnormally steep rate of descent and allowed his superior to fly into the ground unchallenged.

In recent years, cockpit resource management programs have made pilots more aware of the pitfalls of this "nobody's going to tell me how to fly" brand of egotism; even so, post-accident analyses (of cockpit voice recordings, etc.) do occasionally reveal overly deferential first officers who appeared to be aware of developing problems but who failed to speak up assertively, apparently for fear of creating antagonism.

The assumption of defence mechanism theorists is that individuals have stable tendencies both in terms of whether 'healthy' or 'unhealthy' (defensive) coping strategies will emerge under duress, and in terms of precisely which defences are invoked and how much they are relied upon. The Defence Mechanism Test (DMT), developed in Sweden in 1960, is a psychological test which scores ten of these putative mechanisms.[72] The test involves a series of pictures containing both a sympathetic central figure and a threatening peripheral figure. These images are presented repeatedly for very brief but gradually increasing lengths of time: the viewing period is initially subliminal but progressively increases to a full second. Scoring is based on the exposure time needed for the subject to perceive the threat figure. The test is based on the premise that the individual who notices a threat early will devote less time and energy to repression and other psychological defenses, and more to constructive coping responses.

From the point of view of aviation psychologists schooled in the traditions of cognitive psychology, the psychoanalytic approach upon which the DMT is based may seem quaint and unpromising. Indeed, some researchers have voiced serious reservations about the test methodology: for example, there is no actual evidence to show that subjects taking the test actually feel 'threatened' by the pictures. However, as we shall discuss later, Scandinavian research findings leave open the possibility that, in some pilots, psychological defence mechanisms may indeed 'kick in' under stressful circumstances, often with disastrous consequences. It is also possible that the phenomenon of 'anticipatory stress' may be attributable in part to a collapse in psychological defences as reality encroaches (see Chapter 7); if this is true, persons who do not tend to rely on defence mechanisms in the first place could be less susceptible to anticipatory stress.

The Defence Mechanism Test is already used by the Swedish and Danish Air Forces for screening purposes,[23] and appears to have considerable potential for more widespread application. For example, a longitudinal study conducted by the Swedish Air Force found that pilots with undesirable DMT scores were three times more likely to be eliminated from the force, either because of training failures, accidents, or development of psychosomatic ailments, flight related neuroses, or other emotional problems. The test proved to be especially predictive of accident involvement: 'defensive' pilots in this category outnumbered 'nondefensive' pilots by a ratio of 13 to 1.[98]

A follow-up study with a modified scoring system found that pilots who successfully adjusted to flying were eight times more likely to have scored well on the DMT than those who did not; fully 93 percent of those with unfavourable DMT scores did not function well as pilots, as compared to 44 percent those with good scores.[99] Along the same lines, a Danish study found that successful flight trainees in that country's Air Force were five times more likely to have favorable test scores, and that 87 percent of the negative scorers failed to complete training.[129] Similar results have been obtained for both Norwegian parachute jumpers[9] and divers,[139] and for Danish attack divers.[73] In general, Scandinavian research has found a 'good' score on the Defence Mechanism Test to be moderately predictive of healthy adjustment to flying, and a 'poor' score to be very strongly predictive of failure.

However, attempts to replicate these findings in other countries have not been successful: an RAF study, for example, found no relationship between DMT scores and training performance.[141] There may be methodological issues involved, an interesting possibility in light of the fact that in the Norwegian parachute study, also, the DMT had no predictive value during mock tower jumps, only during real jumps from aircraft. A possible interpretation, therefore, is that it is only in very stressful and extreme circumstances that defensive mechanisms impinge upon behaviour and performance, and not in simulations or other training environments.[9,138] Finally, there may be subtle cultural influences that affect the predictive usefulness of the DMT, such that the Swedish version does not 'travel well'.

More general measures of stress tolerance

Trait anxiety. The distinction between state and trait anxiety was introduced in Chapter 1. As already noted, the former is situation specific (and therefore transient), while the latter represents a more general personality trait: the tendency to react to stressful circumstances with increased state anxiety. As such the trait anxious individual could by definition be regarded as 'stress prone', and a nonanxious person as 'stress resistant'. Experimental research bears this out, insofar as persons with high trait anxiety placed in socially threatening conditions have usually reacted with greater state anxiety than their nonanxious counterparts.[55,103,110]

However, the picture is actually somewhat more complicated than this. First, there have been exceptions to the above pattern: Endler and Shedletsky, for example, found no consistent differences in the reactions of high and low trait anxious subjects.[30] Endler suggests that this discrepancy is most likely an effect of the instrument used to measure trait anxiety.[28] Most other studies have employed either the Taylor Manifest Anxiety Scale[136] or Spielberger's State-Trait Anxiety Inventory,[133] both of which are unidimensional measures; the Endler and Shedletsky study assessed trait anxiety by means of the S-R Inventory of Anxiousness,[29] which is a multidimensional instrument. Clearly, it is not enough to define trait anxiety simply as 'that which is measured by the State-Trait Anxiety Inventory' (or any other test); more insights are needed as to the precise nature of trait anxiety, its causes, and its relationship to other personality characteristics.

There is another way in which trait anxiety, however it is measured, does not correlate with a more general vulnerability to stress. In the studies cited above, as hinted, the stressors used were of a particular type, known collectively as 'ego threats'. Ego threats are situations involving social risk, the possibility of personal failure, or damage to self esteem. However, there is another category of threat, that of actual physical danger. Interestingly, response to physical threat is largely unaffected by the presence or absence of trait anxiety:[7,133] as we noted in Chapter 1, for example, while experiments involving the threat of electric shocks do provoke an increase state anxiety, these changes do not correlate with the levels of trait anxiety observed in the test subjects.[56,57,63]

'Hardiness'. Studies of the relationship between personality traits and subjectively experienced stress have most often been concerned with the role of stress in inducing physical illness. As such the model of 'stress' used tends to focus less on cognitive appraisal than on physiological arousal, and on the 'organismic strain' assumed to result from it.[41] One example of such a model that has become familiar to the general public is the 'Type A personality' construct, which posits a link between certain behaviour patterns and an increased incidence of coronary heart disease. Another, more ambitious model, which has been developed in the past decade, is that of the so-called 'hardy personality' described by Kobasa and her colleagues.

This type of individual is said to possess a particular suite of personality traits that mitigate the negative impact of stressful life events and reduce vulnerability to stress related illnesses. The following three characteristics are believed to be significant: 'commitment' (that is, a high degree of emotional involvement in life's activities); a sense of control over the events of one's life; and a positive attitude toward change. Kobasa's own studies have, in fact, linked this cluster of traits to a lower incidence of physical illness,[65-71] although some other investigators have failed to replicate her results.[40,119]

This book, of course, is concerned less with physical health as such than with the effects of psychological stress on cognitive functioning and complex performance. Kobasa's model is nonetheless of interest here because of its applicability to appraisal based concepts of stress. For example, Lazarus and Folkman have suggested that the apparent stress resistance of 'hardy' individuals derives specifically from certain patterns of cognitive appraisal which influence their perception both of the nature and level of threat in a situation.[79] Support for this hypothesis has been found in a study by Rhodewalt and Agustsdottir,[113] who reported a positive correlation between possession of a hardy personality profile, positive appraisal of specific life events, and a general perception that these events were under the individual's personal control. (Nonhardy subjects, in contrast, were more likely to view similar events in their own lives as aversive and not under their control.) Along similar lines, Allred and Smith found that persons who conformed to Kobasa's model of hardiness were more likely than their nonhardy counterparts to remain confident and optimistic during a controlled experiment involving evaluative threat.[3] In general, then, the cognitive correlates of 'hardiness' would appear to be a promising area for future research.

Summary and conclusions

As we have seen, personality research in aviation has a long history, and there is no shortage of personality characteristics that have at one time or another been proposed as being important to flying performance. Some that do appear to have some relevance include achievement motivation, the ability to work well as part of a team, risk taking at appropriate levels (and this level may vary with the type of flight operation), and adequate but not unrealistic amounts of self confidence. In keeping with the theme of the book this chapter has focussed primarily on personality dimensions relevant to the experience of stress, particularly with respect to cognitive appraisal. Those we have particularly touched upon include locus of control, self efficacy, and tolerance of ambiguity, as well as defence mechanisms. While aviation specific research on these variables has been minimal, all four have the potential to make valuable contributions to future applied studies in this area.

One additional issue worth touching upon here concerns the definition of 'personality' and the status of personality 'traits'. Should appraisal variables such as locus of control be regarded as traits or as attitudes? As we discussed earlier, personality *traits* (such as, for example, extraversion) are generally viewed as being fixed, enduring qualities relatively resistant to change, while *attitudes* appear to be somewhat less so. However, no real consensus exists as to the actual relationship between these two constructs, not least since some correlations appear to exist between certain 'attitudes' and 'traits'. Thus, the distinction is somewhat problematic, at least in academic terms. In practical terms, however, it would be interesting to explore the extent to which suboptimal cognitive patterns such as low self efficacy or inappropriate defence mechanisms are amenable to outside intervention. One possibility, for example, is that pilots who are identified as having such patterns could be taught, if not to eliminate them, at least to recognize them and to adopt compensatory strategies of various kinds. In any event, it seems clear that aviation psychology should continue to bene-fit substantially from research on personality.

References

1. Alkov, R.A., Gaynor, J.A., and Borowsky, M.S. (1985), 'Pilot error as a symptom of inadequate stress coping', *Aviation, Space, and Environmental Medicine*, vol. 56, pp. 244-7.

2. Allen, B.P., and Potkay, C.R. (1981), 'On the arbitrary distinction between states and traits', *Journal of Personality and Social Psychology*, vol. 41, pp. 916-28.

3. Allred, K.D., and Smith, T.W. (1989), 'The hardy personality: cognitive and physiological responses to evaluative threat', *Journal of Personality and Social Psychology*, vol. 56, pp. 257-66.

4. Anastasi, A. (1982), *Psychological Testing*, 5th ed., Macmillan, New York.

5. Appley, M.H., and Trumbull, R. (1967), 'On the Concept of Psychological Stress', in Appley, M.H. and Trumbull, R. (eds.), *Psychological Stress: Issues in Research*, Appleton-Century-Crofts, New York.

6. Ashman, A., and Telfer, R. (1983), 'Personality profiles of pilots', *Aviation, Space, and Environmental Medicine*, vol. 54, pp. 940-3.

7. Auerbach, S.M. (1973), 'Trait-state anxiety and adjustment to sur-gery', *Journal of Consulting and Clinical Psychology*, vol. 40, pp. 264-71.

8. Averill, J.R. (1973), 'Personal control over aversive stimuli and its relationship to stress', *Psychological Bulletin,* vol. 80, pp. 286-303.

9. Baade, E., et al. (1978), cited in Goeters and Fassbender (1991).

10. Bandura, A. (1977), 'Self-efficacy: toward a unifying theory of behavior change', *Psychological Review,* vol. 84, pp. 191-215.

11. Bandura, A. (1982), 'Self-efficacy mechanism in human agency', *American Psychologist,* vol. 33, pp. 344-58.

12. Bartram, D., and Dale, H.C.A. (1981), *The EPI as a Selection Test for AAC Pilots,* University of Hull Ergonomics Research Group Report ERG/Y6536/81/8.

13. Beaty, D. (1991), 'The worst six accidents over the last thirty years from the human factors' point of view', *Flight Deck,* 2, pp. 19-25.

14. Berlin, J.I., Gruber, E.V., Holmes, C.W., Jensen, P.K., Lau, J.R., Mills, J.W., and O'Kane, J.M. (1982), *Pilot Judgment Training and Evaluation* (DOT/FAA/CT-82/56), Embry-Riddle Aeronautical University, Daytona Beach, Florida.

15. Besco, R.O. (1991), 'The myths of pilot personality stereotypes', *Proceedings of the Sixth International Symposium on Aviation Psychology,* Ohio State University, Columbus.

16. Bowers, K.S. (1968), 'Pain, anxiety, and perceived control', *Journal of Consulting and Clinical Psychology,* vol. 32, pp. 596-602.

17. Buch, G., and Diehl, A. (1984), 'An investigation of the effectiveness of pilot judgment training', *Human Factors,* vol. 26, pp. 557-64.

18. Cattell, R.B., Eber, H.W., and Tatsuoka, M.M. (1970), *Handbook for the Sixteen Personality Factor Questionnaire (16PF),* Institute for Personality and Ability Testing, Champaign, Illinois.

19. Champion, R.A. (1950), 'Studies of experimentally induced disturbance', *Australian Journal of Psychology,* vol. 2, pp. 596-602.

20. Chan, K.B. (1977), 'Individual differences in reactions to stress and their personality and situation determinants: some implications for community mental health', *Social Science and Medicine,* vol. 11, pp. 89-103.

21. Chidester, T.R., 'Human Factors Research: Narrowing the Extremes of Flight Crew Performance', Lecture presented to the Federation of Behavioral, Psychological and Cognitive Sciences, Washington, DC.

22. Culpepper, B.W., Jennings, C.L., and Perry, C.J.G. (1972), *Psychiatric and Psychometric Predictability of Test Pilot School Performance* (Technical Report 72-390), USAF School of Aerospace Medicine, Brooks AFB, Texas.

23. Dolgin, D.L., Gibb, G.D., Nontasak, T., and Helm, W.R. (1987), *Instructor Pilot Evaluations of Key Naval Primary Flight Criteria,* NAMRL-1331, Naval Aerospace Medical Research Laboratory, Pensacola, Florida.

24. Dolgin, D.L., and Gibb, G.D. (1989), 'Personality Assessment in Aviator Selection,' in Jensen, R.S. (ed.), *Aviation Psychology,* Gower Technical, Aldershot.

25. DuCette, J., and Wolk, S. (1973), 'Locus of control and extreme behavior', *Journal of Consulting and Clinical Psychology,* vol. 39, pp. 253-8.

26. Edwards, A.L. (1959), *The Edwards Personal Preference Schedule,* Psychological Corporation, New York.

27. Ellis, A., and Conrad, H.S. (1948), 'The validity of personality inventories in military practice', *Psychological Bulletin,* vol. 45, pp. 385-427.

28. Endler, N.S. (1975), 'A Person-Situation Interaction Model for Anxiety', in Spielberger, C.D. and Sarason, I.G. (eds.), *Stress and Anxiety,* vol. 1, John Wiley & Sons, New York.

29. Endler, N.S., Hunt, J. McV., and Rosenstein, A.J. (1962), 'An S-R inventory of anxiousness', *Psychological Monographs*, vol. 76, (17, whole no. 536), pp. 1-33.

30. Endler, N.S., and Shedletsky, R., (1973), 'Trait versus state anxiety, authoritarianism, and ego threat versus physical threat', *Canadian Journal of Behavioural Science*, vol. 5, pp. 347-61.

31. Eysenck, H.J., and Eysenck, S.B.G. (1964), *Manual of the Eysenck Personality Inventory*, Hodder and Stoughton, Sevenoaks.

32. Farmer, E.W. (1984), 'Personality factors in aviation', *The International Journal of Aviation Safety*, (September), pp. 175-9.

33. Fine, P.M. and Hartman, B.O. (1968), *Psychiatric Strengths and Weaknesses of Typical Air Force Pilots* (Technical Report 68-121), USAF School of Aerospace Medicine, Brooks AFB, Texas.

34. Folkman, S., Schaefer, C., and Lazarus, R.S. (1979), 'Cognitive Processes as Mediators of Stress and Coping', in Hamilton, V. and Warburton, D.M. (eds.), *Human Stress and Cognition: An Information Processing Approach*, John Wiley & Sons, Chichester.

35. Foushee, H.C., and Helmreich, R.L. (1988), 'Group Interaction and Flight Crew Performance,' in Wiener, E.W. and Nagel, D.C. (eds.), *Human Factors in Aviation*, Academic Press, San Diego.

36. Frenkel-Brunswik, E. (1949), 'Intolerance of ambiguity as an emotional and perceptual personality variable', *Journal of Personality*, vol. 18, pp. 108-43.

37. Fry, G.E., and Reinhardt, R.F. (1969), 'Personality characteristics of jet pilots as measured by the Edwards Personal Preference Schedule', *Aerospace Medicine*, vol. 40, pp. 484-6.

38. Fulkerson, S.C. (1956), *Adaptability Screening of Flying Personnel: Development of a Preliminary Screening Battery*, School of Aviation Medicine, Randolph Air Force Base, San Antonio, Texas.

39. Fulkerson, S.C., Freud, S.L., and Raynor, G.H. (1958), 'The use of the MMPI in the psychological evaluation of pilots', *Journal of Aviation Medicine*, vol. 29, pp. 122-9.

40. Funk, S.C., and Houston, B.K. (1987), 'A critical analysis of the Hardiness Scale's validity and utility', *Journal of Personality and Social Psychology*, vol. 53, pp. 572-8.

41. Gentry, W.D., and Kobasa, S.C. (1984), 'Social and Psychological Resources Mediating Stress-Illness Relationships in Humans', in Gentry, W.D. (ed.), *Handbook of Behavioral Medicine*, Guilford.

42. Goeters, K.-M., and Fassbender, C. (1991), *Definition of Psychological Testing of Astronaut Candidates for Columbus Missions*, German Aerospace Research Department (DLR), Department of Aviation and Space Psychology, Hamburg, Germany.

43. Green, L.R. (1963), *An Exploratory Investigation of the Relationship between Four Personality Measures and Voluntary Resignation from Aviation Training*, US Naval School of Aviation Medicine, Pensacola, Florida.

44. Gregorich, S., Helmreich, R.L., and Wilhelm, J.A. (1989), *The Structure of Cockpit Management Attitudes*, NASA/UT Technical Report 89-1.

45. Gregorich, S., Helmreich, R.L., Wilhelm, J.A., and Chidester, T. (1989), 'Personality Based Clusters as Predictors of Aviator Attitudes and Performance', *Proceedings of the Fifth International Syposium on Aviation Psychology*, Ohio State University, Columbus, Ohio.

46. Griffin, R.G., and Mosko, J.D. (1977), *Naval Aviation Attrition 1950-1976: Implications for the Development of Future Research and Evaluation*, Naval Aerospace Medical Research Laboratory, Pensacola, Florida.

47. Guilford, J.P. (1947), *Printed Classification Tests*, Army Air Forces Aviation Psychology Program Research Report No. 5, US Government Printing Office, Washington, DC.

48. Hamilton, V. (1957), 'Perceptual and personality dynamics in reactions to ambiguity', *British Journal of Psychology*, vol. 48, pp. 200-15.

49. Hamilton, V. (1960), 'Imperception of Phi: some further determinants', *British Journal of Psychology*, vol. 51, pp. 257-66.

50. Hedlund, D.F. (1965), 'A review of the MMPI in industry', *Psychological Reports*, vol. 23, pp. 507-10.

51. Helmreich, R.L. (1984), 'Cockpit management attitudes', *Human Factors*, vol. 26, pp. 583-9.

52. Helmreich, R.L., Sawin, L.L., and Carsrud, A.L. (1986), 'The honeymoon effect in job performance: temporal increases in the predictive power of achievement motivation', *Journal of Applied Psychology*, vol. 71, pp. 185-8.

53. Helmreich, R.L., and Spence, J.T. (1978), 'The Work and Family Orientation Questionnaire: an objective instrument to assess components of achievement motivation and attitudes toward family and career', *JSAS Catalog of Selected Documents in Psychology*, vol. 8, no. 35, ms. 1677.

54. Helmreich, R.L., Wilhelm, J.A., and Gregorich, S. (1988), *Revised Versions of the Cockpit MAnagement Attitudes Questionnaire (CMAQ) and CRM Seminar Evaluation Form*, NASA/UT TR 88-3.

55. Hodges, W.F. (1968), 'Effects of ego threat and threat of pain on state anxiety', *Journal of Personality and Social Psychology*, vol. 8, pp. 364-72.

56. Hodges, W.F., and Spielberger, C.D. (1966), 'The effects of threat of shock on heart rate for subjects who differ in manifest anxiety and fear of shock', *Psychophysiology*, vol. 2, pp. 287-94.

57. Hodges, W.F., and Spielberger, C.D. (1969), 'Digit span: an indicant of trait or state anxiety?' *Journal of Consulting and Clinical Psychology*, vol. 33, pp. 430-4.

58. Jackson, D.N. (1974), *Personality Research Form Manual,* Research Psychologists Press, Goshen, New York.

59. Jackson, D.N. (1984), *Personality Research Form,* Research Psychologists Press, Port Huron, Michigan.

60. Jessup, G., and Jessup, H. (1971), 'Validity of the Eysenck Personality Inventory in pilot selection', *Occupational Psychology,* vol. 45, pp. 111-23.

61. Joaquin, J.B. (1980), *The Personality Research Form and Its Utility in Predicting Undergraduate Pilot Training Performance in the Canadian Forces,* Working Paper 80-12, Canadian Forces Personnel Applied Research Unit, Willowdale, Ontario.

62. Kantor, J., and Bordelon, V. (1985), 'The USAF pilot selection and classification research program', *Aviation, Space, and Environmental Medicine,* vol. 56, pp. 254-7.

63. Katkin, E.S. (1965), 'The relationship between manifest anxiety and two indices of autonomic response to stress', *Journal of Personality and Social Psychology,* vol. 2, pp. 324-33.

64. Keinan, G. (1987), 'Decision making under stress: scanning of alternatives under controllable and uncontrollable threats', *Journal of Personality and Social Psychology,* vol. 52, pp. 639-44.

65. Kobasa, S.C. (1979), 'Stressful life events, personality, and health: an inquiry into hardiness', *Journal of Personality and Social Psychology,* vol. 37, pp. 1-11.

66. Kobasa, S.C. (1982), 'The Hardy Personality: Toward a Social Psychology of Stress and Health', in Suls, J. and Sanders, G. (eds.), *Social Psychology of Health and Illness,* Lawrence Erlbaum Associates, Hillsdale, New Jersey.

67. Kobasa, S.C., Maddi, S.R., and Courington, S. (1981), 'Personality and constitution as mediators in the stress-illness relationship', *Journal of Health and Social Behavior,* vol. 22, pp. 368-78.

68. Kobasa, S.C., Maddi, S.R., and Kahn, S. (1982), 'Hardiness and health: a prospective study', *Journal of Personality and Social Psychology*, vol. 42, pp. 168-77.

69. Kobasa, S.C., Maddi, S.R., and Pucetti, M.C. (1982), 'Personality and exercise as buffers in the stress-illness relationship', *Journal of Behavioral Medicine*, vol. 5, pp. 391-404.

70. Kobasa, S.C., Maddi, S.R., and Zola, M.A. (1983), 'Type A and hardiness', *Journal of Behavioral Medicine*, vol. 6, pp. 41-51.

71. Kobasa, S.C., and Pucetti, M.C. (1983), 'Personality and social resources in stress resistance', *Journal of Personality and Social Psychology*, vol. 45, pp. 839-50.

72. Kragh, U. (1960), 'The Defense Mechanism Test: a new method for diagnosis and personnel selection', *Journal of Applied Psychology*, vol. 44, pp. 303-9.

73. Kragh, U. (1962), 'The prediction of success of Danish attack divers by the Defense Mechanism Test (DMT)', *Perceptual and Motor Skills*, vol. 15, pp. 103-6.

74. Krohne, H.W., and Rogner, J. (1982), 'Repression-Sensitization as a Central Construct in Coping Research', in Krohne, H.W. and Laux, L. (eds.), *Achievement, Stress, and Anxiety*, Hemisphere/ McGraw-Hill, New York.

75. Kuhlen, R.G. (1963), 'Needs, perceived need satisfaction opportunities, and satisfaction with occupation', *Journal of Applied Psychology*, vol. 47, pp. 56-64.

76. Lacey, J.I. (1967), 'Somatic Response Patterning and Stress: Some Revisions of Activation Theory', in Appley, M.H. and Trumbull, R. (eds.), *Psychological Stress: Issues in Research*, Appleton-Century-Crofts, New York.

77. Lacey, J., and VanLehn, R. (1952), 'Differential emphasis in somatic response to stress', *Psychosomatic Medicine*, vol. 14, pp. 73-81.

78. Lazarus, R.S. (1966), *Psychological Stress and the Coping Process*, McGraw-Hill, New York.

79. Lazarus R.S., and Folkman, S. (1984), *Stress, Appraisal, and Coping*, Springer Publishing Company, New York.

80. Lefcourt, H.M. (1976), *Locus of Control: Current Trends in Theory and Research*, Lawrence Erlbaum Associates, Hillsdale, New Jersey.

81. Lefcourt, H.M. (ed.) (1981), *Research with the Locus of Control Construct* (vol. 1), Academic Press, New York.

82. Lefcourt, H.M., Lewis, L., and Silverman, I.W. (1968), 'Internal vs. external locus of control of reinforcement and attention in a decision-making task', *Journal of Personality*, vol. 36, pp. 663-82.

83. Lefcourt H.M., and Wine, J. (1969), 'Internal vs. external control of reinforcement and the deployment of attention in experimental situations', *Canadian Journal of Behavioral Science*, vol. 1, pp. 167-81.

84. Leimann Patt, H.O. (1988), 'The right and wrong stuff in civil aviation', *Aviation, Space, and Environmental Medicine*, vol. 59, pp. 955-9.

85. Lester, L.F,. and Bombaci, D.H. (1984), 'The relationship between personality and irrational judgement in civil pilots', *Human Factors*, vol. 26, pp. 565-72.

86. Lester, L.F., and Connolly, T.J. (1987), 'The measurement of hazardous thought patterns and their relationship to pilot personality', *Proceedings of the Fourth International Symposium on Aviation Psychology*, Ohio State University, Columbus.

87. Lester, L.F., Diehl, A.E., Harvey, D.P., Buch, G., and Lawton, R.S. (1986), 'Improving risk assessment and decision making in general aviation pilots', *Proceedings and Abstracts of the Annual Meeting of the Eastern Psychological Association*, vol. 57, p. 40.

88. Magnusson, D. (1982), 'Situational Determinants of Stress: An Inter-actional Perspective', in Goldberg, L. and Breznitz, S. (eds.), *Handbook of Stress,* Free Press, New York.

89. McGrath, J.E. (1970a), 'A Conceptual Formulation for Research on Stress', in McGrath, J.E. (ed.), *Social and Psychologcal Factors in Stress,* Holt, Rinehart and Winston, New York.

90. McGrath, J.E. (1970b), 'Major Methodological Issues', in McGrath, J.E. (ed.), *Social and Psychologcal Factors in Stress,* Holt, Rinehart and Winston, New York.

91. McFarland, R.A. (1953), *Human Factors in Air Transportation,* McGraw-Hill, New York.

92. Melton, A.W. (1947), *Apparatus Tests: Army Air Forces Aviation Psychology Program Research Report No. 4,* US Government Print-ing Office, Washington, DC.

93. Melton, R.S. (1954), 'Studies in the evaluation of the personality characteristics of successful naval aviators', *Journal of Aviation Medicine,* vol. 25, pp. 600-4.

94. Miller, S.M. (1979), 'Controllability and human stress: method, evidence and theory', *Behavioral Research and Therapy,* vol. 17, pp. 287-304.

95. Millon, T. (1983), *Millon Clinical Mutiaxial Inventory,* Interpretive Scoring Systems, Minneapolis, Minnesota.

96. Myhre, G. (1988), 'Accidents in Fighter Aircraft Caused by "Human Factors": Why do they Occur?' in AGARD Conference Proceedings No. 458, *Human Behaviour in High Stress Situations in Aerospace Operations,* Neuilly-sur-Seine, NATO Advisory Group for Aerospace Research and Development.

97. Nance, J.J. (1986), *Blind Trust,* William Morrow and Company, New York.

98. Neuman, T. (1972), *Cross-Validation of the Defense Mechanism Test by the criterion of passing or failure in basic military flight training*, Report No. FTD-HC-23-1150-72, Wright-Patterson AFB, Ohio.

99. Neuman, T. (1978), *Dimensioning and validation of percept-genetic defence mechanisms: A hierarchical analysis of the behaviour of pilots under stress*, FOA Report C55020-H6 (translated from Swedish by R.E. Williams), Her Majesty's Stationery Office, London.

100. North, R.A., and Griffin, R.G. (1977), *Aviator Selection 1919-1977*, NAMRL SR 77-2, Naval Aerospace Medical Research Laboratory, Pensacola, Florida.

101. Novello, J.R., and Youssef, Z. (1974a), 'Psycho-social studies in general aviation: 1. 'Personality profile of male pilots', *Aerospace Medicine*, vol. 45, pp. 185-8.

102. Novello, J.R., and Youssef, Z. (1974b), 'Psycho-social studies in general aviation: 2. 'Personality profile of female pilots', *Aerospace Medicine*, vol. 45, pp. 630-3.

103. O'Neil, J.F., Spielberger, C.D., and Hansen, D.N. (1969), 'The effects of state anxiety and task difficulty on computer-assisted learning', *Journal of Educational Psychology*, vol. 60, pp. 343-50.

104. Opton, E.M., and Lazarus, R.S. (1967), 'Personality determinants of psychophysiological response to stress: a theoretical analysis and an experiment', *Journal of Personality and Social Psychology*, vol. 6, pp. 291-303.

105. Paine, L., Jr. (1990), 'Nothing mysterious about what makes a good pilot', *Western Flyer*, March, p. 30.

106. Phares, E.J. (1968), 'Differential utilization of information as a function of internal-external control', *Journal of Personality*, vol. 36, pp. 649-62.

107. Phares, E.J. (1976), *Locus of Control in Personality*, General Learning Press, Morristown, New Jersey.

108. Picano, J.J. (1991), 'Personality types among experienced military pilots', *Aviation, Space, and Environmental Medicine,* vol. 62, pp. 517-20.

109. Pines, H.A., and Julian, J.W. (1972), 'Effects of task and social demands on locus of control differences in information processing', *Journal of Personality,* vol. 40, pp. 407-16.

110. Rappaport, H., and Katkin, E.S. (1972), 'Relationships among manifest anxiety, response to stress, and the perception of autonomic activity', *Journal of Consulting and Clinical Psychology,* vol. 38, pp. 219-24.

111. Retzlaff, P.D., and Gibertini, M. (1987), 'Air Force personality: hard data on the right stuff', *Mult. Behav. Res.,* vol. 22, pp. 383-9.

112. Retzlaff, P.D., and Gibertini, M. (1988), 'Air Force Pilot Intelligence, Personality, and Psychological Taxonomy', *Proceedings of the annual convention of the American Psychological Association,* American Psychological Association, Atlanta, Georgia.

113. Rhodewalt, F., and Agustsdottir, S. (1984), 'On the relationship of hardiness to the Type A behavior pattern: perception of life events versus coping with life events', *Journal of Research in Personality,* vol. 18, pp. 212-23.

114. Rokeach, M. (ed.) (1960), *The Open and the Closed Mind,* Basic Books, New York.

115. Rotter, J.B. (1966), 'Generalized expectancies for internal versus external control of reinforcement', *Psychological Monographs,* vol. 80 (whole no. 609).

116. Rotter, J.B. (1975), 'Some problems and misconceptions related to the construct of internal versus external control of reinforcement', *Journal of Consulting and Clinical Psychology,* vol. 43, pp. 56-67.

117. Sanders, M.G., and Hoffman, M.A. (1975), 'Personality aspects of involvement in pilot-error accidents', *Aviation, Space, and Environmental Medicine,* vol. 46, pp. 186-90.

118. Sanders, M.G., Hoffman, M.A., and Neese, T.A. (1976), 'Cross-validation study of personality aspects of involvement in pilot-error accidents', *Aviation, Space, and Environmental Medicine,* vol. 47, pp. 177-9.

119. Schmied, L.A., and Lawler, K.A. (1986), 'Hardiness, Type A behavior, and the stress-illness relation in working women', *Journal of Personality and Social Psychology,* vol. 51, pp. 1218-23.

120. Schulz, P., and Schonpflug, W. (1982), 'Regulatory Activity During States of Stress', in Krohne, H.W. and Laux, L. (eds.), *Achievement, Stress, and Anxiety,* Hemisphere/McGraw-Hill, New York.

121. Seeman, M. (1963), 'Alienation and social learning in a reformatory', *American Journal of Sociology,* vol. 69, pp. 270-84.

122. Seeman, M. and Evans, J.W. (1962), 'Alienation and learning in a hospital setting', *American Sociological Review,* vol. 27, pp. 772-93.

123. Selye, H. (1956), *The Stress of Life,* McGraw-Hill, New York.

124. Selye, H. (1975), *Stress Without Distress,* New American Library, New York.

125. Shalit, B. (1977), 'Structural ambiguity and limits to coping', *Journal of Human Stress,* vol. 3, pp. 32-45.

126. Shannon, R.H., and Waag, W.L. (1972), *Toward the Development of a Criterion for Fleet Effectiveness in the F-4 Fighter Community,* Naval Aerospace Medical Research Laboratory, Pensacola, Florida.

127. Shull, R.N., Dolgin, D.L., and Gibb, G.D. (1988), *The Relationship Between Flight Training Preference and Jenkins Activity Survey Measures,* NAMRL-1339, Naval Aerospace Medical Research Laboratory, Pensacola, Florida.

128. Siem, F.M., Carretta, T.R., and Mercatante, T.A. (1987), *Personality, Attitudes, and Pilot Training Performance*, AFHRL TP-87-36, Air Force Human Resources Laboratory, Manpower and Personnel Division, Brooks Air Force Base, San Antonio, Texas.

129. Sjoberg, L. (1981), 'The value of DMT in the selection of pilots', *Nordisk Psykjologi,* vol. 33, pp. 241-8.

130. Smock, C.D. (1955), 'The influence of psychological stress on the 'intolerance of ambiguity', *Journal of Abnormal and Social Psychology,* vol. 50, pp. 177-82.

131. Spence, J.T., and Helmreich, R.L. (1983), 'Achievement related motives and behavior', in Spence, J.T. (ed.), *Achievement and Achievement Motives: Psychological and Sociological Approaches,* W.H. Freeman & Co., San Francisco.

132. Spence, J.T., Helmreich, R.L., and Holahan, C.K. (1979), 'Negative and positive components of masculinity and femininity and their relationships to self-reports of neurotic and acting out behaviors', *Journal of Personality and Social Psychology,* vol. 37, pp. 1673-82.

133. Spielberger, C.D., Gorsuch, R.L., and Lushene, R.E. (1970), *Manual for the State-Trait Anxiety Inventory,* Consulting Psychologists Press, Palo Alto, California.

134. Strelau, J. (1989), 'Individual Differences in Tolerance to Stress: The Role of Reactivity', in Spielberger, C.D., Sarason, I., and Strelau, J. (eds.), *Stress and Anxiety* (vol. 12), Hemisphere Publishing Corporation, New York.

135. Strongin, G. (1991), Personal communication.

136. Taylor, J.A. (1953), 'A personality scale of manifest anxiety', *Journal of Abnormal Psychology,* vol. 48, pp. 285-90.

137. Ursano, R.J. (1980), 'Stress and adaptation: the interaction of the pilot personality and disease', *Aviation, Space, and Environmental Medicine,* vol. 51, pp. 1245-9.

138. Ursin, H., Baade, E., and Levine, S. (eds.) (1978), *Psychobiology of Stress: A Study of Men,* Academic Press, New York.

139. Vaernes, R. (1982), 'The Defence Mechanism Test predicts inadequate performance under stress', *Scandinavian Journal of Psychology,* vol. 23, pp. 37-43.

140. Voas, R.B., Bair, J.T., and Ambler, R.K. (1957), *Validity of Personality Inventories in the Naval Aviation Selection Program,* NASM-13, Naval School of Aviation Medicine, Pensacola, Florida.

141. Walker-Smith, G.J. (1988), 'The Trials and Tribulations of RAF Defence Mechanism Testing', in *Human Behaviour in High Stress Situations in Aerospace Operations',* NATO AGARD Conference Proceedings No. 458, Neuilly-sur-Seine, France, pp. 18.1-18.6.

142. Wichman, H., and Ball, J. (1983), 'Locus of control, self-serving biases, and attitudes toward safety in general aviation pilots', *Aviation, Space, and Environmental Medicine,* vol. 54, pp. 507-10.

143. Wichman, H., and Oyasato, A. (1983), 'Effects of locus of control and task complexity on prospective remembering', *Human Factors,* vol. 25, pp. 583-91.

7 Fear and stress extremes

Deeply rooted in man's mind is the idea that flying is a supernatural achievement. The sky has held promise and threat [and] it is into this new world without visible limit, already rich in personal and communal legend and superstition, that the flyer enters ... Its special characteristics cannot help but have meaning for his emotional life.
-- Douglas Bond, *The Love and Fear of Flying*

Flying, being an unnatural form of human locomotion, arouses natural human fears.
-- J.M. Ramsden, *The Safe Airline*

This chapter will address the problem of fear and extreme stress reactions among pilots. We will begin by discussing the phenomenon of pilots who suffer from fear of flying, and then move on to some other manifestations of stress, including paralysis of action (the 'frozen pilot syndrome') and anticipatory stress reactions. We will also discuss the problem of combat stress, not only because of its specific effects on military aircrew but also because the study of human behaviour and reactions in this most extreme of stress conditions can provide certain insights into the nature of stress, stress resistance, and performance in more routine circumstances -- both in air operations and, indeed, in everyday life.

Fear of flying

Fear of flying (also known as 'flight anxiety' or 'flight phobia') is an affliction that, in the popular mind, is probably associated more with members of the travelling public than with aircrew. In fact, however, it is a real, if occasional, phenomenon among those who operate aircraft as well as those who merely ride in them. Among the most commonly affected are student pilots: excessive anxiety is a major cause of attrition from flight training programs.[7,38] However, even experienced aviators with a prior history of successful flying have been known to unexpectedly develop phobic reactions.

Nonpilots who are frightened of air travel can, at least, try to arrange their lives so as to avoid or minimize the activity. Professional aviators do not have this option, of course, a fact which poses difficulties not only for them but for their employers. Commercial enterprises, for example, often have a large investment in their pilots, who represent the confidence and competence of the airline. The military, too, can hardly afford to have pilots become emotionally incapacitated during their period of service. As in civilian aviation, there are risks to efficiency and safety in leaving flight operations in the hands of motivationally impaired pilots -- that is, those who would rather not be flying. Moreover, as noted in Chapter 6, dropouts from expensive military flight training represent significant financial losses for taxpayers. For all of these reasons, the phenomenon of flight anxiety is a matter of considerable interest to aviation psychologists and medical personnel.

Symptoms

Anxiety about flying can assume a wide range of overt symptoms. At the behavioural level, the problem may manifest itself as an outright refusal to fly, the reason given being that it is "too dangerous" (or frightening). Alternatively, the pilot may focus not on the real or supposed hazards of aviation itself but on various physical or emotional symptoms which are felt to be incapacitating: he might state, for example, that he would be happy to fly if he could just relax more, or concentrate better, or get more sleep.[71] He may also exhibit an exaggerated worry about such elements as less than ideal weather or minor mechanical difficulties.[67]

In physical terms, the anxious pilot may suffer from any of a wide range of symptoms, including loss of appetite, faintness, rapid heartbeat, excessive perspiration, airsickness, gastrointestinal problems such as cramping or diarrhea, and, as suggested above, insomnia. Psychological manifestations, in addition to a general nervousness, may include nightmares, cognitive impairments such as spatial disorientation or 'mental blocking', and feelings of guilt, foreboding, lack of control, or depersonalization.[55]

In some susceptible individuals the emotional manifestations of flight anxiety can also encompass recognized psychopathologies. These are generally of the neurotic type and include dissociative disorders involving fragmentation of memory systems (amnesia, somnambulism, fugue states);

psychosomatic ailments, that is, physical complaints with origins in emotional stress (headaches, ulcers, dermatitis, asthma, and so forth); and conversion reactions, which are mysterious and dramatic impairments with no discernable organic basis (deafness, inability to speak, loss of feeling or function in certain body parts, unexplained pains).[7] All of these phenomena are considered to be neurotic defenses against anxiety.[76]

Aetiology

Historical perspective. The earliest literature on fear of flying (which dates back to the First World War and hence focusses on military pilots) ascribed flight anxiety to such varied causes as extreme fatigue, poor health, emotional trauma (arising from exposure to aviation accidents), or, more simplistically, to lack of 'nerve'.[3,4,28,54] As the science of psychology grew in sophistication, attention also began to be paid to the role of personality variables, and by the time of the Second World War distinctions were being made between different categories of anxious pilots. Some, it was decided, had neurotic personalities and were prone to anxiety disorders whatever the circumstances; others were fundamentally healthy individuals suffering from phobic reactions brought on by situational factors.[17] Within the latter group, a further distinction was developed between pilots who were merely physically exhausted (for whom the prescribed remedy was rest), and those who had had emotional breakdowns in response to frightening or traumatic experiences associated with flying.[8] This included not only first-hand experiences such as near accidents or 'close calls', but, for example, events that were witnessed or that resulted in the death of a friend.[42,47] However, these studies did not always separate the notion of combat stress from more generalized flight anxiety.

Current views. The postwar years have seen further elaboration of the concept of flight anxiety as a multifaceted phenomenon not explainable by any single aetiology. For example, a review published in 1971 stressed that anxiety in pilots should be analyzed both in terms of the immediate factors precipitating the reaction, and the underlying personality traits likely to increase susceptibility in the first place.[53] In fact, research from the same period suggested that psychological rather than environmental factors constitute the best indicator of the pilot's chances of overcoming flight anxiety.[27] Along similar lines, a somewhat later paper classified flight anxiety into three types: simple fatigue, specific phobic reactions, and more generalized anxiety, noting that the therapeutic outlook was progressively less optimistic for each.[25]

The current consensus on the subject is that a generalized fear of flying is associated with highly anxious personality types, while more focussed reactions are likely to have specific environmental precipitants. It is also worth noting that these environmental precipitants may include factors not directly related to flying, such as sexual conflicts, family problems, and other aspects of the individual's personal life.[47]

Therapeutic approaches

While therapy programs for the flight anxious abound, they have for the most part been designed for members of the public rather than for professional pilots themselves. In general, the most effective of these have involved a variety of behavioural therapies, most often the technique of systematic desensitization.[1,41] Most accounts of this type of therapy have not provided extensive follow-up data, although one by Dennholtz, Hall, and Mann reported an 89 percent success rate that was maintained for three and a half years.[18]

One example of a program aimed specifically at pilots is that of the United States Navy, which has instituted a therapy course for Navy and Marine Corps flight students whose anxiety levels interfere with training.[1] The program incorporates both desensitization and various relaxation techniques; within the course of a three year study, 79 percent of the personnel who received treatment went on to complete their flight training.[7] Interestingly, in this particular study certain personality differences were noted between patients who were successfully treated and those who failed to resume flight training. While neither group evinced any significant psychopathology, the unsuccessful pilots were characterized by low self confidence, a low tolerance for criticism, and difficulties with concentration, as measured by the Minnesota Multiphasic Personality Inventory (MMPI) at the outset of treatment. The explanation offered for their failure to benefit from systematic desensitization is that this therapy is more effective in treating state anxiety than trait anxiety.[12] Indeed, other research has suggested that trait anxious individuals do not respond well to desensitization therapy.[50]

A second factor which distinguished between the pilots who recovered from their fear of flying and those who did not was the nature of the presenting symptoms. Those pilots who suffered primarily from airsickness responded well to desensitization treatment, while patients whose anxiety manifested itself as insomnia, nervousness, or gastrointestinal discomfort were helped less by the therapy. The latter constellation of symptoms (which, as we shall see, is reminiscent of that seen in combat stress) has been characterized as more generalized, more strongly associated with trait anxious personalities, and as being less situation specific (that is, it can be evoked by a wide range of stimuli, both internal and external). Similar treatment outcomes have been observed in other studies of aerophobics, such as those by Rosenthal[58] and Wolpe.[77]

Behavioural extremes

We turn next to two particular characteristics of fear or stress that have received relatively little research attention within the context of aviation. These are *(a)* anticipatory stress, and *(b)* inaction or failure to respond -- phenomena which among aviators are probably associated most often with unusual levels of threat. Pilots love to fly, and almost always look forward to flying with positive emotions. However, anticipatory stress is a phenomenon that has sometimes been recorded among aircrew preparing for important checkrides, combat encounters, and other particularly threatening events; manifestations range from faint unease to trembling, vomiting, and even an outright refusal to fly.

Inaction, or failure to respond, is sometimes described in its acute forms as paralysis or 'freezing', and has been witnessed at some level by many, perhaps most flight instructors. It obviously can have extremely serious consequences in the unforgiving and time critical environment of aviation, and discussion of the phenomenon here may help to stimulate future work on its nature and possible countermeasures.

Anticipatory stress

> *Sore stress of apprehension ... dreading worse designed,*
> *From month to month, trembling and unassured.*
> -- William Wordsworth, *Ecclesiastical Sonnet 37*

In 1976 a (biochemical response based) stress study was reported that was interpreted as showing very marked preflight stress in aircrew of US based EC-135J aircraft.[21] While no data were presented to link this to any performance changes in flight, there is no denying that the simple anticipation

Most people will agree with me that when I say the worst part of any bombing raid is the start. I, for my part, hate the feeling of standing around in the crew rooms, waiting to get into the vans that will take you out to your aircraft. It's a horrible business. Your stomach feels as though it wants to hit your backbone. You can't stand still. You laugh at small jokes, loudly, stupidly ... Sometimes you feel sick and want to go to the lavatory ... the smallest incidents annoy you ... I have always felt bad until the door of the aircraft clangs shut ... then it's all right. Just another job.

-- Wing Commander Guy Gibson, V.C., *Enemy Coast Ahead*

of threat or danger has been associated with decrements in performance of many complex tasks (an example being Carter and Cammermayer's research on simulated chemical warfare medical intervention exercises).[15] Wing Commander Gibson's account of his feelings before bombing raids (see sidebar) relates a commonly reported experience -- high levels of anticipatory anxiety, which, however, melt away once the feared circumstances are actually encountered. Anticipatory stress is not, of course, confined to military environments: it is something that we have all experienced at some level, if only for a wedding speech or final examination. However, considering how disabling it can be, and how critical preflight activities and contingency planning are to flight safety and mission success,[52] anticipatory stress has been the object of surprisingly little systematic field research in aviation. Most studies that do exist tend to be nonaviation laboratory tests of the type where the threat consists of electric shocks.

There was, nevertheless, a period in the mid-1960s when the topic was addressed in several aviation related studies, although electric shock still featured as the 'stressor'. For example, Wherry[75] presented a model of psychological stress which distinguished between stress and 'anticipatory threat stress' that was defined in terms of the potential for physical harm. While stress was, in this model, assumed to be associated with deterioration of performance, anticipatory threat stress was not necessarily so. In fact the anticipation period was said to provide an opportunity for the indi-

Fear and Stress Extremes

201

vidual to adapt behaviour to the upcoming potentially stressful circumstances. Thus, the effect of 'mild' anticipatory threat stress was said to be beneficial, serving to improve performance.

More severe anticipatory stress, however, was viewed as negative in its implications for performance, as it could lead to a deterioration or even complete breakdown in functioning. It was, therefore, considered important to be positive and proactive in controlling the individual pilot's perceptions of the anticipated threat. This could entail the active manipulation of

(a) the perceived probability of the aversive situation or event;

(b) the perceived proximity of the aversive situation or event; and

(c) the perceived degree of unpleasantness of the aversive situation or event.

An empirical test of these 'primary determinants' of anticipatory threat stress was provided by one study that was built around a simulated flight: as the three variables listed above were increased, so performance decreased, consistently with Wherry's model.[16] Another study using Wherry's approach examined the performance of general aviation pilots flying a simulated instrument flight under the threat of electric shock.[19] In one group, errors were linked directly to the administration of shocks, while in the other, errors corrected within five seconds did not attract a shock. Thus, pilots in the second group had a larger measure of control over the 'stressor'. The results were interpreted as supporting the hypothesis that the perceived relevance of one's own performance to the occurrence of events mediates the degree of anticipatory threat stress: perceived control, or rather the lack of it, could be said to constitute a significant 'secondary determinant' of such stress.

The approach adopted by Wherry and his colleagues was in some respects rather advanced for aviation stress studies of the 1960s, and remains so even when compared to many studies today. For example, the researchers recognized that 'threat' was determined by the subject's own perceptions (rather than inhering directly in the experimenter's manipulations). Moreover, they were aware of the need to adopt some theoretical framework for their studies. Considered as a model, however, Wherry's observations appear to be essentially a reiteration of the U-shaped curve hypothesis discussed in Chapter 2 -- that small amounts of stress improve performance and large amounts impair performance. As such it suffers from many of the problems that have traditionally beset proponents of 'U theories', such as the assumption that stress, arousal, and motivation are interchangeable constructs. Nevertheless, these studies represent rare examples of theory based research on anticipatory stress in the context of flying performance.

More recent research, little of it aviation specific, has followed in Wherry's footsteps in attempting to pin down 'primary determinants' of anticipatory stress -- that is, the specific factors which most influence the production of this anxiety. In evaluating this research it is helpful to have a 'real world' aviation example against which to consider the hypotheses. Consider, then, the following true story.

'Janice' was a flight student who stood to be eliminated from the training programme at a large US university if she failed her flight check yet again. She had just received a low grade in history as well, but this didn't worry her; however, she admitted to feeling considerable anticipatory stress about the flight check. Her chosen career, after all, was 'on the line'. More-over, this was not the least of it: she also stood to lose a good deal of money, alienate her parents, and lose face with her peers. What is more, she would have to leave town, which would mean subletting her apartment. Finally, when the day of the flight check arrived, the weather was flyable but not helpful. Janice was allocated her least favourite aircraft and 'Flunk 'em Fred', an (unjustifiably) notorious check pilot. As the appointed time neared Janice became more and more agitated. Finally, she became cer-tain that nothing could save her and feigned illness to cancel the flight.

These events can be analyzed in terms of a number of propositions about anticipatory stress. These are as follows:

1. The more importance accorded to a goal, the more anticipatory stress is generated when that goal is threatened.

2. The greater the number of goals that are threatened, the greater the anticipatory stress that is generated.

3. The greater the extent to which a goal is threatened, the greater the anticipatory stress that is produced.

As a matter of fact these hypotheses have received considerable experi-mental scrutiny. Two Canadian researchers, Paterson and Neufeld, re-viewed the research evidence and found considerable support for the idea that these dimensions are important ones in determining anticipatory stress.[51] A caveat has to be offered concerning the tempting assumption that the most important factor in anticipatory stress is bound to be the severity of the threat, that is, the aversiveness of that which is feared. The time variable, imminence, has a powerful effect which can render threat severity meaningless. This point can be illustrated by our feelings about death. The prospect of death is highly aversive for most people, but we do not suffer undue anticipatory stress about it -- not, that is, until we fear it to be unduly imminent. The more imminent a threatening circumstance is (or strictly, as Wherry was careful to state, *perceived* to be), the greater its capacity to provoke anticipatory stress.

Similarly, it is suggested that the longer the 'lead' time given (that is, the more time elapses between the onset of concern about the feared event and its occurrence), the greater the anticipatory stress when the event becomes imminent. That is, stress may build up or 'incubate' (as Breznitz, an Israeli researcher, has described it).[10] The concept of 'incubation' is roughly opposite to Wherry's concept of 'adaptation', although both are said to take place during the anticipatory period. In one study by Breznitz, for example, subjects informed that they would receive an electric shock exhibited an immediate marked increase in heart rate. After the initial jump, however, heart rate declined, but over time crept back up as the feared event became more imminent. Interestingly, the longer the lead time was, the higher was the final heart rate.[10]

It has been suggested that the causal variable in this effect may not be time, but rather 'emotional workload' -- in other words, worry. Time merely permits worry, allowing the individual to dwell on the source of anxiety for longer. Another variable likely to be relevant here is perception of control during the anticipatory period. Where there are coping strategies available, time can decrease anticipatory stress, while in the absence of control it may permit stress to incubate.[11] A related variable potentially influencing the degree of anticipatory stress is uncertainty about the availability of control when the threatening circumstance arrives. Thus, perceived self efficacy and locus of control, personality variables discussed in Chapter 6 (and touched on again later), also seem likely to be important factors in anticipatory stress.

Finally, in terms of research evidence, the picture remains clouded over the claim that the lower the probability of a specified event's occurrence, the lower the level of anticipatory stress it produces. (This probability was a hypothesized 'primary determinant' of anticipatory stress in Wherry's model). The problem is that at least two variables are involved: the magnitude of the probability itself, and uncertainty over that magnitude.[51] These two elements are easily confounded in experimental studies.

Additional implications. The evidence suggests that anticipatory stress can 'incubate', reaching intense levels prior to actual exposure to the feared circumstances. In aviation this could mean that some aircrew may experience significant levels of stress (perhaps the highest experienced in an entire mission or duty period) before they have ever left the ground. In such cases stress related performance decrements have to be suspected not so much in flight management, airmanship, control, and the like, but in vital preflight activities. Thes activities include flight planning, 'contingency' planning, interpreting weather briefings, evaluating NOTAMS (Notices to Airmen), assessing maintenance status and passenger/cargo load, and, of course, preflight inspection of the aircraft. These are among the most important activities a pilot performs. Indeed, the phrase 'inadequate preflight planning' is a depressingly common one in the conclusions of accident investigation boards.

Many preflight activities are among the most cognitively challenging that a pilot undertakes, involving the selection, integration, and analysis of a considerable body of meteorological, navigational, and systems performance information. Analytical and integrative skills are, as we discussed in Chapter 4, 'fragile' in terms of their vulnerability to stress, and disruption of these during the preparations for flight could obviously have long term consequences as severe as, or more severe than, many of the stress induced cognitive decrements that can occur during flight itself. Despite these considerations, it is difficult to determine from existing research just how serious a problem anticipatory stress represents. We do not know, for example, who is most likely to suffer from anticipatory stress, when it will occur, which activities are affected, or what interventions are effective.

There are also a number of lingering theoretical questions. For example, it is not clear from Wherry's or from subsequent models why or under what circumstances anticipatory stress might 'incubate' and magnify with time, and when it will not. If stress results from the appraisal of demand, coping ability, and importance of success, it is not obvious why this appraisal should change for the worse as an aversive event nears and, in many cases, uncertainty diminishes. A researchable speculation is that psychological defence mechanisms such as rationalization and denial (see Chapter 6) play an important role in altering these appraisals. For example, a 'Janice' might, in the days before her flight check, persuade herself that her proficiency is adequate, perhaps no worse than that of others who have 'scraped through'. She might rationalize that she still has plenty of time to prepare for the flight check, that she might draw a 'Santa Claus' check pilot, or that the weather will be perfect (or, alternatively, not fly-able at all). However, such defences are presumably difficult to sustain as an event draws ever nigh and reality inexorably intrudes. A similar proc-ess can be posited in the account by Wing Commander Gibson presented earlier: as the aircraft is declared servicable, fueled, and 'bombed up', the weather is announced to be adequate, and so forth, the evidence accrues that the combat mission (at that time horribly dangerous by any measure) will indeed take place.

Gibson's account also invites certain questions, however. Gibson was presumably afraid of dying in combat over Germany (sadly, his ultimate fate), not of climbing aboard his Lancaster. Why did his anticipatory stress not continue -- and, for that matter, incubate -- at least until actual combat? The easy answer is that preparing the aircraft and going through the various procedures associated with this provided a sense of control, a way of coping. Had his agitation increased at this point, however (as was reportedly the case with some individuals), we might just as glibly have argued that preparing the aircraft for combat forced attention onto the inescapable threat, stripping away psychological defences and increasing the 'emotional workload'. Indeed, any mechanism purporting to account for Gibson's sudden relief would also have to account for why this is not seen in all individuals. There may even be group differences: there is some evidence, for example, that women suffer less from anticipatory stress than men.[41] Certainly there is a case for studying individual differ-ences in psychological defensiveness, preflight distress, and the perform-ance of important preflight activities.

Stress induced inaction

> I knew exactly what to do, for I had had plenty of experience in instru-ment flying; but for a moment I was paralysed. Enclosed in that small space and faced with a thousand bewildering instruments, I had a moment of complete claustrophobia. I must get out. I was going to crash ... Then I saw the flare path. I dropped back into my seat feeling thoroughly ashamed of myself. (Richard Hillary, *The Last Enemy*)

Occasionally, acute reactive stress may result in partial or complete paraly-sis of action. This phenomenon can arise either in the course of a genuine-ly life threatening emergency or, as Richard Hillary's account of his first night solo suggests, at times of perceived or imagined threat. However, the data on this phenomenon are very incomplete: it is rarely seen in the laboratory or flight simulator since it is very difficult (not to say unethical) to stress individuals to this extent in controlled conditions. Nevertheless, the effect has frequently been observed in real life -- so often, indeed, that the English language has several idioms to describe this immobilization through fear: to be 'rooted to the spot' or even to be 'petrified' (that is, of course, 'turned to stone' by the experience). The phenomenom appears to be different from the 'night shift paralysis' (discussed in Chapter 10) which has been seen in air traffic controllers and which probably has its roots in fatigue, underarousal, and time of day effects.

In the context of flight deck operations, Terry Heaslip[32] and his colleagues at Accident Investigation and Research, Incorporated, of Ottawa have dubbed apparent paralysis of action the 'Frozen Pilot Syndrome', and have pointed out that even highly trained and experienced pilots can be affected by it. The phenomenon is characterized by "fixation of attention on only one (often very minor and irrelevant) aspect of the emergency ... [and] a complete breakdown in rational behaviour and ... logical response" (p. 782). One's orientation towards this problem, and, indeed, whether one seeks to address it through drills, training, selection, or medical screening depends upon which explanatory framework is invoked. Some of the more promising hypotheses will be considered here.

Tonic immobility hypothesis. In common with many other animals, humans occasionally exhibit tonic immobility in the face of serious and unavoidable threat. In contrast to attentive immobility, in which the animal becomes motionless but intensely alert (ears pricked up, etc.), tonic immobility is an unresponsive and extreme reaction to fear, often called shamming death or terror paralysis. In prey animals tonic immobility has been observed to lead to the inhibiting or abandonment of attack by a predator. Moreover, when a predator becomes inattentive to its immobile 'catch', the paralyzed state may be broken suddenly and violently as the prey either bounds away or attacks the predator.

Tonic immobility has been reported by various human groups, from combat fatigued ('shell shocked') soldiers to rape victims.[72] Its symptoms include the rapid onset (and equally sudden termination) of a conscious but 'frozen' state featuring sever motor inhibition, tremor, numbness and reduced pain awareness, reduced body temperature, slowed heart rate, and an inability to speak or even scream. While it is highly likely that extreme states such this do occur, albeit rarely, in terrified aircrew, tonic immobility does not appear to be a plausible mechanism for most reports of 'frozen pilot syndrome'. It is, for example, inconsistent with the observation that minor, irrelevant, or peripheral control actions are often performed, and (ultimately unrealized) intentions or off-task thoughts expressed. For most cases of 'the syndrome' it is probably necessary to explore less biological and more psychological hypotheses.

'Creek but no paddle' hypothesis. Perhaps the most obvious 'explanation' of inaction or paralysis is that it is not a case of stress causing the inability to take appropriate action, but rather of the inability to take action causing stress. Schaffer's neurophysiological hypothesis, for example, posits that stress comes about when a highly motivated person is unable to find an adaptive response to some disruption in the relationship to his or her environment[62] -- or, as George Mandler put it, when there are "no available action or thought structures ... to handle the situation" (p. 191).[43] Mandler has noted how little stress is apparent in highly trained personnel such as astronauts. Such individuals are equipped with sophisticated mental models of their vehicle's systems and dynamics, and they have ready response 'scripts', plans, action sequences, and problem solving strategies for almost any conceivable emergency. To this extent emergencies are virtually reduced to routine (and, therefore, nonstressful) procedures.

Certainly there is experimental evidence for the stress neutralizing effect of expertise. For example, as described in Chapter 4, Stokes has demonstrated that unlike novice pilots, experts -- even those who are trait anxious -- are unaffected by stress in simulated flight decision making tasks. Tuis is true even where stress impairs the pilots' scores on standard cognitive tests.[69] If Mandler's observations are always applicable, then the best -- perhaps the only -- countermeasure to 'frozen pilot syndrome' should be further training, to ensure that no one is ever at a loss for appropriate 'thought structures' and action plans.

Regrettably, the problem is not solved so easily. First, evidence from accident and incident reports frequently shows that in very stressful circumstances, even trained personnel may fail to implement the simplest procedures (such as the rejected takeoff procedure -- see sidebar overleaf). It is clearly implausible to ascribe such failures to the absence of appropriate 'thought structures' or action plans. Moreover, it may be that one or more stress related mechanisms, such as those discussed below, may be implicated in the original failure to generate or implement a timely action plan. Not all cases of apparent 'freezing' need be caused by the same mechanisms, but some of the likely, or least, possible mechanisms can be considered on the basis of what is already known.

Toronto International Airport, 26 June, 1978: An Air Canada DC-9 attempted to take off but an emergency developed which required an RTO (rejected takeoff). This procedure requires that the RTO be declared and within three seconds to have all decelerative forces deployed. The captain, an experienced ex-military pilot, failed to call the RTO for his First Officer instead beginning the procedure by retarding the throttles. After this he took no further action, "staring straight ahead" according to the First Officer. In response to this inaction the First Officer intervened, setting reverse thrust. The captain then belatedly declared the RTO by calling "Reject Buckets" (for reverse thrust). The captain did not apply effective brake pressure either immediately or at any time during the incident. Instead he started to fumble with a peripheral control as the aircraft approached the end of the runway at 250 feet per second. The First Officer finally intervened again, applying maximum braking some eight seconds and 2000 feet of runway since the start of the RTO. The aircraft overran the end of the runway at 70 knots and crashed into ground obstacles, killing and injuring a number of passengers. The main fuel tanks ruptured but there was no fire. Postaccident analysis showed that timely braking alone, without spoilers or thrust reversers, would have prevented the crash.

-- Condensed from accounts by Heaslip[32] and McLeod[44]

Attention and memory effects. The symptoms of the 'syndrome' noted by Heaslip and his colleagues[32] could, in part, be an extreme manifestation of cognitive tunnelling (see Chapter 3) combined with the complete disruption of inferential processes in (a presumably reduced capacity) working memory. Certainly anecdotal reports are often consistent with this, taking the 'all I could see/hear' form (e.g., "all I could see was the altimeter unwinding, I didn't notice the fuel was still off").

Nevertheless, while these processes may be present to varying extents, this is obviously not a comprehensive or satisfying explanation of the paralysis effect. Among other intriguing elements unexplained is the reason that attention is sometimes focussed, apparently perversely and maladaptively, upon *irrelevant* peripheral details instead of the central, most urgent task. Indeed, one of the more curious, intriguing and often reported features of the phenomenon is the intrusion of, sometimes ludicrous, thoughts.* This is difficult to reconcile with Easterbrook's hypothesis discussed in Chapter 3 -- the notion that attentional narrowing evolved to exclude unnecessary extraneous and peripheral information.[20]

Disruption of prioritizing effects. Another possibility is suggested by Simmel's observation that, in the air, recognizing that a threat exists and correctly assessing the threat can be two rather different matters.[64] That is, pilots sometimes overassess the dangers of a situation and prioritize their actions accordingly, and sometimes underassess. Underassessment of a threat may lead to the assumption that more resources (for example, time, fuel, and so forth) are available than in fact is the case. Under such circumstances, rather than averting the imminent mishap the pilot may, for example, waste time attempting to diagnose a failure (or, as flight instructors say, worrying too much about how you got into the mess and not enough about how to get out of it). Similarly, time may be wasted improving the cabin environment (e.g., turning on air vents), or removing aversive stimuli (e.g., turning off warning horns). To the observer who *has* correctly assessed the urgency of the situation, or to the post hoc investigator, such activities seem absurdly inappropriate, beside the point, and tantamount to action paralysis.

Shifts from 'automatic' to 'controlled' processing. In an often cited paper, Schneider and Shiffrin distinguished between two modes of cognitive processing.[60] Well-learned activities and routines (for example, proficient touch typing, or stick-and-rudder control in a conventional aircraft) are largely accomplished using a sort of mental autopilot whose functioning is efficient, fast, accurate, and requires little conscious effort or attention. Like any autopilot, however, it is inflexible, 'blind', and cannot rapidly adapt to novel demands.

Many emergencies are, of course, novel situations for a pilot, or at least are novel (even improbable) combinations of previously experienced circumstances or events. These require controlled processing -- a flexible, adaptive, but slow and error prone cognitive mode that is more demanding of mental resources such as conscious attention and memory capacity (for example, 'one finger' typing, or control of a damaged or abnormally responding aircraft). A sudden change of circumstances, then, could re-

---

* One of the authors suffered a punctured tyre in a blizzard en route to a fancy dress party. As the vehicle spun uncontrollably in the road the only thought in mind was "I'm going to die dressed as a pirate".

quire a rapid shift in cognitive mode. The shift itself may be momentarily disruptive or disorienting, requiring time to 'gather ones thoughts', i.e., to direct attention to the relevant features of the situation, recall procedures and other pertinent information, and integrate the information necessary to effect control or render a decision.

However, under real or perceived threat, the additional mental resources necessary for controlled processing are the very ones diminished by stress. Attention may be restricted and working memory capacity reduced (or effectively so by the intrusion of non-task related self referential thoughts -- e.g., "This can't be happening to me" or "I'm going to die and I didn't put the cat out"). Indeed, the domination of thought by 'worry work' may act as an effective signal jammer and prevent the changeover from automatic processing, causing the perseveration of behaviour sometimes commented on by observers ("He just continued the approach as though nothing were wrong...").

Anxiety reduction and psychological defences. The British Army Personnel Research Establishment's *Pilot's Guide to Stress and Performance* warns that among the mental processes that can lead to error is an 'anti-anxiety' strategy, so to speak, in which "incoming information is modified in such a way as to reduce anxiety." (p. 4) What the guide appears to be referring to is the phenomenon of psychological defence mechanisms, which were discussed in Chapter 6 along with a number of other personality traits and mental habits thought to mediate the experience of stress. As we noted there, the question of whether psychological defence mechanisms are considered adaptive or, ultimately, maladaptive depends in part on the situations in which they come into play.

The point to be made here is that in particularly extreme and traumatic conditions (such as during certain flight deck emergencies or in combat situations), the tendency to censor or adapt one's perceptions to preserve some mental equilibrium probably increases. For example, the kind of denial illustrated in the Riyadh airliner fire (see sidebar on p. 174) could result in inaction that is tantamount to paralysis or 'freezing'. Heaslip and his colleagues speculate that the 'frozen' pilots in the incidents they considered were obsessively focussing upon matters which served in some fashion only to relieve their anxieties, despite having no practical value in averting impending disaster.[32]

Certainly there are mechanisms for this. Recall, for example, that the perception of control is an important variable influencing the amount of stress experienced: the belief that one has some control over the stress producing situation has been shown to reduce anxiety, even if that belief is ill founded.[26,35] In light of this it is understandable that pilots may find comfort in tinkering, albeit ineffectually, with equipment or instruments that *can* be controlled -- even if they have no relevance to the problem at hand. Norman Milgram notes, for example, that this appears as a coping strategy in combat: "However inconsequential or ineffective certain behaviors may be in fact, they may be effective at least for the short haul in permitting the individual to function and sustain a sense of perceived control of the problem and of oneself" (p. 16).[46]

Before leaving the topic of stress induced inaction for a consideration of combat stress, we turn briefly to one of the least understood and most neglected dimensions of situational awareness, the perception of time.

Temporal distortions

> *The Zero whipped upward in a violent loop, and for an eternity of a split second it seemed that I would meet the [cliff] wall just as the Airacobra had.*
>
> -- Saburo Sakai, *Samurai*

While 'situation awareness' has become a very fashionable research term and topic over the past few years in aviation psychology, the temporal dimension of that awareness has received much less attention than, for example, the spatial dimension. Indeed, it has received very little scrutiny at all. However, a pilot overestimating the duration of an event might, among other effects, perceive himself or his flight deck colleagues as oddly inactive or 'frozen' during the unfolding of the event. A pilot underestimating the duration of an event might not see himself as unduly inactive, but might be perceived that way by others not sharing his particular temporal distortion.

At the very least, temporal distortions would be likely to bias aircrew reports (accident and incident reports, combat debriefings, etc.). In some circumstances, however, time distortion is also likely to have substantive long term implications. Consider, for example, the decision to eject or not to eject from an aircraft, and the decision to fire or not to fire at what might be an attacking enemy: in both cases an accurate perception of the amount of time available is of critical importance.

Much of the evidence for temporal distortion is anecdotal -- we have all heard accounts of traumatic events in which 'everything seemed to happen in slow motion', despite the brevity of the event. The general belief is that perceptions of time tend to be distorted in stressful situations, most often of an extreme or traumatic nature. As a matter of fact, there is laboratory evidence for just such effects: for example, in an early study by Falk and Bindra electric shocks were associated with significant overestimation of time periods.[22]

It has been suggested that two factors influence human perception of time -- external (or environmental) elements, and internal (or endogenous) elements.[30] A number of candidates for 'internal clock' mechanisms have been considered -- heart rate and respiration, blood pressure, and so on; however, none has exhibited the expected association with subjective temporal flow,[59] although body temperature may have the most potential in this respect.

One possible environmental factor is the degree of novelty and/or complexity in the array of stimuli presented to the observer. However, as Peter Hancock has pointed out, theoreticians have differed over the rather fundamental matter of whether such complexity (poorly defined as it is) is associated with subjective time compression or with expansion.[30] Interestingly, questionnaire data from Air Force pilots surviving ejection reflects this theoretical confusion, with some pilots reporting that time seemed to slow down while others maintained that it speeded up.[13,14]

The topic of temporal distortion is one which combines great theoretical interest and operational importance with significant methodological problems for research. Nevertheless, if we are not prepared to simply avert our gaze from a significant dimension of situational awareness, and a significant potential source of reporting bias, perception of time is a nettle that must be grasped.

Combat stress

When the foeman bares his steel, we uncomfortable feel.
-- W.S. Gilbert, *The Pirates of Penzance*

Combat stress, it has been suggested, "is different from the other stress factors in that it is a combination of other stressors" (Backer and Orasanu,[5] p. 9). From the viewpoint encouraged by the stimulus based literature on stress, which tends to examine one discrete 'stressor' at a time, this statement is correct. However, the everyday stress of workaday life is often a combination of factors also. For example, if we consider a fatigued and 'burned out' airman in a low morale unit, separated from his wife and facing a serious flight deck emergency, we could could just as easily be referring to a commercial pilot in a bankrupt domestic airline as an officer on a combat mission in some faraway war. (Indeed, evidence presented in the section on stress and employee-management relations in Chapter 11 makes it clear that this comparison is by no means a frivolous one).

In the light of this, the difference between combat stress and the stress experienced by civilians might be considered more a matter of degree than of kind, although, given the prevalence of psychiatric 'casualties' in everyday life (depressions, anxiety states, phobic states, and so forth), even this may not always be true. Thus, we believe that a consideration of combat stress is doubly interesting, both as a phenomenon in its own right and (although caution in generalizing must be exercised) as something of a model of, or at least a source of clues to, complex multistressor processes in general.

What is meant by combat stress?

Combat stress (or, in more stimulus based terms, *the reaction to* combat stress) is a condition that has historically gone under many names. These range from the quaint term 'nostalgia' used in seventeenth century Europe and in the American Civil War (from the homesickness component of stress often evident in war weary soldiers), to 'shell shock' -- the First World War term that embodied the prevailing notion that exposure to explosions traumatized the nervous system. Later, under the influence of Freudian psychology, the term 'war neurosis' became fashionable, in keeping with the view that combat provoked the reemergence of subconscious conflicts dating back to infancy. Victims of shell shock and war neurosis were frequently viewed as being deficient in some way -- lacking 'character' -- and thus being predisposed to 'nerves' or even cowardice.

In the Second World War the terms 'battle stress', 'combat exhaustion' and 'combat fatigue' became common, and reflected a move away from assumptions of defective personality and toward the view that the battlefield environment engendered a particular form of weariness.[65,73] However even in this conflict, terms such as LMF ('Lack of Moral Fibre' -- see p. 222) were still used and continued the tradition of pejorative, personality based conceptions of combat stress. More recently psychologists have favoured more neutral terminology: 'combat stress', 'combat stress reaction', and 'acute combat reaction' are now more usual names.

What exactly is the condition?

Combat stress reaction should really more accurately be described as a group of conditions, a constellation of symptoms which may not occur all together in any single individual. In fact, no two cases are likely to be identical. As with fear of flying, somatic symptoms may include loss of appetite, headaches, weight loss, insomnia, trembling, pallor, sweating, and gastric upsets, as well as palpitations, numbness, and outright paralysis or even blindness. On the other hand, there may be the merest nervous tic (the 'twitch' as it was known to RAF aircrew in the Second World War). Emotional symptoms often include apathy, depression, irritability, weepiness, lethargy, or withdrawal. Behavioural components can range from restlessness or an increased startle response to ranting, fleeing, or hiding. Cognitive disturbances may include decision paralysis, inability to concentrate, unresponsiveness, communication difficulties (speechlessness), and forgetfulness or even frank amnesia. In a 1991 Israeli study, about half of the combat stress cases analyzed were polymorphic, that is, had multiple symptoms. Among the most frequently observed symptoms were anxiety and depression, with anxiety tending to turn to depression across the time course of the condition.[78]

In summary, combat stress reaction is not mere fatigue or exhaustion, but neither is it simple fear, anxiety, neuroticism, or any other recognized clinical condition. It is, as the Bartemeier Commission put it in 1946, more a "temporary psychological disorganization out of which ... various more definite and more familiar syndromes evolve" (p. 422).[6] Interestingly, from the standpoint of the discussion of arousal, stress, and performance in Chapter 2, this psychological disorganization can manifest itself both in terms of very high adrenergic arousal (panic, flight, and so forth), very suppressed adrenergic arousal (withdrawal, stupor, depression) or, as the list of symptoms suggest, almost any state in between.

How is combat stress brought about?

A number of important surveys of combat stress casualties followed the Second World War, which, despite no shortage of more recent conflicts, remains the source of much of the best, 'classic' literature on combat stress. In one such survey it was concluded that aerial combat was a particularly stressful activity.[29] Case studies within this survey revealed that major breakdowns could be caused not only by a single, very traumatic event, but also by prolonged exposure to more minor tribulations, or by prolonged exposure suddenly followed by a more traumatic event.[56] What these experiences appear to have in common, be they brief or prolonged, is that they undermine and ultimately destroy the protective illusion of safety that humans tend to have in everyday life and which they carry into battle.[63] (See the discussion of psychological defence mechanisms in Chapter 6). It is interesting to note that non-combat related clinical studies suggest that depressed individuals suffer from 'depressive realism', a pessimistic but, in probabilistic terms, all too accurate assessment of the real risks of everyday life. By comparison, normal (that is, nondepressive) individuals are 'professional Pollyannas' -- that is, they appear to have an outlook on life that has a positive bias, a viewpoint characterized by an unrealistic but psychologically functional overestimation of their safety and control over events.[2]

In war, at least three 'defensive' cognitive strategies are said to underpin the continuation of this comforting illusion. The first is the 'myth of invulnerability', the conviction that others may fail or fall but not I. Indeed, for many people both in and out of combat (young flight students, for example), life seems so robust, and the prospect of personal oblivion so unreal, that the notion of one's personal mortality seems curiously remote and intellectual. The second 'crutch' is the belief that the group's leadership (commander, captain, instructor, etc.) is essentially infallible and omnipotent. This combines with the third belief, that is, that the group or organization, the full awesome range of resources deployed in support of you and your comrades, cannot fail to cocoon you against harm.[33,63,65]

Enemy action, however, has the potential not only to penetrate this cocoon of materiel but also to penetrate the cognitive armour that these beliefs provide. In combat, the individual may come to believe that not only is life fragile and cheap, but that the odds of personal survival are slim (an actuarial reality in some air warfare). He may find that his leaders exhibit monumental incompetence or are powerless to help him, and he may come to the conclusion that 'all the king's horses and all the king's men' are still unable to intervene to retrieve a situation.

The stripping away of the combat flier's psychological defences takes place, of course, in circumstances often characterized by *multiple stressors* -- that is, in circumstances in which acute stress events are superimposed upon chronic conditions, involving fatigue, deprivation, danger and the cumulative emotional toll of losing comrades. The beleaguered pilots of the RAF during the Battle of Britain in 1940, for example, fought exhausted, day after day for months, returning to home bases subject to constant air raid alarms and actual bombing attacks. In such conditions it is hardly surprising that sometimes even the prospect of combat, or indeed, of any further aversive event, may be sufficient to provoke a stress response.

Vulnerability to combat stress

Given the conditions that combat brings (high uncertainty, deprivation, and emotional trauma), it is hardly surprising that, as several surveys have indicated, more or less anyone involved in combat is a potential psychiatric casualty. However, there has been a rather slow moving clinical debate (spanning several decades) concerning the role of premorbid psychosocial factors in the aetiology of stress reaction in combat personnel. Some researchers have argued that there is little evidence that predispositional factors (personality, family history, etc.) predict combat stress reactions.[66] Others believe that their own research results do indeed suggest that family problems, relationship difficulties, adjustment at school, and the like predispose individuals toward becoming psychological casualties of war.[61]

American research immediately after the Second World War suggested that intelligence and education did serve as 'protective' factors associated with reduced susceptibility to combat stress reaction.[70] Studies by Israeli researchers in the 1970s and 1980s provide evidence that is generally consistent with this, emphasizing the importance of educational level, military rank, and intelligence in resistance to combat stress.[24,49] The Israeli findings on rank are intriguing, since studies conducted during the Vietnam war, both on infantry and B-52 bomber crews, indicated that the secretion of the adrenal hormone 17-OHCS (one of the many putative biochemical 'markers' of stress) was significantly greater in team leaders than in their subordinates. It was concluded that leaders experienced more stress than their men (as opposed to coping less well),[9] a judgement that is consistent with the view discussed in Chapter 10 ('Stress in air traffic control') that responsibility for others increases stress.

That leaders sometimes exhibit less tendency to succumb to combat stress reactions could be a function of their greater perceived control, as discussed below, perhaps combined with stronger social inhibition of visible stress reactions. On the other hand, the reading of the hormone assay results as indicating elevated stress levels may be simplistic and unreliable, an example of a naive physiological stress model (as discussed in Chapter 1), and an oversimplistic view of arousal (as examined in Chapter 2).

Indeed, some of the results in this series of studies are consistent with this view. For example, the 17-OHCS levels of helicopter ambulance (Medevac) crews operating out of Tan Son Nhut did not vary consistently with whether the crews had been under fire or not, or even whether they had been flying or not. If, as observed, monitored physiological changes bore no relationship to whether or not aviators were experiencing extremely dangerous low level sorties, it is difficult to place great confidence in their usefulness in discriminating between the stress levels experienced by different B-52 crew members.[9]

Some research results lead to interesting, and somewhat surprising, counterintuitive conclusions about vulnerability to combat stress disorders. Airmen who have experienced injury, or survived crashes and bailouts, may show a remarkable willingness to return to combat flight status.[*] The correlation between rated combat efficiency and emotional stability may be quite low (in the range of 0.20 to 0.30 in many cases).[40] One example of this was that of a group of 150 successful combat fliers; fully half of them were found to have either a personal or family background of emotional instability, but not one dropped out of combat duty because of stress.[31]

The importance of perceived control. Samuel Stouffer and his colleagues, writing of combat and its aftermath in the Second World War, noted that despite a high casualty rate US fighter pilots reported the least fear of any US combat aircrew and were particularly willing to accept additional tours of duty. Bomber pilots, however, showed rather less alacrity in signing up for more combat, and other bomber crew members (such as navigators and radio operators) were even less enthusiastic.[70] Likewise, the RAF observed that Bomber Command air gunners tended to report the most fear of any RAF aircrew. It is interesting to note that this ranking, from fighter pilot down to air gunner, also represents a scale of control. Fighter pilots had great autonomy and freedom of action: with their fast and responsive aircraft they could engage the enemy or break off and flee, and they actively contributed to the unfolding of events. Bomber pilots captained their relatively unwieldy aircraft but were otherwise very restricted, having to stay in formation (US), or in the bomber stream (RAF), and keeping to a predetermined route, come flak or fighter. Bomber crews, in turn, had rather less control than the bomber pilot, while gunners could do little more than 'sit tight' for the entire trip unless and until they were attacked.

---

[*]Although there can be organizational and social reasons for this, as we shall see.

As we have seen from discussions in several other chapters, perceived control is an important variable thought to mediate individuls' stress response, a notion that has considerable experimental support.[26,35]

While the amount of control an individual feels that he has in any situation is often a function of environmental circumstances (being pinned down in a foxhole, or strapped into a bomber, for example), the sense of control is not beyond the influence of the individual. Important variables 'protecting' aircrew from stress, probably via the sense of control that they bring, appear to be competence and confidence. The Allied fighter pilots who exhibited such stress resistance, for example, were then, as now, among the most well-trained, proficient, and confident of military personnel. Combat efficiency was best predicted by flying skill in the Second World War, and subsequent studies with groups as diverse as bomb disposal operators and astronauts appear to reinforce the message: confidence in one's own competence is an effective stress countermeasure.[56] Recent research conducted by one of the authors and discussed in Chapter 3 has provided experimental evidence that it may be the quality of the pilot's internalized representation (of the airspace, his aircraft systems, and so forth) -- in other words, the sophistication of his 'mental model' -- that confers both decision making proficiency and stress resistance. In this study, one personality measure usually considered to be relevant to this, trait anxiety, had no apparent effect upon expert performance, while non-aviation specific cognitive functions (such as memory and spatial ability) were equally affected by stress in both expert and novice aviators.[68]

Self efficacy and combat stress. The combination of actual competence and a belief or confidence in this competence often seen in experts recalls the idea of self efficacy discussed in Chapter 6. In fact, perceived self efficacy is a concept that has been utilized as a mediating variable to predict combat performance. There is empirical evidence for the claim that personnel suffering from combat stress do, indeed, exhibit lower perceived self efficacy scores.[74] However, the causal relationship is not clear: it has not been demonstrated whether lower perceived self efficacy contributes to the breakdown in combat effectiveness, or is itself a result of it. Level of perceived self efficacy appears to be conceptually little different from the degree of match between perceived demand and perceived coping resources (discussed in Chapter 1 under transactional models of stress and represented diagrammatically in Chapter 2). More specifically, it appears to map onto Lazarus's notion of 'secondary appraisal', where primary

appraisal is concerned with the evaluation of the threat itself, and secondary appraisal with an evaluation of ones ability to cope with the threat.[39]
In this view, to consider perceived self efficacy (or lack thereof) as being
either a causal antecedent or a result of combat stress may be to risk circu-
larity or even a category error, since it can be argued that perceived self
efficacy simply labels an important mechanism of stress: the metacognitive
evaluation of situational demand versus resources to cope. A very similar
argument can be made about the concept of 'confidence expectancy', a
construct that is closely related to perceived self efficacy. Confidence
expectancy refers to the subjective probability of personal injury or death
that an individual assigns to a situation on the basis of prior experience.
Again, this construct represents an expression of the 'match/mismatch'
cognitive appraisal theory of stress; there is evidence that questionnaires
intended to index confidence expectancy and administered prior to exposure to the stressful situation can predict performance under stress.[34]

Morale and group cohesion. Earlier we referred to the beleaguered pilots
of the Battle of Britain era RAF, about six hundred of whom held off most
of the German Luftwaffe through the summer and early autumn of 1940.
Considering the extraordinary circumstances of the time -- fatigue, danger,
and uncertainty, including the expectation of invasion any day (perhaps
paratroops on the airfields), the rate of psychiatric casualties in Fighter
Command at that time appears to have been remarkably low. In contrast,
despite appalling losses morale seems to have been extraordinarily high.
With fine aircraft, the world's most advanced interception system (the
newly developed radar), and a belief in their cause (not to speak of a private slang and an unwritten raffish dress code), the fighter squadrons
developed an *esprit de corps* which has become legendary. In other words,
as military formations these squadrons had quite remarkable group cohesion, a factor now recognized as an important variable in controlling the
incidence of combat stress casualties.

As Patricia Backer and Judith Orasanu have pointed out in an excellent
literature review on stress and training in the military, the group cohesion
concept stemmed from work conducted at the Massachussetts Institute of
Technology not long after the Battle of Britain was fought. The concept
includes notions of unity, morale, teamwork, role clarity, loyalty, and a
sense of belonging, purpose, and empowerment. Regrettably, however,
much of the literature on group cohesion has neither been consistent nor
statistically sound, although studies conducted since 1988 tend to reinforce

the view that unit cohesion is indeed strongly predictive of military performance and directly linked to the number of combat stress casualties.[5]

Combat exposure and stress in aircrew: a case study

During the Second World War the Flying Personnel Research Committee (FPRC) of the British Ministry of Defence produced a series of papers on operational stress in aircrew. The personnel most frequently scrutinized were the crews of the Royal Air Force Bomber Command. In the years 1943 and 1944 these bomber crews experienced tours of duty that were among the most harrowing of that or any other war, involving the repeated long range nighttime penetration of well-defended enemy airspace. This involved manning a bomber, whose initial weight largely comprised high exposives, incendiaries, petrol, and hot engines, while being shot at by anti-aircraft guns and night fighters. The crews had to endure long flights in cramped conditions and subzero temperatures in the full knowledge that the chances of surviving a tour of operations (thirty missions) were slim indeed, sometimes as low as 10 percent.[23]

The effect of this upon the physical and psychological well-being of the aircrew was studied with a view to determining the risks of 'nervous breakdowns' and the optimal length of a tour of operations, an issue which again became a topic of controversy during the Vietnam War. A report that emerged from FPRC in November 1944 examined three variables which were taken as indices of stress: weight loss, liability to psychological disorders, and sickness rates.[57] Operational crews were contrasted with crews in Operational Training Units, such that the same amount of flying had been accomplished by each group over the selected time period.

Altogether some seven thousand aircrew were studied. Weight data were recorded along with height and age data, and among operational crews were broken down by number of missions flown. Liability to sickness was indexed by measuring attendance on sick parade, while liability to psychological disorders was indexed by referrals for neuropsychiatric treatment. Results indicated that significant weight loss occurred in the aircrew of operational squadrons but not of Operational Training Units. However, the loss occurred in the first third of the tour of duty, subsequently stabilizing at a slightly recovered value until the end of the tour. These losses were not related to selective elimination in combat by age or height. An apparent increase in sickness, also in the first third of the tour, was not statistically significant. However, a significant increase in the rel-

> *I knew three crews during the Battle of Berlin who obviously were in bad shape because of fatigue and should have been rested. Two didn't survive. One of the crews had several close calls and the pilot was a nervous wreck. On one trip they were hit by Flak and the navigator and wireless operator were injured. On another trip they were sprayed with shells from a night-fighter. One shell came through the windshield right in front of the pilot -- the shoulder of his jacket was sliced through. He was not injured but his journey home was a nightmare because of the blast of air through the hole in the windscreen and manhandling a Lancaster which had some of its controls damaged. It was obvious that this crew had had its nine lives and was so shattered by fatigue and tension that there was little chance of them surviving if they continued to operate. They were not rested and they perished.*
>
> *-- Pilot Officer Joe Sheriff (cited in Middlebrook,[45] p. 315)*

ative liability to psychological disorders was observed, again in the first 30 percent of operational missions. It was concluded that there are palpable stress effects as aircrew undergo their 'baptism of fire', but that deterioration halts and well-being stabilizes at lower but acceptable levels as operational hours continue. On the other hand, postwar American studies of US bomber crews provided results that are not consistent with this. US data suggested that the more missions a crew had completed, the less willing the flyers were to sign up for another tour of combat duty, and the more they sought lower risk operations. In other words, fear and anxiety appeared to be directly related to length of exposure to combat.[62]

One confounding factor that could be proposed for the RAF study relates to selective pressures arising from the high losses in the 1943-1944 night bomber offensive. Those in the operational group were necessarily those who had survived; it might be argued that perhaps these aircrew had mental and physical characteristics that were superior to those of comrades who had 'failed to return'. In fact, however, this is unlikely. First, bombers such as the Lancaster carried seven crew members, and loss of the aircraft frequently resulted in loss of the entire crew; the process was therefore highly unselective. Second, most evidence is consistent with the discouraging conclusion that skill, courage, and experience provided little protection to night bomber crews in the skies over Germany. Losses were random and indiscriminate. The methodological approach of this study, therefore, was probably adequate given its objectives and the state of knowledge at the time.

A second problem is more intransigent, however, and highlights the dangers of relying too heavily on physiological measures and their correlates (e.g., rates of reporting sick). Such indices of stress are said to 'stabilize' after the initial increase in stress related symptoms. Both research and anecdotal evidence, however, suggest that combat stress is not moderated by prolonged exposure to battle but rather builds chronically.[75] However, in the wartime RAF, very severe sanctions were at hand for aircrew who too readily admitted to or could not conceal dysfunctional levels of stress. These sanctions included having one's papers stamped "LMF" in red (Lack of Moral Fibre, i.e., cowardice) and being transferred away from friends and comrades as an AC2 (aircraftman second class) to a more menial ground based job in another unit, never to return. Given this, it is possible that 'stabilization' in some of the overt symptoms, such as rates of presenting on sick parade or reporting psychiatric problems to the Medical Officer, conceal the buildup of chronic anxiety. One behavioural correlate of decreased morale, for example, was the rate of early or premature returns from a raid as war-weary crews found reasons to turn back, and there is evidence that the rate of early returns from raids increased steadily throughout the seven month Berlin offensive.[45] Indeed, there are numerous subtle chronic symptoms characteristic of 'burnout' (see also Chapter 10) which are ignored only at the risk of losing aircrew.

The results from most studies of combat stress exposure published in the four decades following the Second World War reinforce the contention that the intensity of fighting and its duration are indeed the most important factors associated with the emergence of 'battle fatigue', rather than the individual's 'moral fibre' or any other predisposing personality factors.[66] (A good deal of this research, however, is concerned more with post-traumatic stress disorder -- that is, with the psychological sequelae of combat -- than with combat stress itself.[73])

Conclusion

Fear of flying has sometimes been simply written off as the nervous over-reaction of the unduly timid. It is seen in an unflattering light as not quite reasonable or even irrational, a flight 'phobia', which, except for intractable cases, should be amenable to therapeutic intervention. For a 'condition', however, flight anxiety has been oddly impervious to economical description, appearing to be multifaceted and arising in the context of diverse precursors or 'causes'. Fear of flying and combat stress have much in common. Combat stress reaction has historically been regarded in an even more unflattering light, having at times been looked on as evidence of cowardice, lack of 'character', or more recently as an understandable overreaction of vulnerable (inadequate, perhaps?) personalities who with appropriate intervention might still be returned to battle. As with flight anxiety, there is some evidence of predisposing personality traits: for example, the profile said to stereotype military pilots (egotistical, highly confident, conformist) has been suggested as being linked with maladaptive psychological defence mechanisms (see Chapter 6). Overall, however, while there is some evidence that stress in general may be mediated by certain personality traits, beliefs, and attitudes, persons of all psychological types are likely to be vulnerable to the effects of *severely* stressful conditions, and the diversity of symptoms and their precursors is impressive.

Against this backdrop, the question we wish to raise concerns, as it were, the burden of proof. That is, which set of observations need explanation: the fearfulness of the minority, or the relative fearlessness of the majority? Observers from another planet might well note that human beings are a remarkably unafraid, indeed, a downright courageous species, delighting in high speeds, novelty, conflict and risk. Everyday examples of courage, resolution and fortitude abound, while cowardice and timidity are strongly proscribed. In human society, 'bearing up' is expected. Bravery is a norm. These same aliens might further record, with puzzlement, that what fear humans do have is distributed with curious disregard to threat potential. Many humans are far more afraid of spiders and snakes than they ought to be, and far less afraid than they ought to be of careening about at sixty miles per hour without wearing seat belts. From this perspective the more challenging question is not why some people are flight anxious, but why most of us, most of the time, are so sanguine about committing our fragile bodies to the stratosphere at 600 miles an hour. The rationalist or statistical reply -- that people know that airline fatalities are rare -- is not persuasive. Spider bite fatalities are also rare.* People fear street murder, a low probability demise that receives tremendous news coverage, but they don't fear diabetes or pneumonia, rather likely killers

---

*As rare as football pools or lottery jackpots. Probability theory, our planetary neighbours might conclude, is not a human strong point.

that receive little or no coverage. Like street murder, aviation accidents and combat casualties attract graphic news coverage. We fly (and join the Air Force) anyway.

There is, we believe, a unifying construct underpinning human willingness to fly, go into combat, or indeed to bungee jump, scuba dive, or race motorcycles. A clue to this was discussed in the section on how combat stress is brought about, that is, the concept of 'depressive realism', which we described as a pessimistic but, in probabilistic terms, accurate assessment of the real risks of everyday life. A corollary is that normal, nondepressed individuals walk through life in a (protective) state of 'optimistic unreality', systematically overestimating the control that they have over events and unconsciously downplaying the risks. This sense of control is buttressed by a number of variables. These probably include, but are not limited to, confidence in society, faith in the power and integrity of organizations and institutions (including goverment, aircraft manufacturers, and airlines), trust in the competence and protective power of leadership and colleagues, and a belief in the efficacy of one's own training and capabilities (see also 'Automation Complacency' in Chapter 12). Together these beliefs confer a sense of security tantamount to invulnerability. To this extent, the curious courage exhibited by humans comes from the sense that each of us is 'plugged into' a vastly broader pool of coping resources than our own. Our courage is cultural and societal rather than merely personal.

Some light is thrown on this by circumstances that place events beyond the personal influence of the individual. The unease felt by many airline passengers[*] probably relates to the surrender of (any possibility of) personal control of events. In most cases, however, the remainder of the belief system is intact, and, together with social pressure to conform, affords sufficient defence against levels of anxiety that would change overt behaviour to the extent of being labelled 'phobic'. Perhaps what we observe in cases of flight anxiety, combat stress reaction, and some cases of stress induced inaction is a breakdown in these (for want of a better term) 'cultural' defences, and in some cases their replacement by nonadaptive psychological defence mechanisms.

This interpretation is certainly consistent with the success of therapy for focussed conditions such as airsickness, and the resistance of more generalized flight anxiety to treatment. Therapy probably cannot compensate very readily for lost confidence in friends, colleagues, leaders, and institutions

---

[*]The authors have, on several occasions, witnessed the spontaneous outbreak of applause upon touchdown after quite normal airline flights.

or society. This view is also consistent with the very varied aetiologies noted in the literature on flight anxiety and combat stress, for the undermining of 'cultural' defences, the destabilizing of the interlocking structure of supportive beliefs about a benign and protective society, may proceed from many points. For one individual, a precipitating factor might be distrust of a society seen as unjust, unstable, and crime ridden, while for another a history of negative life events might be involved. For some, the experience of a single 'close call' provokes an acute sense of mortality, sometimes linked to a realization that, in extremis, one may be quite alone.

Flight anxiety, like combat stress, may flourish where company policy (airline, military formation, etc.) seems unsupportive or downright hostile, leaders incompetent or self seeking, and colleagues undependable, low spirited, and cowed. Indeed, evidence presented in Chapter 11 suggests that company instability and employee/management conflict are among the most potent contributors to pilot stress. In Chapter 10, as well, evidence points to the crucial role of management in the stress experienced by air traffic controllers. Historically, manifestations of flight anxiety and combat stress, and official responses to them, may tell us us more about the contemporary society and its institutions than about the stress casualties themselves. Taking all these clues together, the message may be that the prevention of stress casualties, in peace or war, lies to a great extent in perceptions of the qualities of our society, its organizations, processes, and leadership.

This still leaves the issue of training and expertise and the extent to which these can mitigate the effects of stress in the inevitably imperfect world of airlines, flying schools, and military squadrons. Heaslip and his colleagues[32] call for more training to counter the 'frozen pilot syndrome', and more training is certainly welcome. Nevertheless, as we stated earlier, whether training or selection is the answer (and what sort of training or selection) depends very largely upon how one models the problem.

Further training is certainly indicated for those crew members who have training deficiencies or whose knowledge is poorly consolidated to the point that they lack self confidence. We reviewed evidence that individual competence, and confidence in that competence (perceived self efficacy) were potent counters to stress. Moreover, we noted that the quality of the internalized relationships, the 'mental model' or representation of the knowledge domain was a specific aspect or outcome of training that appeared to convey stress resistance, irrespective of trait anxiety. A sophisticated mental model provides a paddle for every creek, as it were, protects against reversion to slow controlled processing, and unifies and provides coherence for the repertoire of situational experiences that underpin recognition primed decision making (the long term memory decision making strategy described both by Stokes[68,69] and Klein[36] -- see Chapter 4). We think it most likely that attempts to train this in a stressed environment will simply damage and delay the process. Equally importantly, crew members should be trained to recognize flight anxiety or stress induced inaction on the part of their flight deck colleagues, and to intervene if necessary in a timely way, just as they are trained (in cockpit resource management courses) to assert control in the case of the physical incapacitation of fellow crew members.

Among aircrew who are, or are projected to be, trained to a uniformly high standard of performance, further training is not likely to make the difference between stress induced inaction and an appropriate response, or between acute combat stress reaction and well-being. Selection appears to be the most promising avenue in this case. Moreover, there seems to be a good case for attempting to select out, quite specifically, those individuals whose coping style in extremes of stress may be defensively maladaptive. Here the experience of certain European air forces, particularly in Sweden,[48] could be brought to bear on the problem. Specifically, assessment tools which do what the Defence Mechanism Test[37] (see Chapter 6) tries to do could conceivably have applications even for airline pilot screening, and might over time provide a useful database from which to evaluate several of the hypotheses discussed in this chapter.

References

1. Aitken, J.R., and Benson, J.W. (1984), 'The use of relaxation/desensitization in treating anxiety associated with flying', *Aviation, Space, and Environmental Medicine*, vol. 55, pp. 196-9.

2. Alloy, L., and Abramson, L. (1988), 'Depressive Realism: Four Theoretical Perspectives', in Alloy, L. (ed.), *Cognitive Processes in Depression*, Guilford Press, New York.

3. Anderson, H.G. (1919), 'The Psychology of Aviation', in *The Medical and Surgical Aspects of Aviation*, Oxford University Press, London.

4. Armstrong, H.G. (1939), *Principles and Practice of Aviation Medicine*, Williams and Wilkins Co., Baltimore.

5. Backer, P.R., and Orasanu, J.M. (1992), 'Stress and performance training: A review of the literature with respect to military applications', Paper presented at the Annual Meeting of the American Educational Research Association, San Francisco, California.

6. Bartemeier, L.H. (1946), 'Combat exhaustion', *Journal of Nervous and Mental Disease*, vol. 104, pp. 359-425.

7. Benson, J.W., and Aitken, J.R. (1985), 'Psychological differences noted in aircrewmembers undergoing systematic desensitization and their subsequent functioning', *Aviation, Space, and Environmental Medicine*, vol. 56, pp. 238-41.

8. Bond, D.C. (1952), *The Love and Fear of Flying*, International Universities Press, New York.

9. Bourne, P.G. (1970), *Men, Stress and Vietnam*, Little, Brown & Co., Boston.

10. Breznitz, S. (1967), 'Incubation of threat: duration of anticipation and false alarm as determinants of the fear reaction to an unavoidable frightening event', *Journal of Experimental Research in Personality*, vol. 2, pp. 173-9.

11. Breznitz, S. (1971), 'A study of worrying', *British Journal of Social and Clinical Psychology*, vol. 10, pp. 271-9.

12. Carr, J.E. (1978), 'Behavior therapy and the treatment of flight phobias', *Aviation, Space, and Environmental Medicine*, vol. 49, pp. 1115-9.

13. Carson, D.M. (1982), 'Temporal distortions and the ejection decision', *Flying Safety*, vol. 38, pp. 8-28.

14. Carson, D.M. (1983), 'Temporal distortions and the ejection decision: an update', *Flying Safety*, vol. 39, pp. 5-7.

15. Carter, B.J., and Cammermayer, M. (1985), 'Emergence of real casualties during simulated chemical warfare training under high heat conditions', *Military Medicine,* vol. 150, pp. 657-65.

16. Curran, P., and Wherry, R.J. (1967), 'Some secondary determiners of psychological stress', *Aerospace Medicine,* vol. 38, pp. 278-81.

17. Davis, D.B. (1945), 'Phobias in pilots', *Military Surgery,* vol. 105, p. 11.

18. Dennholtz, M.S., Hall, L.A., and Mann, E. (1978), 'Automated treatment for flight phobia: a three-and-one-half year follow-up', *American Journal of Psychiatry,* vol. 135, pp. 1340-3.

19. Drinkwater, B.L., Cleland, T., and Flint, M.M. (1968), 'Pilot performance during anticipatory physical threat stress', *Aerospace Medicine,* vol. 39, pp. 994-9.

20. Easterbrook, J.A. (1959), 'The effect of emotion on cue utilization and the organization of behavior', *Psychological Review,* vol. 66, pp. 183-201.

21. Ellis, J.P., Jr., Hartman, B.O., Bollinger, R.R., and Garcia, J.B., Jr. (1976), 'Flight-induced changes in human amino acid excretion', *Aviation, Space, and Environmental Medicine,* vol. 47, pp. 1-8.

22. Falk, J.L., and Bindra, D. (1954), 'Judgement of time as a function of serial position and stress', *JEP,* vol. 47, pp. 279-82.

23. Frankland, N. (1965), *The Bombing Offensive Against Germany,* Faber & Faber, London.

24. Gal, R. (1986), 'Unit morale: from a theoretical puzzle to an empirical solution: an Israeli example', *Journal of Applied Social Psychology,* vol. 16, pp. 549-64.

25. Girodo, M., and Roehl, J. (1978), 'Cognitive preparation and coping self-talk: anxiety management during the stress of flying', *Journal of Consulting and Clinical Psychology,* vol. 46, pp. 978-89.

26. Glass, D.C., and Singer, J.E. (1972), *Urban Stress,* Academic Press, New York.

27. Goorney, A.B., and O'Connor, P.J. (1971), 'Anxiety associated with flying: a retrospective survey of military aircrew psychiatric casualties', *British Journal of Psychiatry,* vol. 119, pp. 159-66.

28. Gotch, O.H. (1919), 'The Aero-Neurosis of War Pilots', in *The Medical and Surgical Aspects of Aviation,* Oxford University Press, London.

29. Grinker, R. R., and Spiegel, J.P. (1945), *War Neuroses,* The Blakiston Company, Philadelphia and Toronto.

30. Hancock, P.A., and Carson, D.M. (1987), 'The time trap: temporal incongruencies under stressful conditions', *Aviation, Space, and Environmental Medicine.*

31. Hastings, D., Wright, D., and Glueck, B. (1944), *Psychiatric Experiences of the Eighth Air Force,* Josiah Macy Foundation, New York.

32. Heaslip, T.W., Hull, N., McLeod, R.K., and Vermij, M. (1991), 'The Frozen Pilot Syndrome', *Proceedings of the Sixth International Symposium on Aviation Psychology,* Ohio State University, Columbus.

33. Hess, A. (1980), 'Psychological Reactions During War and their Treatments', unpublished report, Israeli Air Force.

34. Keinan, G. (1986), 'Confidence Expectancy as Predictor of Military Performance under Stress', in Milgram, N.A. (ed.), *Stress and Coping in Time of War: Generalizations from the Israeli Experience,* Brunner/Mazel, New York.

35. Keinan, G. (1987), 'Decision making under stress: scanning of alternatives under controllable and uncontrollable threats', *Journal of Personality and Social Psychology,* vol. 52, pp. 639-44.

36. Klein, G.A. (1989), 'Recognition-Primed Decisions', in Rouse, W. (ed.), *Advances in Man-Machine Systems Research*, vol. 5, JAI Press, Inc., Greenwich, Connecticut, pp. 47-92.

37. Kragh, U. (1960), 'The defense mechanism test: a new method for diagnosis and personnel selection', *Journal of Applied Psychology*, vol. 44, pp. 303-9.

38. Krahenbuhl, G.S., Darst, P.W., Marett, J.R., Reuther, L.C., Constable, S.H., Swinford, M.E., and Reid, G.B. (1981), 'Instructor pilot teaching behavior and student pilot stress in flight training', *Aviation, Space, and Environmental Medicine*, vol. 52, pp. 594-7.

39. Lazurus, R.S. (1966), *Psychological Stress and the Coping Process*, McGraw-Hill, New York.

40. Lepley, W. (ed.) (1947), *Psychological Research in the Theaters of War*, USAAF Psychology Research Report 17, US Government Printing Office, Washington, DC.

41. Levy, R.A., Jones, D.R., and Carlson, E.H. (1981), 'Biofeedback rehabilitation of airsick crew', *Aviation, Space, and Environmental Medicine*, vol. 52, pp. 118-21.

42. Lifton, R.J. (1953), 'Psychotherapy with combat fliers', *U.S. Armed Forces Medical Journal*, vol. 4, pp. 525-32.

43. Mandler, G. (1967), invited commentary, in Appley, M.H. and Trumbull, R. (eds.), *Psychological Stress: Issues in Research*, Appleton-Century-Crofts, New York.

44. McLeod, R.K. (1993), personal communication.

45. Middlebrook, M. (1988), *The Berlin Raids*, Viking, New York.

46. Milgram, N.A. (1986), 'An Attributional Analysis of War-Related Stress: Modes of Coping and Helping', in Milgram, N.A. (ed.), *Stress and Coping in Time of War: Generalizations from the Israeli Experience*, Brunner/Mazel, New York.

47. Morgenstern, A.L. (1967), 'Phobic reactions to flying', *Int. Psychiatric Clin.*, vol. 4, pp. 155-75.

48. Neuman, T. (1978), *Dimensioning and Validation of Percept-Genetic Defence Mechanisms. A hierarchical analysis of the behaviour of pilots under stress,* FOA Report C55020-H6, Translated from Swedish by R.E. Williams, 1985. Her Majesty's Stationery Office, London.

49. Noy, S., Nardi, C., and Solomon, Z. (1986), 'Battle and Military Unit Characteristics and the Prevalence of Psychiatric Casualties', in Milgram, N.A. (ed.), *Stress and Coping in Time of War: Generalizations from the Israeli Experience,* Brunner/Mazel, New York.

50. O'Connor, P., and Lister, J. (1973), 'Results of behavior therapy in flying phobias', *Advisory Group for Aeronautics Research and Development*, vol. 133, pp. 15-29.

51. Paterson, R.J., and Neufeld, R.W.J. (1987), 'Clear danger: situational determinants of the appraisal of threat', *Psychological Bulletin,* vol. 101, pp. 404-16.

52. Pepitone, D., King, T., and Murphy, M. (1988), 'The Role of Flight Planning in Aircrew Decision Performance', presented at the Society of Automotive Engineers Annual Aerotech Conference, Anaheim, California.

53. Perry, C.J.G. (1971), 'Aerospace Psychiatry', in Randel, H.W. (ed.), *Aerospace Medicine,* Williams & Wilkins, Baltimore.

54. Pilmore, F.U. (1919), 'The nervous element in aviation', *Naval Medical Bulletin,* vol. 13, pp. 457-78.

55. Rabinowitz, S., and Hess, A. (1984), 'Fear of flying: an Israeli Air Force short case report', *Aviation, Space, and Environmental Medicine,* vol. 55, pp. 316-8.

56. Rachman, S.J. (1990), *Fear and Courage,* 2nd ed., W.H. Freeman & Co., New York.

57. Reid, D.D. (1944), 'Some Measures of the Effect of Operational Stress on Bomber Crews', Flying Personnel Research Committee Report No. 605. Reprinted in Dearnley, E.J., and Warr, P.B. (eds.) (1979), *Aircrew Stress in Wartime Operations*, Academic Press, London.

58. Rosenthal, T. (1978), 'Stimulus modality and aerophobics: cautions for desensitization therapy', *Aviation, Space, and Environmental Medicine*, vol. 49, pp. 115-9.

59. Schaefer, V.G., and Gilliland, A.R. (1938), 'The relation of time estimation to certain physiological changes', *Journal of Experimental Psychology*, vol. 23, pp. 545-52.

60. Schneider, W., and Shiffrin, R.M. (1977), 'Controlled and automatic human information processing: I. Detection, search and attention', *Psychological Review*, vol. 84, pp. 1-66.

61. Segal, R., and Margalit, C. (1986), 'Risk Factors, Premorbid Adjustment, and Personality Characteristics of Soldiers with Refractory Combat Stress Reactions', in Milgram, N.A. (ed.), *Stress and Coping in Time of War: Generalizations from the Israeli Experience*, Brunner/Mazel, New York.

62. Shaffer, L.F. (1951), 'Fear in Combat and Its Control', Working Group on Human Behavior Under Conditions of Military Service, Department of Defense, Research and Development Board, Washington, DC.

63. Shaw, J.A. (1983), 'Comments on the individual psychology of combat exhaustion', *Military Medicine*, vol. 148, pp. 223-5.

64. Simmel, E.C., Cerkovnik, M., and McCarthy, J.E. (1987), 'Sources of Stress Affecting Pilot Judgment', *Proceedings of the Fourth International Symposium on Aviation Psychology*, Ohio State University, Columbus.

65. Solomon, Z. (1993), *Combat Stress Reaction: The Enduring Toll of War*, Plenum Press, New York and London.

66. Solomon, Z., Noy, S., and Bar-On, R. (1986), 'Who Is at High Risk for a Combat Stress Reaction Syndrome?' in Milgram, N.A. (ed.), *Stress and Coping in Time of War: Generalizations from the Israeli Experience,* Brunner/Mazel, New York.

67. Sours, J.E., Ehrlich, R.E., and Phillips, P.B. (1964), 'The fear of flying syndrome: a reappraisal', *Aerospace Medicine,* vol. 35, pp. 156-66.

68. Stokes, A.F., Belger, A., and Zhang, K. (1990), *Investigation of Factors Comprising a Model of Pilot Decision Making: Part II. Anxiety and Cognitive Strategies in Expert and Novice Aviators,* University of Illinois Aviation Research Laboratory, Savoy.

69. Stokes, A.F., Kemper, K.L., and Marsh, R. (1992), *Time-Stressed Flight Decision Making: A Study of Expert and Novice Aviators,* University of Illinois Aviation Research Laboratory, Savoy.

70. Stouffer, S.A., Lumsdaine, A.A., Lumsdaine, M.H., Williams, R.M., Smith, M.B., Janis, I.L., Star, S.A., and Cottrell, L.S. (1949), *The American Soldier: Combat and Its Aftermath,* vol. 2, Princeton University Press, New Jersey.

71. Strongin, T.S. (1987), 'A historical review of the fear of flying among aircrewmen', *Aviation, Space, and Environmental Medicine,* vol. 58, pp. 263-7.

72. Suarez, S.D., and Gallup, G.G. (1979), 'Tonic immobility as a response to rage in humans: a theoretical note', *Psychol. Record.,* vol. 29, pp. 315-20.

73. Weaver, S.F., and Stewart, N.K. (1988), 'Factors Influencing Combat Stress Reactions and Post-Traumatic Stress Disorder: A Literature Review', Technical Report 791, US Army Research Institute for the Behavioral and Social Sciences.

74. Weisenberg, M., Schwarzwald, J., and Solomon, Z. (1991), Effects of combat stress reaction and posttraumatic stress reaction on perceived self-efficacy in battle, *Military Psychology,* vol. 3, pp. 61-71.

75. Wherry, R.J. (1966), 'Model for the study of psychological stress', *Aerospace Medicine,* vol. 37, pp. 495-9.

76. White, R.W., and Watt, N.F. (1973), *The Abnormal Personality,* 4th ed., Ronald Press Company, New York.

77. Wolpe, J., Brady, J., Serber, M., Agras, S., and Liberman, R., (1973), 'The current status of systematic desensitization', *American Journal of Psychiatry,* vol. 130, pp. 961-5.

78. Yitzhaki, T., Solomon, Z., and Kotler, M. (1991), 'The clinical picture of the immediate combat stress reaction (CSR) in the Lebanon war', *Military Medicine,* vol. 156, pp. 193-7.

8 Fatigue in flight operations

I'm so tired, I haven't slept a wink
I'm so tired, my mind is on the blink.
-- Lennon and McCartney

Ye be wearied and faint in your minds.
-- Hebrews 12:13

Fatigue, it has long been recognized, affects the mind and emotions as well as the body. The issue of fatigue is, therefore, an important one in any discussion of pilots' cognitive performance. This is perhaps most obvious where aircrew fatigue is implicated in aviation accidents, but it is relevant not only to considerations of public safety but to pilot efficiency and well-being. A review of the subject, however, shows a decided lack of consensus as to how fatigue should be measured or, indeed, defined. Since no widely accepted definition of fatigue currently exists, each investigator typically supplies his or her own,[18] one result being that studies of pilot fatigue vary so much in both criteria and methodology that they are often difficult to compare with one another.

One researcher, for example, reports that pilots performing flight simulator tasks make the largest number of errors between midnight and 6:00 a.m.[40] Another looks not at errors made on laboratory equipment but at accident statistics in the real world, and concludes that a key predictor of fatigue related accident involvement is the amount of flying the pilot has done in the preceding twenty-four hours.[9] A third evaluates fatigue by observing aircrew members in various work environments and asking them whether they feel tired. Clearly, these investigators have different ways of approaching the subject of pilot fatigue and, probably, different ways of defining it. To integrate and draw conclusions from such disparate data, we need to have a clear model of what fatigue is and how it is properly assessed.

235

The nature of fatigue

The word 'fatigue' is, like the word 'stress', an umbrella term that encompasses many meanings. The phrase *physical fatigue*, for example, may refer variously to muscle soreness, oxygen debt, or to more systemic feelings of tiredness caused by sleep deprivation, illness, or poor nutrition (see sidebar). *Mental fatigue* is typically associated with tasks demanding intense concentration, rapid or complex information processing, and other high level cognitive skills. Examples of flight operations likely to engender this type of fatigue might include single pilot night instrument approaches at unfamiliar airports, or air combat maneuvering exercises. Alternatively, mental fatigue may arise from prolonged (if less intense) activity -- particularly those requiring sustained alertness such as maritime search patrols or long haul low level pipeline inspection flights. Yet another state which might be included in this category of fatigue is that of boredom, particularly when it results from repetitive or monotonous activity (see Chapter 12). Finally, one may speak of *emotional fatigue* or 'burnout' -- that is, the wearying effect of working under trying conditions or performing psychologically disagreeable tasks. (The association of this type of state with fatigue is borne out in the language, as when we speak of being 'tired of' the same old grind, or 'worn out by' constant bickering.)

Newark International Airport, New Jersey, June, 1992: We overshot the initial level off altitude by 500 feet. The Standard Instrument Departure (SID) calls for an initial level off at 5,000 feet. However, the SID had been amended that morning to 2,500 feet but we did not notice this.

Crew meals had been removed from the aircraft. We were hungry, weak and had no opportunity to acquire a nutritional meal. Our judgement may have been impaired with a lack of nutritional sustenance. There are many trips where we fly a total of eight hours or more and are on duty for fourteen to sixteen hours without access to a morsel of food. This, in my view, poses a serious decrement to safety.

-- NASA Aviation Safety Reporting System (Accession No. 215225)*

---

*It is interesting to compare this first officer's account of the incident with that of his captain (Accession No. 214452), which appears on p. 355.

This account of fatigue 'types' is not intended to serve as a formal taxonomy, but merely to convey some idea of the scope of the word as it is commonly used. While it can be informative to describe fatigue in terms of locus (body, mind, emotions) and assumed cause (intense workload, prolonged workload, and so forth), this approach to the subject also has significant limitations.

First, the distinction between physical and mental fatigue can become somewhat muddy in the real world. Some conditions (for example, sleep deprivation) are clearly associated with both physical and mental depletion; in any case, the distinction between mind and body is increasingly recognized as being at best somewhat blurred, and at worst artificial and misleading. As for 'classifying' fatigue according to the various factors that can give rise to it, there are obvious logical pitfalls inherent in defining any phenomenon in such a manner: it does not follow that if (for example) sustained effort causes fatigue, it is therefore a *kind* of fatigue. Rather than attempting to compile a comprehensive catalogue of fatigue 'types', then, it may be more useful to consider the various criteria by which fatigue is recognized.

Houston, June, 1991: We requested runway 12 Right for departure. The tower cleared us to "position and hold 12 Right". We were running the checklist and I taxied onto runway 17. The tower cleared us for takeoff and about 500 feet down the runway the controller said "You're on 17 but that's OK, you're cleared for takeoff." I was the captain and accept full responsibility for the occurrence. Our airline is in Chapter 11 bankruptcy and all pilots are flying an average of ninety plus hours per month with eight days off and no schedules. Everyone is fatigued and 'burned out'. I know the FAA says it's legal to work these schedules but they are not the ones flying them. I think the duty regulation under Federal Aviation Regulations Part 135 should be changed.

[ASRS called this reporter for further details: reporter emphasized that his company's financial straits have put a lot of pressure upon all the employees through excessively long work days and resultant fatigue. Reporter believes that companies take undue advantage of their employees under the current set of rules.]

-- NASA Aviation Safety Reporting System (Accession No. 182481)

Subjective criteria

One way to assess fatigue is simply by personal report: just as a person who perceives that he has a headache, does, by definition, in fact have one, so a person who *feels* tired *is* tired. Certainly this approach accords with the way the concept is applied in ordinary discourse. When an individual states that he is fatigued, we do not say, "Oh? Prove it!" But we sometimes seek to clarify the source and nature of the fatigue by asking questions such as, "Have you had a long day? Been jogging too much? Going to bed late? Working night shifts?" Similarly, from the standpoint of empirical research it may, of course, be useful to know whether a pilot 'feels tired' after performing a particular flight operation, and some studies do employ self reported assessments as one way of measuring fatigue.

Whether such reports are meaningful, consistent, or generalizable is, of course, another matter: although attempts have been made to correlate subjective assessments of fatigue with objective measures,[69] their validity has been called into question.[19] Despite these limitations, it could be argued that subjective measures have a certain inherent appropriateness, since some aspects of fatigue are not fully amenable to empirical quantification.

Functional criteria

Another way of looking at fatigue is to examine its practical effects -- that is, the associated decrease in work efficiency or increase in the number and severity of errors made. For example, a tired pilot might increasingly fail to notice nearby aircraft in an timely manner; this drop in vigilance could be (and generally is) interpreted as a sign of fatigue. The advantage of this approach to fatigue is obvious: performance decrement is observable, quantifiable, and, most of all, operationally relevant. The use of performance decrement as an index of fatigue can be further justified by observing that in many cases the purpose in studying fatigue in the first place is to identify the errors associated with it, so as to forestall catastrophic accidents. An argument can certainly be made, then, for studying these errors directly rather than probing more deeply into abstract conceptual models of fatigue.

There are two important pitfalls, however, in working solely from this kind of applied framework. One problem is definitional, the other practical. First, there is a tendency among many researchers to regard performance decrement as the defining quality of fatigue -- a synonym, even -- rather than as one manifestation of it. One critic of this view[18] notes, for example, that fatigue is often characterized along the lines of "decreased ability" or "a common state whereby a person fails to meet a previous standard on a repeated task" (p. 1133). While utilitarian definitions of this sort are adequate for some purposes, the dangers of circular reasoning should be obvious. The practical problem arises from the difficulty in associating performance decrements exclusively with fatigue: there are, of course, innumerable other causes of performance decrement apart from fatigue (e.g., hunger, intoxication, anxiety, lack of motivation), just as there are other effects of fatigue apart from performance decrement (e.g., physiological and neurological changes).

Approaches to fatigue assessment

Accident investigation

Nonstandardized approaches. One approach to the assessment of fatigue in aviation has been to study existing accident and incident reports with a view to determining which are fatigue related, and why. While this method might appear to provide a direct source of practical and highly relevant information on the subject, it also has some significant limitations, as the following example helps to illustrate.

In a project conducted under the auspices of Battelle Memorial Laboratories in California, Lyman and Orlady[53] reviewed over two thousand incident reports received by the Aviation Safety Reporting System (ASRS), which, as described in the preface, collects confidential reports of aircraft incidents (that is, near accidents). While fewer than 4 percent of the reports explicitly mentioned pilot fatigue as a factor, the authors suggested that the real incidence of fatigue related error may have been substantially higher, given that many of the other factors cited, such as inattention and miscommunication, could themselves have been effects of fatigue. Using broader criteria, Lyman and Orlady estimated the true rate of fatigue involvement in ASRS reported incidents to be over 21 percent. However, as noted in the preface ASRS reports should not be regarded as statistically representative, and just as there is probably more actual crime than reported crime, the real rate of fatigue related incidents may well be appreciably higher.

One consideration to be borne in mind regarding the reports is that they were not standardized in any way: they were generated by the pilots involved and were necessarily subjective, and their format, style, level of detail, and general perspective varied widely. Similar problems are likely to exist with any analysis based around existing data and reports, whether they are written by pilots (as in this particular study) or by government accident investigators (as with some other reviews). The level of sophistication regarding cockpit fatigue may vary, attitudes may vary, even definitions may vary.

A second methodological difficulty connected with retrospective accident analyses is that they generally include no statistical controls. It is, therefore, difficult to form reliable inferences about cause and effect. Lyman and Orlady maintain, for example, that 21 percent of the incidents in the ASRS database involved pilot fatigue. Even if we accept this figure, there is no way of knowing how many pilots with comparable fatigue levels were *not* involved in incidents during the same time period.

A third limitation of this type of study is that fatigue related error can have more than one source. As noted already, fatigue may stem variously from the demanding nature of the task being performed, from long hours on the job, from lack of sleep, or from any number of other factors such as physical stressors or illness. Often, of course, more than one factor may be present, and the investigator or researcher can only speculate as to which, if any, are significant. The following account, originally cited by Borowsky and Wall,[9] exemplifies this problem:

> A helicopter on an SAR (search and rescue) mission crashes into the ocean while flying at night in rain showers; causal factor -- pilot error compounded with possible vertigo and disorientation. Post mishap investigation revealed that although the pilot had slept 27.5 hours in the past four days, only 4.5 had been within twenty-four hours of the crash and that had been from 6:45 a.m. to 11:15 a.m. Another possible causal factor was found to be that the pilot had spent the nine hours prior to the mishap in an alert status, five of which were spent in the cockpit of the alert aircraft.

In this account, not one but several conditions conducive to fatigue are in evidence. They include task difficulty (resulting from poor visibility due to the darkness and rain), extended time on duty, lack of sleep, and operating at night. (As will be discussed subsequently, mental alertness and efficiency tend to be lower at this time). The authors' purpose in noting the time of day that sleep had occurred is to suggest that it was not an appropriate time in the pilot's internal sleep/wake cycle, and that what little sleep he did obtain may therefore have been of poor quality. They further suggest that he may have been suffering from circadian desynchronization (see p. 253, and also the following chapter). Any or all of these circumstances *may* have contributed to the accident; needless to say, however, no amount of hindsight or speculation can provide definitive answers.

Standardized approaches. It is, however, possible to explore these variables at the statistical level with the aid of a more structured reporting system. A report by Borowsky and Wall[9] did just this, using data on naval aircraft mishaps obtained in collaboration with the Naval Safety Center. The reports, which were completed by flight surgeons, contained detailed information concerning pilots' activities prior to accidents in which they were involved, with an emphasis on circumstances often associated with fatigue. These included the number of hours worked within the previous twenty-four and forty-eight hour periods, as well as the number of hours spent flying, the number of missions flown, and the number of hours slept within the same periods.

Other data collected included the number of hours spent continuously awake before the accident, the number of hours continuously on duty, the number of hours in the cockpit, and the duration of the most recent sleep episode. Significantly, a distinction was made between those pilots who were found to be at fault in the accidents and those who were not, although the authors suggest that pilots not involved in accidents at all might have constituted a stricter control group. Other data included aircraft type, and overall accident rates (that is, the number of accidents relative to the total number of flights) at different times of the day. This approach made it possible to identify which variables showed an actual statistical association with mishaps.

Of all these variables, only two showed a significant correlation with accident liability. One was the number of hours worked in the preceding twenty-four: pilots who had been on duty for more than ten hours had a higher accident rate than those who had worked less than than amount. The other factor proved to be time of day: flights departing between 9:00 a.m. and 6:00 p.m. were statistically less likely to involve mishaps than those beginning either before or after that period.

This does not mean that such factors as amount of prior sleep should be considered irrelevant to aircrew fatigue. Borowsky and Wall suggest a number of possible reasons for the small number of significant correlations, which, not incidentally, point up some of the challenges faced by all researchers in this area. One reason, as already noted, may lie in the nature of the control group; the use of different statistical analyses might also alter the findings. A more important possibility, however, is the likely presence of uncontrolled variables. Borowsky and Wall mention several connected with operations, including weather, speed, and the purpose of the flight.

They also suggest strongly that disruptions to the sleep/wake cycle may affect fitness for duty, citing research to the effect that attempts to sleep at an unaccustomed time of the day may not be entirely successful. For example, aircrew on nighttime assignments who are scheduled to sleep during the day may not necessarily be able to take full advantage of the time allotted to them, either in terms of the quantity or quality of sleep.[36] (The issue of biological rhythms and pilot fatigue is one that Borowsky and Wall, writing in the early 1980s, lacked the data to fully evaluate. It will, however, be addressed at some length, both in this chapter and in the one that follows.)

In summary, the study of accident (and incident) reports represents one method of investigating pilot fatigue. These reports are clearly useful as a source of anecdotal information, and can help to identify promising areas for empirical research. They are also valuable for the insights they can furnish as to likely causes of pilot fatigue, particularly when considered at the statistical level. However, research of this type has significant limitations, including the difficulty of furnishing data about the effects of fatigue on specific aspects of flying performance.

Performance testing

Another way of investigating fatigue is via the use of controlled laboratory experiments. This allows researchers to observe specific performance effects under various conditions. For the purposes of the present discussion this category of research may be divided into two types: relatively general, domain independent, or 'abstract' investigations of individual cognitive functions, and more operationally oriented tests that attempt to approximate the complexity of actual flight operations.

General tests. The general literature on fatigue related performance decrement is considerable. Many studies in this area involve such simple tasks as card sorting, basic mathematical calculations, tracking an object displayed on a computer screen, and the like. Nonspecialists may question the relevance of such abstract tests as these to the aviation environment when it is possible to observe flying performance directly in an aircraft or flight simulator. However, as we discussed in Chapter 2, flying performance, like human intelligence, does not lend itself well to simple unidimensional or 'global' assessments; it cannot be reduced to a single, measurable skill or ability. Rather, it is a complex skill involving an entire suite of cognitive functions, and one way to study complex operations is to break them down into their various component tasks and analyze each one separately. Another advantage to using simple tasks is that performance tends to be relatively easy to quantify.

Aviation specific tests. Research into the effects of fatigue on flying performance has also made use of more ecologically valid settings such as flight simulators. These tests, when well designed, can also lend themselves to quantification. An example can be seen in one study that was conducted in an F-104 simulator.[40] The subjects, who were all experienced pilots, were given a starting point and told to fly a circular pattern at a specific speed and altitude. The task was complicated by the presence of a simulated 200-knot wind which continually changed direction, and also by flight incidents built into the program (a sudden weight increase and a sudden drag increase). Performance was measured by the number of deviations from the preestablished range, altitude, and speed parameters, as well as by recovery time following any such deviations.

This approach to assessing pilot fatigue obviously differs from more domain independent laboratory tests, in that it measures not general cognitive functions but performance of specific flight tasks. However, the fact that the task is performed on a simulator and constrained in certain ways makes it possible to evaluate performance objectively and consistently.[*] We now turn from a general discussion of the ways in which fatigue is defined and investigated in the aviation world to a more specific description of the activities and situations that cause fatigue. These may be divided into factors related to the activities themselves (time on task, high workload), and factors related to the persons performing the activities (sleep deprivation, circadian rhythm effects).

---

[*]We note, parenthetically, that the purpose of the study was to determine whether performance varied at different times of the day and night, and under conditions of circadian desynchronization. As a matter of fact it did: specific findings will discussed subsequently.

Sustained effort ('time on task')

According to the classical view originally proposed by Bartlett,[3] fatigue can be described as a set of measurable changes in performance arising from extended time on task (that is, duration of activity). Implied is a more or less linear, or at least monotonic, decrement in performance the longer the activity is performed. This perspective, while useful, is now thought to be overly simplistic. Studies of driving error, for example, suggest a variety of complex patterns in the role of time on task in bus and long distance truck accidents. In the domain of flight operations, as well, Bartlett's model does not appear adequate to explain the patterns of fatigue that occur in complex, real world operations. This can be seen, for example, in the results of a review conducted by the Boeing Commercial Aircraft Company,[49] which examined fatigue related errors and scheduled time on duty using data from the Aviation Safety and Reporting System. Boeing researchers, in collaboration with the ASRS office, conducted structured telephone interviews with fifty-two respondents who had indicated fatigue as a factor in the incidents they reported. The results indicated that, far from increasing as the day progressed, the number of incidents tended to

---

New Jersey, December, 1990: Flying the morning after a minimum crew rest (and the morning after our airline had declared Chapter 11 bankruptcy) we landed in Newark after a flight up from Washington National in marginal VFR conditions. There are two taxiways entering our ramp from the inner -- RH and RK. Many times before my captains have entered the ramp via RH after being assigned RK, as this captain did twice previously during this trip. This is seldom a problem as both taxiways enter the same ramp. This time we were assigned RH. My head was down momentarily while reading the after-landing checklist, and when I looked up the captain was taxiing across the concrete median south of taxiway RH, momentarily disoriented. I asked, "Is this a taxiway?" He slowed, looked around, and replied "I guess it isn't," and continued across to the ramp. Fortunately, the aircraft was light and the concrete did not buckle, the aircraft was not damaged, and nothing further happened. I was tired and the captain had seemed quite distracted during the whole trip (day three of a three day trip).

-- NASA Aviation Safety Reporting System (Accession No. 165100)

peak in the middle of the duty period and decrease thereafter. The incident rate also decreased on a day to day basis, occurring most often at the beginning of the duty week and least often at the end. Most surprising, over 40 percent of the incidents studied occurred within the first two hours of scheduled flying time; two-thirds of these took place within the first hour. (The implications of this particular finding will be discussed later in this chapter, in the discussion of time of day effects.)

Sleep deprivation

Insufficient sleep represents another potential source of pilot fatigue, and one with particular implications for flight safety. Sleep deprived individuals are, of course, more likely to become drowsy or even doze off on the job; this can obviously have catastrophic consequences in the dynamic, unforgiving environment of an aircraft cockpit. However, lack of sleep can also affect performance in a number of additional, less drastic ways (some of which may overlap with other kinds of fatigue effects).

How little is too little?

While it might be assumed that a sleep deprived person can self evidently be defined as one who feels sleepy, there is actually more than one way of looking at the issue; perhaps surprisingly, there is no particular consensus among sleep researchers as to how much sleep is truly optimal. Modern surveys indicate that adults in our society typically sleep about seven or seven and a half hours per night; on the other hand, one team of investigators, in a paper provocatively entitled 'Are we chronically sleep deprived?', points out that in the early twentieth century people commonly slept nine hours per night.[68] Studies also show that people allowed to wake up as late as they like typically sleep for an additional two hours or more beyond the usual seven;[2,28,67] moreover, this 'extra' sleep does not shorten the amount of time slept on the following night.[22] (The same effect has been observed with daytime naps: they do not appear to diminish subsequent nighttime sleep.[21])

Implicit in these observations is the idea that a desire or capacity for sleep can be taken as evidence of actual need for sleep -- that a person who feels sleepy is, ipso facto, suffering from sleep 'deprivation'. This assumption can be challenged on several points. First, while drowsiness is

US Flight Time Limitations and Rest Requirements: Scheduled Operations

(a) A crewmember [may not fly] in scheduled operations or in other commercial flying if that crewmember's total flight time in all commercial flying will exceed --

(1) 1,200 hours in any calendar year.

(2) 120 hours in any calendar month.

(3) thirty-four hours in any seven consecutive days.

(4) eight hours during any twenty-four consecutive hours for a flight crew consisting of one pilot.

(5) eight hours between required rest periods for a flight crew consisting of two pilots qualified under this part for the operation being conducted.

(b) Except as provided at (c) in this section, no flight crewmember may accept an assignment for flight time during the twenty-four consecutive hours preceding the scheduled completion of any flight segment without a scheduled rest period during that 24 hours of at least the following:

(1) nine consecutive hours of rest for less than eight hours of scheduled flight time.

(2) ten consecutive hours of rest for eight or more but less than nine hours of scheduled flight time.

(3) eleven consecutive hours of rest for nine or more hours of scheduled flight time.

(c) A crewmember may be scheduled for less than the rest required in paragraph (b) of this section or may reduce a scheduled rest under the following conditions:

(1) A rest required under paragraph (b)(1) of this section may be scheduled for or reduced to a minimum of eight hours if the flight crewmember is given a rest period of at least ten hours that must begin no later than twenty-four hours after the commencement of the reduced rest period.

(2) The same applies if the crewmember is given a rest period of at least eleven hours that must begin no later than twenty-four hours after the commencement of the reduced rest period.

-- Condensed from FAA (1992) Federal Aviation Regulations (FAR) Part 135 (Air Taxi and Commercial Operators), paragraph 135-265.

most marked in sleep deprived individuals, it can also occur in those engaged in boring or monotonous activities. Second, the experience of sleepiness is linked not only to the amount of prior sleep obtained but also to internal biological rhythms (to be discussed), and it is quite common to feel drowsy at certain times of the day even when well rested.[55] On the other side of the coin, it has been demonstrated that most individuals can adapt to a regime of six hours of sleep per night without ill effects.[37] As researchers Carskadon and Roth[11] have pointed out, therefore, an obvious question to ask when considering adequacy of sleep is, adequate for what purpose? They go on to note that the very concept of inadequate sleep presupposes that there is also such a thing as adequate sleep, and, moreover, that this can be defined; a related question concerns the overall purpose of sleep. Perhaps surprisingly, researchers do not universally agree even on these fundamental matters, and these ambiguities should be borne in mind when applying findings from sleep research to applied settings.

Performance effects of sleep deprivation

Research on the performance effects of sleep deficit dates back to the 1890s, when three subjects at the University of Iowa psychology laboratory remained continuously awake for nearly eight days, performing a series of mental and psychomotor tasks at regular intervals.[59] The effects reported for these individuals have been replicated a number of times in the intervening century (by, for example, Kleitman[46]). These effects have included progressive deterioration in such areas as working memory, sensory acuity, and motor speed. Many effects of fatigue are still not well understood; for example, while it has been suggested that tired or sleepy individuals become increasingly likely to engage in risk taking behaviour (presumably to finish tasks quickly), substantive evidence on this point is lacking. However, several of the more well-researched performance effects will be described in detail below.

Vigilance effects. Tasks requiring sustained attention (vigilance) and rapid reaction time are particularly sensitive to the effects of inadequate sleep.[37,61] In fact, tests involving these skills have often been used as a general marker for diminished response capacity in sleepy individuals.[60] This fact has significant implications for flight safety: many aviation contexts require the crew member to remain consistently alert, often under rather monotonous conditions, but also to respond immediately to occasional (and unpredictable) changes or stimuli (see also Chapter 12). For example, manual (nonautopilot) IFR flight requires both continuous scanning of the instrument panel and rapid response to a variety of cues, an activity that can become particularly demanding in single-pilot or nighttime operations. VFR flight requires steady and consistent attention to the external airspace so as to avoid other aircraft, especially in conditions of heavy traffic; in terminal control areas pilots must in addition be alert to instructions from air traffic control. Air combat maneuvers also require uninterrupted concentration, as do operations involving prolonged vigilance such as pipeline patrols. All of these operations may be compromised if the pilot is suffering from inadequate sleep.

Lapsing. The particular sensitivity of vigilance tasks to sleep loss may be largely explained by the phenomenon of 'blocks'[5] or 'lapses'.[76] These are transient, intermittent episodes marked by a complete loss of awareness and failure to respond to external stimuli. They are also referred to as 'microsleeps',[57] as they have been shown to be accompanied by EEG changes normally associated with stage 1 sleep.[6] Microsleeps may be as brief as one to ten seconds in length,[14,31,58,62,77] but generally increase both in number and duration as sleep deprivation continues.[76] In the cockpit, of course, even a brief loss of awareness may have serious consequences (as one pilot has remarked, a microsleep may lead to a very long sleep indeed). Lapsing may also spell the difference between success and failure in certain operations requiring sustained vigilance, such as pipeline patrols and aerial rescue searches: in many cases, once an item of information is missed there is no second chance to obtain it.

Cognitive slowing. Slower responses to task demands and stimuli have been observed for a variety of cognitive tasks, including mental arithmetic,[17,51,70] logical reasoning,[1] and tracking.[56] Some sleep researchers have assumed that slowed performance arises not through any particular changes in cognitive processing but merely because of lapses (which can be expected to reduce *overall* response speed). It is true that one typical effect of sleep deficit is a greater unevenness in performance (as opposed to a monotonic decline), with greater decrement and variability at the bottom of an individual's performance range than at the top.[16] This pattern would tend to confirm the presence of lapses; however, cognitive slowing may also represent an additional phenomenon in its own right.[15,52]

Springfield, Illinois, April, 1992: Following a reduced rest (eight hours) after more than a fourteen hour duty day, we were beginning our first takeoff of the day [in a twin turboprop commuter]. As we were cleared for takeoff, I called for the before takeoff checklist: "Air flows OFF; Speed levers HIGH." The first officer called out, "OFF AND HIGH" and advanced the power levers for target torque. I realized shortly after we had reached 70 knots that the engine speed levers were in the "LOW" position and consequently engine RPM was low. I advanced the RPM levers and the takeoff continued without incident.

It could have turned out differently. We were both extremely fatigued and easily distracted. I don't know why my first officer didn't advance the speeds or why I failed to notice that they hadn't been advanced until late into the takeoff roll. But I think long duty days and minimum legal rests were certainly contributing factors.

As long as Part 135 carriers are allowed to schedule pilots to fly fatigued they will do so. Line pilots fear using the word fatigue to schedulers because they fear disciplinary action. My company's viewpoint is that if it is legal you should be able to do it. To prevent this kind of inattentive inaction type of incident requires pilots to be mentally alert. The only way any scheduling changes will occur is if the FAA changes its rest requirement policy. Right now the rest requirements are really an accident waiting to happen.

-- NASA Aviation Safety Reporting System (Accession No. 206269)

Related to the phenomenon of cognitive slowing is the observation that in most areas of performance, sleep deprivation tends to have a more marked effect on speed than on accuracy. This has been observed in a wide variety of tasks, including logical reasoning and others noted above. The speed/accuracy tradeoff has sometimes been interpreted in terms of a deliberate strategy on the part of the person performing the task.[15] However, an exception to this pattern occurs when the nature of the task is such that the individual has no way of slowing down: then, errors begin to increase, or items are missed entirely. (Tasks such as these are referred to as 'work paced', as opposed to 'self paced' -- vigilance tasks are an example.) Although this phenomenon, too, has at times been attributed simply to lapsing,[76] later analyses have interpreted it in terms of actual cognitive slowing.[75]

San Francisco, August, 1991: I was about to embark on the seventh leg of a trip and had been on duty for more than twelve hours. My captain called in fatigued, but I did not. I was pressured to continue because the company president had informed my Chief Pilot that because I am still on (my new hire) probation that I should be careful not to call in fatigued or sick. Although the flight from San Francisco to San Luis Obispo was uneventful, when I arrived I felt as though I had been in a microsleep during the flight because I did not remember segments of it. I feel that the company should use probation as a means of weeding out employees who have poor performance and not as a means to pressure pilots to fly unrealistic schedules.

As I am writing this I am on a trip that is two days long. The first day is normal, but my layover is eight hours and four minutes followed by a seven leg day that has a duty time of thirteen hours and twenty-two minutes. This second day is unrealistic and I am scared that if I call in fatigued I could lose my job. Yet I am also scared that I will be flying physically and mentally tired.

-- NASA Aviation Safety Reporting System (Accession No. 188094)

Memory effects. Sleep loss also appears to have negative effects on memory. Short term memory problems have been linked to lapsing during encoding[61] and to attention deficit during memorization.[20] Long term memory decrements are not as readily attributed to lapsing. In one study, no effect was found on the recall of information acquired before the sleep loss, but both immediate and delayed recall were impaired when the stimulus material was presented after the individual had already become deprived of sleep.[74]

Another issue concerns the amount of sleep deprivation required before memory problems begin to surface. In many of the existing studies, memory difficulties are not apparent before the subject has remained continuously awake for thirty hours or more.[15] This does not tell us what to expect from more chronic sleep deficit (where sleep is curtailed over a period of days rather than eliminated outright), although this type of situation is presumably at least as common among aviators. In general, much remains unknown about the nature and extent of sleep related memory deficit.

Sensitivity to time on task. As discussed earlier in this chapter, task duration is one factor that influences fatigue levels generally, even in people who are not short of sleep. That is, there is a tendency for performance to deteriorate the longer a task is performed. Under sleep deprivation this effect becomes more pronounced: in fact, one recent review[15] describes task duration as "the most powerful determinant of lapsing and decreased performance in a sleepy person" (p. 108). Although the sleep deprived individual may be able to sustain normal levels of performance for brief periods of time, deterioration sets in faster than it would in a well-rested person, and is also more severe. The amount of time required for this to occur depends on many factors, including the person's level of familiarity with the task, the complexity of the task, and the degree to which stimuli are predictable. The nature of the task is also significant: while some kinds of vigilance tasks may be maintained for an hour,[72] performance involving sustained attention and frequent reactions may deteriorate within ten or fifteen minutes under sleep deprivation.[30,66,73] One study has even shown performance decrement after one minute.[34]

Time of day factors (circadian rhythms)

Working round the clock or at odd times of the day can result not only in sleep deprivation but also in disturbance of the sleep/wake cycle and other biological rhythms. This type of internal disruption is perhaps most typically associated with travel across multiple time zones ('jet lag'). However, even normal, undisrupted internal rhythms can have a marked effect both on the subjective perception of fatigue and on its manifestations (i.e., performance). Briefly stated, humans function better at some times of the day than others, and the lowest level of performance tends to occur at times normally spent sleeping, that is, during the night. As will be discussed below, this effect occurs independently of the amount of sleep the individual has had: it has been well documented even in persons who are not suffering from sleep deprivation at all.

It should be obvious that this phenomenon has marked implications for flight safety. For example, a military pilot roused unexpectedly at 4:00 a.m. might experience suboptimal flying performance less because of inadequate sleep than because mental efficiency is naturally low at this time. Similarly, a commercial airline pilot on an overnight flight who has slept earlier in the day to compensate for the anticipated lack of nighttime sleep may still find that she does not function well in the early hours of the morning. Nevertheless, research into aircrew fatigue has not, historically, been very successful in differentiating the effects of internal biological rhythms from fatigue caused by lack of sleep or by workload factors. Because confusion on this matter is so widespread, the distinction will be discussed in some depth here.

The nature of circadian rhythms

Most physiological functions are cyclical in nature: that is, they exhibit either a pattern of activity that repeats itself at regular intervals, or some type of oscillation in magnitude that is also self repeating. Some of these intervals are very brief: cycles of brainwave activity, for example, are measured in fractions of seconds, and heartbeat and respiration are also of limited duration. The human menstrual cycle, in contrast, lasts several weeks. A very large number of physiological processes, however, adhere to a cycle of approximately one day and are referred to as *circadian rhythms*. The most familiar and observable circadian rhythm is that of sleeping and waking, but there are daily fluctuations in many other less noticeable physical processes as well. These include body temperature, blood pressure, heart rate, sensory acuity, adrenal gland output, brain neurotransmitter levels, cell division, hormone levels, sensitivity to pain and other stressors, and drug efficacy and toxicity.[33] As Klein, a well-known researcher in this area[44] has put it, "The sleep-wake cycle is but a part of the 'circadian rhythm' phenomenon, not its cause" (p. 224).

Interestingly, biological rhythms can also affect an individual's ability to cope with external stressors: certain stimuli are more likely to be perceived as stressful at some times of the day than at others. Loud noise, for example, is associated with a significantly greater performance decrement in the early morning than at other times; this general effect may have cntributed to the findings of the Boeing study cited earlier concerning early morning incident rates.[49] Noted sleep researcher Simon Folkard has also noted that in any consideration of the causes of stress, time of day effects merit particular attention since, unlike many other external variables, they cannot be avoided.[24]

The oscillations of these physiological functions are regulated by what has traditionally been described as an 'internal clock'. (Actually, it is now accepted that there are two separate clocks, each controlling different physiological functions; see p. 257, and also the following chapter.) A significant feature of this clock is that its phase length is not precisely twenty-four hours long: that is, it is not inherently identical to the time interval established by the earth's rotation. In practice, however, daily physiological rhythms do manage to remain synchronized to the cycle of night and day, because the internal clock is responsive to time cues in the external environment which keep it 'on course'. These cues are referred to as *zeitgebers* (German for 'time givers'). One obvious zeitgeber, as already indicated, is the light/dark cycle; some others, such as mealtimes, are socially determined and may vary from one culture to another. Cognitive awareness of clock time can also act as a zeitgeber. An individual whose circadian rhythms are synchronized to a given set of environmental time cues (for example, a particular time zone) is said to be *entrained* to that environment. Conversely, abrupt transposition to a different set of cues produces a state known as *circadian desynchronization*. (As already noted, when this transition is occasioned by travel to another time zone, it is popularly known as jet lag.)

Although the distinction is not always explicitly acknowledged in aviation literature, the subject of circadian rhythms and fatigue can be said to involve two separate issues. On the one hand there are the effects of normal, undisrupted circadian rhythms on everyday functioning, or what are sometimes termed time of day effects. On the other hand there are the effects of desynchronized rhythms occasioned by rapid flight across multiple time zones. Much of what has been written about pilots and biological rhythms tends to confound these two phenomena; we have therefore adopted the opposite approach and will reserve our discussion of desynchronization for Chapter 9.

Circadian rhythms and performance

Physiological rhythms are known to correlate significantly with mental and psychomotor performance: simply stated, humans function better at some ' times of the day than at others. In fact, these natural ups and downs can assume considerable importance in demanding environments such as aviation, where pilots are sometimes pushed to the limits of their abilities and where the cost of error can be extremely high. In point of fact, several analyses of aircraft accident and incident reports have shown that error rates exhibit distinct trends over the course of the day. For example, an examination of accidents within the Israeli Air Force[64] revealed that the daytime accident rate was highest during the first hour after awakening in the morning, decreased thereafter until late afternoon, and rose again during the evening: a pattern highly consistent with the daily performance curve observed in laboratory studies. Nighttime accidents were not included in the study, but another review, this one of incidents in the ASRS database, indicated that the largest number of fatigue related errors occured between midnight and 6:00 a.m.[53] This, too, accords with the results of experimental studies of daytime and nighttime cognitive functioning.

Of course, all studies of fatigue in 'real world' operational contexts need to be scrutinized quite carefully for the possible presence of confounding variables. As already noted, pilot fatigue has many causes, and it is not always easy to divorce time of day effects from other fatigue factors. Considering the higher error rate observed after midnight, for example, it could be argued that a pilot flying at this time is more likely to be suffering from some degree of sleep deprivation than one completing a daytime assignment. Visibility is also of course lower after dark, making the task of flying more demanding. As for the reported increase in accidents in the late afternoon and evening, perhaps this is simply an effect of accumulated fatigue at the end of a working day. Another example of a time of day factor unrelated to circadian rhythms is that of air traffic density, which can naturally be expected to vary at different times.

These questions have been addressed in controlled laboratory studies in which subjects perform a given task repeatedly at different points in the day (and night). This allows changes in performance to be monitored without interference from external variables. In many studies of this type the tests used are fairly simple, for example, card sorting,[35] digit summation, and symbol cancellation.[43] These tests are used as indicators of basic mental skills that are necessary in a wide range of more complex tasks; they include psychomotor performance,[42] vigilance,[35] reaction time,[44] and logical reasoning.[23]

Such studies indicate that many aspects of human efficiency and performance follow a distinct and well-documented pattern of highs and lows through the course of the day. This performance curve is similar across a wide range of tasks (although there are some variations and exceptions). In general terms, however, efficiency has been shown to improve steadily throughout the morning, peak at some point in the afternoon or early evening, and fall off sharply after midnight, reaching a low point at approximately 4:00 a.m. The level of performance is therefore lowest at night, during the traditional sleep period, but begins to rise again as morning approaches; the cycle then repeats itself.[41]

The pattern is not, however, confined to simple laboratory tasks; it has also been documented in connection with complex operations such as aviation. An example can be seen in the F-104 simulator study cited earlier,[40] in which experienced pilots completed a brief but demanding mission at three hour intervals throughout a twenty-four hour period. As noted already, performance was measured in several different ways (by deviations from predetermined speed, altitude, and range requirements, as well as by recovery time when deviations occurred). Although some differences were observed among the various parameters, when these were averaged the overall performance at different times of the day closely echoed that reported for simpler, more 'artificial' laboratory tasks: a relatively high error rate was observed in the morning, which progressively decreased until about 3:00 p.m.; errors then started to increase again and reached their highest frequency between 3:00 and 6:00 a.m.

It should be obvious from this that the lower level of functioning observed during the night is not attributable solely to lack of sleep or to cumulative fatigue. First, it is not necessary to remain awake all night for the effect to occur: the same performance curve is evident when subjects sleep normally except during actual testing. Second, performance does not degrade in a linear fashion the longer the individual is deprived of sleep: even persons who have remained awake throughout the night experience an upswing in alertness and efficiency as morning approaches, rather as if sleep had actually taken place. This early morning increase in arousal may be a common occurrence among pilots performing overnight flights.[33]

In fact, the same familiar daily performance curve can even be observed in individuals who are kept awake for very extended periods. Even after a number of days without sleep, performance on a variety of tasks continues to drop during the night and rise again in the daytime. The cumulative effect of sleeplessness is visible in the form of an overall downward trend superimposed on this pattern, but even after several days of continuous wakefulness, performance continues to fall at the customary bedtime hour and improve markedly in the morning.[27]

Research difficulties. As the preceding discussion indicates, it is possible, at least in theory, to study circadian performance rhythms in isolation from other fatigue factors (sleep deprivation, workload), so that the practical effects of these rhythms can be better understood. In practice, of course, fatigue variables tend to occur in combination. For example, a private pilot returning home in the evening after a long day in the cockpit would probably experience both fatigue from extended flying and a natural 'energy low', although sleep deprivation would be unlikely. A military pilot performing a nighttime sortie might also function at a less than optimal level and, perhaps, suffer from loss of sleep; he may in fact feel quite fatigued subjectively even if he does not spend many hours in the cockpit. A commercial pilot completing a lengthy overnight flight may experience all three fatigue factors, as may a military pilot on a 'sustained operation'. This confluence of factors can obviously create difficulties for the researcher who wishes to study the effects of circadian rhythms in applied settings such as aviation. Another practical difficulty lies in the complexity of flight tasks.

Perhaps for these reasons, human performance investigators who do specialize in real world operations have not tended to give the role of circadian rhythms a great deal of independent consideration, and most available literature is not marked by a sophisticated grasp of the subject. In the field of aviation, the majority of research on circadian rhythms has been concerned with desynchronization -- that is, with the effects of flight across multiple time zones. This is, of course, a separate and important topic, but it is also a particularly complex one. Pilots performing such flights suffer not only from the effects of unusual work hours and other fatigue factors (extended duty periods, sleep deprivation), but also to internal physiological disruptions which may be quite fatiguing in their own right. The complexity of this issue has distracted attention somewhat from the effects of circadian rhythms in other operational contexts, and has muddied the field with respect to interactions between circadian performance variation and other factors such as sleep deprivation. To help make the distinction clear, this chapter will confine itself to discussing normal, undisrupted circadian rhythms and their effects on flying.

Background to the problem. An historical look at the manner in which the study of circadian performance rhythms developed may shed additional light on the way the subject is approached today. Diurnal variations in physical and mental performance were first observed in the late nineteenth century, and engaged the attention of educational and (later) industrial psychologists interested in predicting the level of performance to be expected at different times of the school day or work shift. (It was thought, for example, that optimal times of day could be identified for the teaching of various academic subjects.) While a few researchers did attempt to identify natural diurnal rhythms in (for example) physiological functions[50] and mental efficiency,[4] most investigators in the late nineteenth and early twentieth centuries adhered to the more traditional view that mental fatigue and associated performance decrements were directly related to the degree and duration of effort expended. Relatively few studies examined performance rhythms as a separate biological entity divorced from working conditions, and those that did were marred by a number of methodological difficulties such as uncontrolled practice effects and a failure to differentiate time of day effects from the cumulative effects of fatigue.[26,48]

The first well-controlled studies of the relationship between biological rhythms and human performance were made by Nathaniel Kleitman.[45,46] Using simple perceptual-motor tasks, Kleitman obtained extensive documentation of the general daily performance curve described already (that of increasing efficiency throughout the first half of the day and decreasing efficiency thereafter). However, he also identified an extremely close correlation between this pattern and core body temperature: as performance improved, so did temperature, and vice versa. In fact, the two values matched one another so closely and consistently that Kleitman concluded that they must be causally linked, and theorized that changes in the level of mental functioning were a direct effect of variations in basal metabolism. Kleitman even went so far as to suggest that body temperature could be used as a direct index of mental efficiency, thus bypassing completely the use of actual performance testing.[47]

These ideas have not been entirely borne out by subsequent research. First, in Kleitman's time it was generally assumed that all circadian oscillations were regulated by a single 'internal clock'. However, more recent studies by chronobiologists indicate that physiological rhythms are controlled by two separate but linked oscillatory systems, each of which controls different functions.[65] This finding raises new questions about the temperature and performance rhythms observed by Kleitman -- were they really entrained to one another, as he believed, or was each separately entrained to the same external cues?[78] It now appears that the latter is the case: while temperature and performance rhythms are normally in synchrony, they can under certain conditions be decoupled from one another.* These developments notwithstanding, Kleitman's conclusions regarding

---

*For that matter, there is nothing unique about temperature, as task performance can be correlated with an entire suite of metabolic and other physiological functions. Temperature was adopted as the traditional index because it is both stable and easy to measure; those functions requiring blood or urine sampling can be assessed only at intervals, while temperature readings can be obtained more or less continuously.

body temperature and mental efficiency have enjoyed a certain tenacity over the years;[18,25] as noted previously, the disciplines of cognitive psychology and chronobiology have evolved somewhat independently of one another.

Exceptions to the usual circadian performance curve. It has also been observed that research on performance rhythms has been perhaps unduly influenced by Kleitman's emphasis on perceptual-motor functioning;[24] the fact that these relatively simple skills do follow a single, well-replicated circadian pattern has encouraged many researchers to assume that more complex cognitive operations will do the same.[10,12,35] Even some apparently simple skills, however, fall outside the usual curve.

Working memory. Performance on working memory tasks, for example, has been shown to peak at or before noon and decrease thereafter. This pattern has been observed in studies using a wide range of working memory tests.[23] The reason for this effect has not been definitively established; there may be a negative correlation between memory processes and arousal level. It has also been speculated that one aspect of the memory function may include the 'clearing' of stored information and that this function may improve throughout the day (as do most other simple cognitive skills); if this is the case, efficient clearing of information might actually impede working memory.[32] It should also be remembered that working memory is an important component of many other cognitive tasks, and that decrements to this function may have far-reaching effects.

Time estimation. Time estimation, important in many aviation operations, also does not follow the usual pattern of improvement throughout the day. Indeed, not all researchers agree as to whether a circadian pattern exists at all for this faculty.[7,12] Laboratory induced changes in body temperature have been shown to bring about corresponding changes in time estimation, but studies of natural circadian variations have failed to yield a coherent picture, and the process is not well understood. It is possible that more than one internal clock may be involved in time estimation.[54]

Individual variation. The picture is further complicated by the fact that marked individual variation exists in the rhythms themselves. It is a commonplace that some people are most efficent and productive during the morning hours, while others perform their best work in the evening or even late at night. Although physiological research on so-called 'morning types' and 'evening types' has failed to find a high degree of variation in temperature rhythms,[13,39] more significant differences have been observed in performance. One study, for example, identified a group of extreme 'morning types' who did not follow the commonly reported pattern of improvement throughout the day, and a group of extreme 'evening types' who failed to show the typical evening performance decrement.[38] As this phenomenon is not well understood at present, it is difficult to integrate into a predictive model of circadian performance rhythms. It has, however, been observed that evening types tend to cope more easily with time zone changes and unusual work hours, and that this factor could be useful for the planning of duty schedules.[29]

More well-defined personality variables also appear to influence circadian rhythmicity. An early study found, for example, that extraverts and introverts experience peak performance at different times of the day.[8] A subsequent study then demonstrated that the relevant factor in this phenomenon was the dimension of impulsivity: the performance of impulsive individuals improved throughout the day, while that of low impulsives did not, and in some cases even declined.[63]

Yet another factor influencing circadian rhythmicity appears to be the age of the individual. For example, a study of sleep loss in flight crews conducted by NASA Ames Research Center found that pilots over forty involved in long haul flight operations incurred an average of 3.5 times more sleep loss per day than their younger counterparts.[29] This is most likely because age interacts with the 'morningness/eveningness' distinction described above: persons tend increasingly to become morning types as they grow older. Thus, this variable too may have useful personnel and scheduling applications.

Conclusion

It is an understatement to say that the study of fatigue is a complex subject; the area of circadian rhythms and skilled performance has been marked by particular inconsistency, even confusion. One difficulty is that even investigators who specialize in performance rhythms have not yet developed a clear and comprehensive picture of time of day effects, a model that can be applied predictively to a variety of complex tasks. Aviation researchers, while acknowledging the probable importance of time of day effects in flying performance, have had relatively little to say of a more specific nature (other than to assess the effect of prolonged wakefulness and transmeridian travel upon sleepiness).

It is worth reiterating here that operating an aircraft does not depend on a single, measurable (and degradable) skill. Rather, as discussed in Chapters 3 and 4, flying requires an integration of many skills: working memory, vigilance, spatial ability, and psychomotor functioning, to name but a few. Because it is simpler to analyze the effects of sleeplessness, stress, and diurnal variation on each skill separately, the studies designed to assess these skills have tended to use fairly simple, domain independent tasks that can be monitored in the laboratory. This research is not without implications for performance in multitask operations such as aviation, but it has yet to be incorporated into an actual working model applicable to the whole flight task. Also, data are still lacking on the effects of circadian rhythms on more complex cognitive functions relevant to aviation, such as decision making and information retrieval.

References

1. Angus, R.G., and Heslegrave, R.J. (1985), 'Effects of sleep loss on sustained cognitive performance during a command and control situation', *Behavior Research Methods, Instruments, and Computers,* vol. 17, pp. 55-67.

2. Aserinsky, E. (1969), 'The maximal capacity for sleep: rapid eye movement as an index of sleep satiety', *Biological Psychiatry,* vol. 1, pp. 147-59.

3. Bartlett, F.C. (1943), 'Fatigue following highly skilled work', *Proceedings of the Royal Society,* Series B, vol. 131, pp. 247-57.

4. Bergstrum, F.G. (1894), 'An experimental study of some of the conditions of mental activity', *American Journal of Psychology,* vol. 43, pp. 230-45.

5. Bills, A.G. (1931), 'Blocking: a new principle of mental fatigue', *American Journal of Psychology,* vol. 43, pp. 230-45.

6. Bjerner, B. (1949), 'Alpha depression and lowered pulse rate during delayed actions in a serial reaction test: a study of sleep deprivation', *Acta Psychologica Scandinavica,* vol. 19 (Suppl. 65), pp. 1-93.

7. Blake, M.J.F. (1967), 'Time of day effects on performance in a range of tasks', *Psychon. Science,* vol. 9, pp. 349-50.

8. Blake, M.J.F. (1971), 'Temperature and Time of Day', in W.P. Colquhoun (ed.), *Biological Rhythms and Human Performance,* London, Academic Press, pp. 109-48.

9. Borowsky, M.S., and Wall, R. (1983), 'Naval aviation mishaps and fatigue', *Aviation, Space, and Environmental Medicine,* vol. 54, pp. 535-8.

10. Broughton, R. (1975), 'Biorythmic variations in consciousness and psychological functions', *Canadian Psychological Review,* vol. 16, pp. 217-39.

11. Carskadon, M.A., and Roth, T. (1991), 'Sleep Restriction', in T.H. Monk (ed.), *Sleep, Sleepiness and Performance,* John Wiley & Sons, New York.

12. Colquhoun, W.P. (1971), 'Circadian Variations in Mental Efficiency', in W.P. Colquhoun (ed.), *Biological Rhythms and Human Performance,* London, Academic Press, pp. 39-107.

13. Colquhoun, W.P. (1979), 'Phase shift in temperature rhythm after transmeridian flight, as related to pre-flight phase angle', *International Archives of Occupational and Environmental Health,* vol. 42, pp. 149-57.

14. Dement, W.C., and Mitler, M. (1974), 'An Introduction to Sleep', in Petre-Quadens, O. and Schlag, J. (eds.), *Basic Sleep Mechanisms,* Academic Press, New York, pp. 271-96.

15. Dinges, D.F., and Kribbs, N.B. (1991), 'Performing while sleepy: effects of experimentally-induced sleepiness', in Monk, T.H. (ed.), *Sleep, Sleepiness, and performance,* John Wiley & Sons, New York.

16. Dinges, D.F., Orne, M.T., Whitehouse, W.G., and Orne, E.C. (1987), 'Temporal placement of a nap for alertness: contributions of circadian phase and prior wakefulness', *Sleep,* vol. 10, pp. 313-29.

17. Dinges, D.F., Whitehouse, W.G., Orne, E.C., and Orne, M.T. (1988), 'The benefits of a nap during prolonged work and wakefulness', *Work and Stress,* vol. 2, pp. 139-53.

18. Dodge, R. (1982), 'Circadian rhythms and fatigue: a discrimination of their effects on performance', *Aviation, Space, and Environmental Medicine,* vol. 53, pp. 1131-6.

19. Drew, G.C. (1979), 'An Experimental Study of Mental Fatigue', in Dearnaley, E.J. and Warr, P.B. (eds.), *Aircrew Stress in Wartime Operations,* Academic Press, New York.

20. Elkin, A.J., and Murray, D.J. (1974), 'The effects of sleep loss on short-term recognition memory', *Canadian Journal of Psychology,* vol. 2, pp. 23-36.

21. Evans, F.J., Cook, M.R., Cohen, H.D., Orne, E.C., and Orne, M.T. (1977), 'Appetitive and replacement naps: EEG and behaviour', *Science,* vol. 197, pp. 687-9.

22. Feinberg, I., Fein, G., and Floyd, T.C. (1980), 'EEG patterns during and following extended sleep in young adults', *Electroencephalography and Clinical Neurophysiology,* vol. 50, pp. 467-76.

23. Folkard, S. (1975), 'Diurnal variation in logical reasoning', *British Journal of Psychology,* vol. 66, pp. 1-8.

24. Folkard, S. (1983). 'Diurnal Variation', in Hockey, G.R.J. (ed.), *Stress and Fatigue in Human Performance,* John Wiley & Sons, New York, pp. 245-72.

25. Fort, A., Harrison, M.T., and Mills, J.N. (1973), 'Psychometric performance: circadian rhythms and the effect of raising body temperature', *Journal of Physiology,* vol. 231, pp. 114-5.

26. Freeman, G.L., and Hovland, C.I. (1934), 'Diurnal variations in performance and related physiological processes', *Psychological Bulletin,* vol. 31, pp. 777-99.

27. Froeberg, J., Karlsson, C.G., Levi, L., et al. (1972), Circadian variations in performance, psychological ratings, catecholamine excretion, and diuresis during prolonged sleep deprivation', *International Journal of Psychobiology,* vol. 2, pp. 23-36.

28. Gagnon, P., DeKoninck, J., and Broughton, R. (1985), 'Reappearance of EEG slow waves in extended sleep with delayed bedtime', *Sleep,* vol. 8, pp. 118-28.

29. Gander, P.H., Nguyen, D., Rosekind, M.R., and Connell, L.J. (1993), 'Age, circadian rhythms, and sleep loss in flight crews', *Aviation, Space, and Environmental Medicine,* vol. 64, pp. 189-95.

30. Glenville, M., Broughton, R., Wing, A.M., and Wilkinson, R.T. (1978), 'Effects of sleep deprivation on short duration performance compared to the Wilkinson Auditory Vigilance Task', *Sleep,* vol. 1, pp. 169-76.

31. Guilleminault, C., Billiard, M., Montplaisir, J., and Dement, W.C. (1975), 'Altered states of consciousness in disorders of daytime sleepiness', *Journal of the Neurological Sciences,* vol. 26, pp. 377-93.

32. Hamilton, P., Wilkinson, R.T., and Edwards, R.S. (1972), 'A Study of Four Days Partial Sleep Deprivation', in Colquhoun, W.P. (ed.), *Aspects of Human Efficiency: Diurnal Rhythms and Loss of Sleep,* The English Universities Press, London, pp. 101-13.

33. Hawkins, F.H. (1987), *Human Factors in Flight,* Gower Technical Press, Aldershot, Hants.

34. Heslegrave, R.J., and Angus, R.G. (1985), 'The effects of task duration and work-session location on performance degradation induced by sleep loss and sustained cognitive work', *Behavior Research Methods, Instruments, and Computers,* vol. 17, pp. 592-603.

35. Hockey, G.R.J., and Colquhoun, W.P. (1972), 'Diurnal Variations in Human Performance: A Review', in Colquhoun, W.P. (ed.), *Aspects of Human Efficiency: Diurnal Rhythm and Loss of Sleep,* The English Universities Press, London, pp. 1-23.

36. Holley, D.C. (1974), *Circadian Desynchronization and the Sleep-Wake Cycle*, Department of Biological Sciences, San Jose State University, California.

37. Horne, J. (1988), *Why We Sleep*, Oxford University Press, New York.

38. Horne, J.A., Brass, C.G., and Pettit, A.N. (1980), 'Circadian performance differences between morning and evening 'types', *Ergonomics*, vol. 23, pp. 29-36.

39. Horne, J.A., and Ostberg, O. (1977), 'Individual differences in human circadian rhythms', *Biological Psychology*, vol. 5, pp. 179-90.

40. Klein, K.E., Bruener, H., Holtmann, H., Rehme, H., Stolze, J., Steinhoff, W.D., and Wegmann, H.M. (1970), 'Circadian rhythm of pilots' efficiency and effects of multiple time zone travel', *Aerospace Medicine*, vol. 41, pp. 125-32.

41. Klein, K.E., and Wegmann, H.M. (1980), *Significance of Circadian Rrhythms in Aerospace Operations*, AGARDograph No. 247, NATO-AGARD, Neuilly-sur-Seine.

42. Klein, K.E., Wegmann, H.M., and Bruener, H. (1968), 'Circadian rhythm in indices of human performance, physical fitness, and stress resistance', *Aerospace Medicine*, vol. 39, pp. 512-8.

43. Klein, K.E., Wegmann, H.M., and Hunt, B.I. (1972), 'Desynchronization of body temperature and performance circadian rhythm as a result of outgoing and homegoing transmeridian flights', *Aerospace Medicine*, vol. 43, pp. 119-32.

44. Klein, K.E., Wegmann, H.M., Athanassenas, G., Hohlweck, H., and Kuklinski, P. (1976), 'Air operations and circadian performance rhythms', *Aviation, Space, and Environmental Medicine*, vol. 47, pp. 221-30.

45. Kleitman, N. (1933), 'Diurnal variations in performance', *American Journal of Physiology*, vol. 104, pp. 449-56.

46. Kleitman, N. (1963), *Sleep and Wakefulness*, University of Chicago Press, Chicago.

47. Kleitman, N., and Jackson, D.P. (1950), 'Body temperature and performance under different routines', *Journal of Applied Physiology*, vol. 3, pp. 309-28.

48. Lavie P. (1980), 'The search for cycles in mental performance', *Chronobiologia*, vol. 7, pp. 247-56.

49. Logan, A.L., and Braune, R.J. (1991), 'The Utilization of the Aviation Safety Reporting System: A Case Study in Pilot Fatigue', *Proceedings of the Sixth International Symposium on Aviation Psychology*, Ohio State University, Columbus.

50. Lombard, W.P. (1887), 'The variations of the normal knee jerk, and their relation to the activity of the central nervous system', *American Journal of Psychology*, vol. 1, pp. 5-71.

51. Loveland, N.T., and Williams, H.L. (1963), 'Adding, sleep loss, and body temperature', *Perceptual and Motor Skills*, vol. 16, pp. 923-9.

52. Lubin, A. (1967), 'Performance under Sleep Loss and Fatigue', in Kety, S.S., Evarts, E.V., and Williams, H.L. (eds.), *Sleep and Altered States of Consciousness*, Williams and Wilins, pp. 506-13.

53. Lyman, E.G., and Orlady, H.W. (1980), *Fatigue and Associated Performance Decrements in Air Transport Operations*, (NASA Contract NAS2-10060), Batelle Memorial Laboratories, Mountain View, California.

54. Minors, D.S., and Waterhouse, J.M. (1981), *Circadian Rhythms and the Human*, John Wright & Sons, Bristol.

55. Monk, T.H. (1991), 'Circadian Aspects of Subjective Sleepiness: A Behavioural Messenger?' in Monk, T.H. (ed.), *Sleep, Sleepiness and Performance*, John Wiley & Sons, New York.

56. Mullaney, D.J., Kripke, D.F., Fleck, P.A., and Johnson, L.C. (1983), 'Sleep loss and nap effects on sustained continuous performance', *Psychophysiology,* vol. 20, pp. 643-51.

57. Murray, E.J. (1965), *Sleep, Dreams, and Arousal,* Appleton-Century-Crofts, New York.

58. Naitoh, P., and Townsend, R.E. (1970), 'The role of sleep deprivation research in human factors', *Human Factors,* vol. 12, pp. 253-7.

59. Patrick, G.T., and Gilbert, J.A. (1896), 'On the effects of loss of sleep', *Psychological Review,* vol. 3, pp. 469-83.

60. Pivik, R.T. (1991), 'The Several Qualities of Sleepiness: Psychophysiological Considerations', in Monk, T.H. (ed.), *Sleep, Sleepiness and Performance,* John Wiley & Sons, New York.

61. Polzella, D.J. (1975), 'Effects of sleep deprivation on short-term recognition memory', *Journal of Experimental Psychology,* vol. 104, pp. 194-200.

62. Pressman, M.R., and Fry, J.M. (1989), 'Relationship of autonomic nervous system activity to daytime sleepiness and prior sleep', *Sleep,* vol. 12, pp. 239-45.

63. Revelle, W., Humphreys, M.S., Simon, L., and Gilliland, K. (1980), 'The interactive effect of personality, time of day, and caffeine: a test of the arousal model', *Journal of Experimental Psychology: General,* vol. 109, pp. 1-31.

64. Ribak, J., Ashkenazi, I.E., Klepfish, A., Avgar, D., Tall, J., Kallner, B., and Noyman, Y. (1983), 'Diurnal rhythmicity and air force flight accidents due to error', *Aviation, Space, and Environmental Medicine,* vol. 54, pp. 1096-9.

65. Rutenfranz, J., Aschoff, J., and Mann, H. (1972), 'The Effects of a Cumulative Sleep Deficit, Duration of Preceding Sleep Period and Body-temperature on Multiple Choice Reaction Time', in Colquhoun,

W.P. (ed.), *Aspects of Human Efficiency: Diurnal Rhythms and Loss of Sleep,* The English Universities Press, London, pp. 217-30.

66. Tilley, A.J., and Wilkinson, R.T. (1984), 'The effects of a restricted sleep regime on the composition of sleep and performance', *Psychophysiology*, vol. 21, pp. 406-12.

67. Verdone, P. (1968), 'Sleep satiation: extended sleep in normal subjects', *Electroencephalography and Clinical Neurophysiology,* vol. 24, pp. 417-23.

68. Webb, W.B., and Agnew, H.W. (1975), 'Are we chronically sleep deprived?' *Bulletin of the Psychonomic Society,* vol. 6, pp. 47-8.

69. Weber, A., Jermini, C., and Grandjean, E.P. (1975), 'Relationship between objective and subjective assessment of experimentally induced fatigue', *Ergonomics,* vol. 18, pp. 151-6.

70. Wilkinson, R.T. (1961), 'Interaction of lack of sleep with knowledge of results, repeated testing, and individual differences', *Journal of Experimental Psychology,* vol. 62, pp. 263-71.

71. Wilkinson, R.T. (1965), 'Sleep Deprivation', in Edholm, O.G. and Bacharach, A.L. (eds.), *Physiology of Survival,* Academic Press, London, pp. 399-430.

72. Wilkinson, R.T. (1968), 'Sleep Deprivation: Performance Tests for Partial and Selective Sleep Deprivation', in Abt, L.E. and Riess, B.F. (eds.), *Progress in Clinical Psychology: Dreams and Dreaming,* Grune and Stratton, New York, pp. 28-43.

73. Wilkinson, R.T., and Houghton, D. (1982), 'Field test of arousal: a portable reaction timer with data', *Human Factors,* vol. 24, pp. 487-93.

74. Williams, H.L., Gieseking, C.F., and Lubin, A. (1966), 'Some effects of sleep loss on memory', *Perceptual and Motor Skills,* vol. 23, pp. 1287-93.

75. Williams, H.L., and Lubin, A. (1967), 'Speeded addition and sleep loss', *Journal of Experimental Psychology*, vol. 73, pp. 3313-7.

76. Williams, H.L., Lubin, A., and Goodnow, J.J. (1959), 'Impaired performance with acute sleep loss', *Psychological Monographs: General and Applied*, vol. 73, pp. 1-26.

77. Williams, H.L., Tepas, P.I., and Morlock, H.C. (1962), 'Evoked responses to clicks and electroencephalographic stages of sleep', *Science*, vol. 138, pp. 685-6.

78. Winget, C.M., DeRoshia, C.W., Markley, C.L., and Holley, D.C. (1984), 'A review of human physiological and performance changes associated with desynchronosis of biological rhythms', *Aviation, Space, and Environmental Medicine*, vol. 55, pp. 1085-96.

9 Transmeridian flight

The times they are a-changin'.

-- Bob Dylan

The previous chapter discussed the issue of pilot fatigue and considered some of the various ways in which fatigue can come about. As we noted, fatigue often arises not from a single cause but through a confluence of factors which, unfortunately, can sometimes be rather difficult to isolate (at least outside of a laboratory setting). One effect of this circumstance is that practical research on fatigue related performance decrement in aircrew cannot always be readily generalized from one setting to another.

This chapter will present a more detailed discussion of aircrew fatigue in one particular operational context, that of long haul flights across multiple time zones. As a situation conducive to pilot fatigue, this type of flight operation has probably received more study than any other. Certainly it presents particular challenges to pilots: sources of fatigue encountered on transmeridian flights may include not only all of those enumerated in Chapter 8, but also the factor of circadian desynchronization (jet lag). The challenge presented by this combination of circumstances can indeed have significant implications for pilot well-being, effective personnel management, and indeed public safety.[18]

We will begin by reviewing the fatigue factors that can affect all pilots, not just those on transmeridian flights. The first of these relates to work-load intensity -- the level of difficulty of the operation being performed. A second factor is time on task, that is, fatigue engendered by extended duty periods. Since flights across multiple time zones are by definition lengthy (at least, in most aircraft), this is an important issue to consider in connec-

The lack of sleep I feel now, at eleven o'clock in the morning, is a grain of sand compared to the mountain that will tower over me when dawn breaks tomorrow. Past dawns I've flown through come forward in memory to warn me what torture the desire for sleep can be.... How wonderful it would be if this really were a dream, and I could lie down on a cloud's soft, fluffy quilt and sleep. I've never wanted anything so much... I'd pay any price -- except life itself. But life itself is the price.

I've lost command of my eyelids. When they start to close, I can't restrain them. They shut, and I shake myself, and lift them with my fin gers. I stare at the instruments, wrinkle forehead muscles tense. Lids close again regardless, stuck tight as though with glue...every cell of my being is on strike, sulking in protest, claiming that nothing, nothing in the world, could be worth such an effort ... all I want in life is to throw myself down flat, stretch out -- and sleep....

During long ages between dawn and sunrise, I'm thankful we didn't make the Spirit of St. Louis a stable plane.... Now that I'm dreaming and ridden by sleep, its veering prods my senses.... Here it's well into midday and my mind's still shirking, still refusing to meet the problems it undertook so willingly in planning for this flight. Are all those months of hard and detailed work to be wasted for lack of a few minutes of concentrated effort? Has landing at Le Bourget become of so little import that I'll trade success for these useless hours of semiconscious relaxation? No; I must, I will become alert, and concentrate, and make decisions.... I shake my head and body harshly. I flex arms and legs, compress muscles of chest and stomach, stamp feet on floor boards, bounce up and down, jam the stick forward to to throw my weight against the belt, jerk it back to press myself tightly to the seat and floor. I'll break this spider web of sleep! *-- But -- but -- what I need most of all is breath -- b-r-e-a-t-h -- The instrument board is vague -- like evening twilight -- My brain swims --*

-- Charles Lindberg, *The Spirit of St. Louis*

tion with pilots performing them. Another general source of fatigue is sleep deprivation; in the case of long haul transmeridian flights this may occur either in the course of the flight itself (in the case of overnight flights) or afterwards, when the change in time zone may make it difficult to 'catch up' on sleep. A fourth fatigue factor consists of time of day effects -- the normal fluctuations in alertness and efficiency associated with circadian rhythms. These, too, can occur on short haul as well as long haul flights; however, the latter may present an additional complication in that changes in time zone can make it difficult for the pilot to predict when periods of fatigue and sleepiness are likely to occur.

Circadian desynchronization (jet lag)

A fifth cause of aircrew fatigue, and one which particularly affects pilots travelling across multiple time zones, is disruption of circadian rhythms or desynchronization. Most people probably think of desynchronization as consisting primarily of a mismatch between the internal sleep/wake cycle and the external environment. Certainly the popular term 'jet lag' tends to be equated with waking and sleeping at unaccustomed or inappropriate times, and it is well known that attempts to sleep on schedule may be unsuccessful under such conditions. However, the symptoms associated with desynchronization also include hunger at unusual times, digestive disturbances such as queasiness and constipation, and miscellaneous aches and pains. Chills can occur, as body temperature now drops during waking hours instead of during sleep. Psychological symptoms include confusion, irritability, and other mood impairments, as well as a general loss of mental efficiency. Difficulties with time and distance estimation have also been noted, as well as psychomotor performance degradation, headaches, and anxiety.[40]

Desynchronization and the human organism

The dual oscillatory system. One reason why the effects of multiple time zone travel can be so far-reaching may relate to the finding that there are not one but two internal 'clocks' or oscillatory systems. There appears to be one system which governs activity and arousal rhythms (i.e., the sleep/wake cycle), and a different one which controls the cycle of body temperature and a number of other physiological and endocrine rhythms. Although these two systems are separate from one another, they normally operate in synchrony because they are both entrained to the same external time cues or zeitgebers (see Chapter 8, p. 253). However, they tend to react in different ways and at different rates when the zeitgebers are disrupted in some manner -- as, for example, by travel to a new time zone. The rhythm that governs body temperature is fairly stable: in experiments where individuals are placed in caves or other environments without time cues, the length of the cycle -- called the *period length* -- varies only between about twenty-three and twenty-seven hours. The sleep/wake cycle, however, is more labile and can under artificial conditions be entrained to 'days' ranging anywhere from eighteen to thirty-three hours in length. Even so, the two systems are not entirely independent of one another, insofar as temperature phase affects sleep onset and duration.[4]

Effects of desynchronization. The range of physiological functions affected by desynchronization is quite extensive. They include the rhythms of body temperature, cardiovascular and metabolic functioning, electrolyte excretion, urinary output, a variety of endocrine functions, and, of course, sleep rhythms, including patterns of REM sleep.[14,29,33] However, there are also changes in the *patterns* exhibited by the various circadian rhythms, over and above their shift toward the new time environment. Changes have been observed, for example, in the range of oscillation of various functions (that is, the degree of difference between high and low points, of, say, body temperature), in mean values (values averaged over twenty-four hours), in the speed with which maximum and minimum values are reached, and in a number of other parameters.[21]

Furthermore, although circadian rhythms do gradually normalize and adjust to the new environment, they do not all do so at the same rate. Following a six-hour shift to the east, for example, the sleep/wake cycle may adjust within two or three days, while the temperature cycle might require five days, and the cycle of cortisol excretion, eight days.[40] An example of this can be seen in a laboratory isolation study described by sleep researcher Timothy Monk and his colleagues,[25] in which a six-hour phase shift was artificially imposed on a group of eight subjects. During the ten days following the shift, some physiological functions, including temperature rhythms and rapid eye movement sleep, adjusted to the new schedule in a steady, progressive manner. Certain other variables, however, including sleep duration and perceived sleepiness, adapted in fits and starts. This appeared to indicate the presence of two separate processes working in competition with one another.

As a matter of fact, different rhythms may even adjust in different *directions*. That is, some may adapt by speeding up until they are in phase with the new time zone, while others may be adjusting by slowing down until the previous day's time cues have 'caught up'. Resynchronization by partition, as this phenomenon is known, occurs most commonly in time shifts of over six hours.[16] In general, normal phase relationships cannot be reestablished until *each* biological rhythm has become entrained to the new environment. The term 'desynchronization', therefore, actually refers to two separate phenomena: lack of synchrony between internal rhythms and the external environment, and lack of synchrony among the various rhythms themselves.

Desynchronization in aircrew

It is all too easy to assume, as Dinges[7] has noted, that "because the plane can be made ready to fly at a moment's notice, at any hour of the day or night, the pilot can also be made ready to perform his or her critical skills at any time". Of course, this is not the case. The effects of rapid time zone travel on aircrew have been studied since the early 1950s, and there is by now a significant body of literature on the physiological changes that this engenders. Surprisingly little is known, however, about specific effects of transmeridian travel on human performance in general or pilot performance in particular.[12] One reason for this is undoubtedly the complex nature of fatigue and the many meanings of the term. Chapter 8 discussed some of the most common sources or 'types' of fatigue that affect all aircrew; needless to say, any or all of these factors may be present on long haul transmeridian flights as well as on shorter operations.

In fact, as we have pointed out, such flights may be particularly vulnerable to some of these other fatigue agents, with the phenomenon of circadian desynchronization simply representing yet another variable in an already complex picture. It is, however, a variable for which we have no evolutionary adaptations, and one which points up in sharp focus some of the intransigent vulnerabilities in complex human-machine systems.

Consider the case of a pilot who has just completed a flight from, say, San Francisco to Frankfurt. The flight departed on the previous day at 2:00 p.m. San Francisco time, and has arrived at 10:00 a.m. Frankfurt time; the time difference between the two cities is nine hours. The pilot will typically now have one or two days off before reporting for duty again. While it is obviously important to obtain adequate sleep during this period so as to be well rested for the next flight, the pilot may well find that it is not easy to do so. Time cues such as sunlight and the activity level of the local population may make it difficult to sleep according to San Francisco time, while his own internal rhythms may leave him feeling wakeful when nighttime arrives in Frankfurt. Although he will probably start to adapt to the new time zone as the layover period progresses, the potential for lingering sleep deficit is obvious. The problem may well be exacerbated in subsequent layovers as the pilot is subjected to further abrupt time changes: he might, for example, fly on to New Delhi (a time shift of another 4 1/2 hours) and quite likely yet a third destination before returning to San Francisco a week after his initial departure.

Even someone who was not exposed to any other fatigue inducing circumstances might find it difficult to obtain adequate rest under such circumstances. In fact, however, desynchronization in aircrew does not tend to occur in a vacuum, divorced from other causes of fatigue. It might even be said that the presence of additional fatigue factors is probably the rule rather than the exception. The pilot we just described, for example, has several possible reasons to feel tired when he arrives in Frankfurt, beyond the circumstance of having crossed nine time zones. Most obviously, he has probably been more or less continuously awake since some time the previous morning and may well be suffering somewhat from lack of sleep. Second, it is 1:00 a.m. in San Francisco, the pilot's home base -- a time when he is normally approaching the lowest level of mental efficiency and alertness, with or without the added complication of sleep deprivation. Third, he has been flying for the past thirteen hours, and the overall length of time that he has been on duty is even longer. Fourth, he has just been involved in landing the aircraft, one of the most demanding phases of the flight. Moreover, as already suggested, factors such as these may become magnified later in the duty week, as the pilot's circadian rhythms become increasingly disoriented and sleep deficit accumulates.

Perhaps because these various factors do tend to occur simultaneously, much existing research on aircrew fatigue has been relatively unsuccessful at distinguishing between them in the context of specific flight operations. Instead, the tendency has been to concentrate on the overall functioning of pilots in real-world operations. There is, for example, a sizable amount of quite specific data concerning the amount and quality of sleep obtained on particular duty and layover schedules within particular flight itineraries, together with assorted measures of physiological functioning; this research has presumably informed such matters as the scheduling of mandatory rest periods between flights. However, until recently little effort has been devoted to analyzing the factors affecting pilot functioning under these circumstances, or to providing an overview of pilot rest requirements.

The United States National Transportation Safety Board's analysis of the accident involving China Airlines Flight 006 (see sidebar) illustrates some of the difficulties that confront investigators who seek to understand the genesis of aircrew fatigue. It also points up the pitfalls of measuring 'fatigue' primarily in terms of a single variable -- in this case, the amount of sleep obtained in the hours immediately preceding the flight. The NTSB report states that the captain was not unduly fatigued at the time of the accident, but this assessment may well be oversimplistic. His failure adequately to monitor the instruments, for example, could be indicative of a drop in vigilance level. The same is true of his overreliance on the auto-pilot.

Vigilance decrement is, in fact, a typical fatigue effect, one which is particularly associated with insufficient sleep. Also, the captain's preoccu-

---

On February 19, 1985 China Airlines Flight 006, a Boeing 747, was en route from Taipei, Taiwan, to Los Angeles, California. While cruising at 41,000 feet over the Pacific Ocean some 300 miles northwest of San Francisco the No. 4 engine lost power. During the attempt to recover, the aircraft rolled right, nosed over, and entered an uncontrollable descent of over 30,000 feet. The aircraft was finally stabilized at 9,500 feet and the flight diverted to San Francisco. Although it landed safely, the 747 had suffered major structural damage, and two persons received serious injuries.

The probable cause of the accident, the National Transportation Safety Board determined, was the captain's preoccupation with the in-flight malfunction, overreliance on the autopilot, and failure to monitor properly the aircraft's flight instruments, resulting in loss of control. The Board also noted that the aircraft had been airborne for some ten hours and had traversed several time zones. The loss of control occurred around 0214 Taiwan local time, that is, about four to five hours after the captain had been accustomed to going to sleep. The Board initially theorized, therefore, that his ability to obtain, assimilate, and analyze all the data presented to him could have been impaired. Ultimately, however, the Board concluded that the captain was alert to the situation as it developed. Among the points noted were (i) the captain had had five hours of rest during the flight; (ii) he had slept for two hours during this period; and (iii) he had been at his duty station for three hours when the upset occurred. Thus, it was concluded, the captain may not actually have been sleep deprived.

-- Condensed from NTSB Report AAR-86/03

pation with the inflight malfunction may have been indicative of difficulty with divided attention, another common effect of fatigue. In fact, the basis for the NTSB's conclusion is unclear. The accident occurred at a time of night when the captain may well have been less than fully alert; also, he had recently returned from a layover in Saudi Arabia and could have been suffering from residual effects of circadian desynchronization. Clearly, the picture can be a confusing one.

Models of aircrew rest requirements. In general, regulations governing pilot duty and rest periods have been derived more from heuristics and 'rules of thumb' than from a full awareness of the many factors affecting the quality of rest and of subsequent flying performance.[15] Nevertheless, several attempts have been made to construct general, predictive models of rest requirements that could be applied widely in the scheduling and management of aircrew activities.

These models consist in general of mathematical formulas with weightings assigned to various factors considered to contribute to fatigue.[39] The earlier versions, which date from the 1970s, were actually developed for the benefit of passengers wishing to avoid 'jet lag', and take into account such variables as the duration of the flight, the number of time zones crossed, and departure and arrival times,[3] as well as flight direction (eastbound or westbound) and the age of the individual.[17]

Subsequent models developed specifically for aircrew engaged in multiple long distance flights have added such factors as the presence, number, and spacing of nighttime flights to be completed, the total number of flights in the itinerary, layover length, and the duration of the itinerary,[24] as well as the average number of duty hours per day.[23,30] The mathematical operations conducted on these variables have also become increasingly complex. One relatively recent example runs as follows:

$$Iw = T + 1/2N + Ctr + Clo * Ctz$$

where Iw is a so-called 'workload index', T refers to duty hours, N to night duty hours, Ctr to the coefficient for number of transits, Clo to the coefficient for preceding layover time, and Ctz to the coefficient for the number of time zones crossed in the preceding flight. The coefficients range between 1 and 3 and are derived from earlier models; the computation is repeated for each segment of the flight itinerary.[39] This model, like its predecessors, was determined through a combination of empirical data on pilot fatigue and inferences concerning the causes of this fatigue, and is admittedly somewhat speculative in nature.

Indeed, to identify every one of the factors that might affect pilots' ability to cope with the stresses of long distance flight, sleep deprivation, and desynchronization is clearly no simple task, not least because a number of important factors that ought to go into such formulations are either unpredictable, subject to change, or not easily observable in the first place. First, individuals vary along a number of relevant parameters, not all of which lend themselves readily to external observation. These include the length of the circadian cycle, the level of sensitivity to external time cues, and personal habits and preferences with regard to social activities, exposure to daylight, and other environmental synchronizers.[15] Second, a variety of circumstances prevailing in the layover location (for example, light and noise conditions) may influence the amount and quality of rest obtained; such factors may not always be known in advance. Third, static formulations of pilot workload capacity are based on predictions of sleep periods rather than on the actual amount of rest obtained, and a strong case could be made for a more dynamic formula adaptable to real-world experience on a day-to-day basis.

Accurate weighting of variables is also a problematic endeavour, since their relative importance may vary for different individuals, and since they may also have synergistic effects upon one another. It has been argued, in fact, that there are inherent limitations to the very notion of determining aircrew sleep requirements by means of a mathematical equation. One team of researchers[15] has recently expressed the opinion that "the timing and quality of sleep obtained by flight crews is the product of a subtle and dynamic interplay between [many] factors and cannot be captured by any simple predictive algorithm" (pp. 33-34); they go on to suggest that future approaches to the problem might incorporate a computer based 'intelligent scheduling assistant'.

We would tend to agree that the number of relevant variables is such that they could be manipulated more easily with the aid of expert systems technology. However, it is also clear that the present fund of information on aircrew sleep requirements needs to be expanded before such a system can be implemented. In particular, a more detailed analysis is needed of the factors that bear upon these requirements; otherwise, computer systems will be no better at weighting the variables than humans currently are. An important task presently facing researchers, therefore, is additional data collection, done with a view toward identifying general patterns that can be applied predictively. Fortunately, the past few years have seen several well-designed studies that should make substantial contributions toward achieving this goal. The next section of this chapter will provide an overview of aircrew rest patterns and discuss some of the recent findings in this area.

Aircrew sleep/wake patterns and the factors that affect them

Duty schedules

In the world of commercial aviation, a primary determinant of aircrew sleep patterns following long distance transmeridian flight is, of course, the duty schedules within which the pilots operate. These schedules are in turn constrained by legal restrictions on the maximum length of duty shifts and the minimum length of subsequent rest periods. However, these regulations are by no means universal or consistent. In 1983 Hans-Martin Wegmann and his colleagues at the Institute for Aerospace Medicine in Cologne conducted a review of scheduling guidelines in nine different countries, and found substantial variations from one country to another.[38] Some were structured in terms of the total length of a duty period, while others considered only the time spent in actual flight. Most took into account the degree of workload expected on a given shift, but opinions varied as to which conditions were associated with heavy workload. For example, one type of operation commonly regarded as being particularly demanding was night flying, but in the various countries studied the period of time defined as 'night' varied in length from as few as six hours to as many as twelve.

In general, however, there appeared to be a consensus to the effect that individual crew members should not be on duty for more than fourteen continuous hours. For demanding conditions such as nighttime flying this maximum is generally reduced to between nine and eleven hours; if relief crew are available it may be increased to as many as eighteen hours. In any event this would appear to constitute an unusually long working day when contrasted with the work shifts typical of most other professions. Moreover, it has been pointed out that in many cases the time spent travelling between home and airport augments the day even further. On many occasions, in fact, pilots going to sleep after a long flight have been awake for periods well in excess of twenty-four hours.

Dallas, Texas, April, 1989: We were a cabin and cockpit crew, over-worked and fatigued to the point of unsafe conditions. The cabin crew's duty day started at XX55. The day consisted of long flights of continuous service with no breaks all night long, including ten minimum turns. As the night progressed, we became more tired due to bad weather over Houston, our final destination. We circled over Houston for approximately forty-five minutes. Then, because of the intensity of the storm and radar problems, we were forced to divert to Austin, Texas. We continued our service, answered questions and tended to passenger needs. By the time we landed in Austin, we had had a long, hard strenuous night. We held on the ground in Austin for one hour, twenty-five minutes, answering passenger questions about possibly being put up for the night in Austin. When we discovered there were no hotel rooms available for our seventy-five passengers and our crew, our captain decided to make another attempt for Houston.

We changed aircraft (one with better radar) and persevered to Houston again. This time we circled around the storms approximately one hour. This time we left Austin at YY00 and without success -- unable to land in Houston. The passengers were irritably uneasy, hungry and tired from the strenuous night. We continued our service, reassuring the passengers and tending to their needs. Consequently we had three people who spoke no English whatsoever and a retarded teenager traveling by herself. She would scream on the takeoffs and landings and during the storms. We had to give special attention to these people. As we served, our hands were shaking with exhaustion, our minds fatigued from the intense night, with no breaks for a meal or from the passengers.

On arrival in Dallas, our captain requested the crew (cockpit and cabin) be replaced due to fatigue, mental and physical. I called our scheduling department. Scheduler quoted from our contract that we had to stay on the plane for one hour, then work another one hour flight to Houston. I was shocked because we were at a crew base where they could replace us. We had been on duty at this point in excess of fourteen intense hours, and they told us to work two more hours! I called scheduling back and told them that due to our exhaustion, fatigue, we could not function in any emergency and we must be replaced. Scheduling replaced us but my cabin crew has been unduly suspended for seven working days, approximately two weeks of work, for making a decision for the safety of the passengers and our own. Our company in flight department has been unfair and unconcerned about our extensive fatigue and the safety of our passengers.

-- NASA Aviation Safety Reporting System (Accession No. 110833)

Stipulated rest periods also varied widely from one country to another. Minimum off-duty time ranged from as few as six hours to as many as sixteen, and in some countries was based on the length of the preceding flight (which was multiplied by 2 or 4). Other factors sometimes taken into account included the number of takeoffs and landings completed and the presence of various adverse flying conditions. Some countries required that rest periods include nighttime hours so as to better facilitate sleep; others did not. The additional fatigue to be expected from crossing multiple time zones was also only occasionally taken into account.

It might be assumed from this lack of consistency that regulations governing rest and duty schedules are to a large extent arbitrarily (or politically) conceived, with only minimal regard for the actual needs of aircrew. This is probably an exaggeration: as Wegmann states, many differences are more likely the result of varying procedural and operational conditions in the countries concerned, and it would be unwarranted to assume that basic safety considerations are routinely ignored. Nevertheless, the point can still be made that flight schedules appear to be determined more by local 'rules of thumb' than by science -- or at any rate that they were in 1983. The report expresses particular concern about the lack of attention paid to circadian rhythmicity and to the difficulties engendered by flights across multiple time zones; as noted already, however, substantial progress has been made since then toward establishing the kind of research base that can correct this situation. Even recently, however, researchers have noted that despite the large volume of data available on aircrew fatigue and the mass of regulations governing layover periods en route, surprisingly little is known about the extent to which these mandated rest periods actually mitigate the effects of desynchronization.[2]

Studies of aircrew rest patterns

Early research on human adaptation to long haul transmeridian flight tended to take one of two forms. Several studies were conducted which relied upon sleep logs completed by pilots themselves; these included records of sleep onset and wakeup times as well as subjective assessments of sleep quality.[30,32] In another type of study, postflight sleep was monitored in laboratories with the aid of electroencephalographic and other physiological measures.[13,22,36] This approach obviously had the advantage of objectivity and also provided more detailed data on such parameters as the type of sleep (REM versus NREM), sleep latency (elapsed time between the first attempt at sleep and actual sleep onset), and the number of awakenings within a sleep period. However, these studies were initially conducted not on pilots but on passenger volunteers, who were not restricted from sleeping en route and who were, in general, relatively unaccustomed to rapid travel across multiple time zones. These factors limited the applicability of such research to the operational needs of aircrew.[20]

Not until relatively recently, in fact, have the tools and methods of sleep research been applied to active aircrew. The first effort in this direction was undertaken in the mid-1980s, in the form of a rather ambitious international program of research sponsored by the National Aeronautics and Space Administration and carried out by teams of researchers from the United States, Britain, Germany, and Japan. Within this cooperative framework, aircrew layover rest and activity patterns were studied at a variety of locations using a standardized experimental protocol.[20] In each study, pilots completed flights across seven to nine time zones and then checked in, not to a hotel as per usual, but to a laboratory where their sleep was monitored continuously with the use of polysomnographic equipment. In addition, the Multiple Sleep Latency Test (MLST)* was administered at regular intervals during pilots' waking hours. In addition to the core procedure observed in all of the studies, individual research teams also collected several types of ancillary data, including, for example, information concerning circadian phase as evidenced by rectal temperature and urinary catecholamine output.

The data obtained were quite consistent across the various studies, and a number of recommendations were presented.[19] First, as has been observed elsewhere, westbound flights generally produced fewer sleep disturbances than eastbound flights. Pilots on a forty-eight hour layover following a westbound flight typically experienced two nights' sleep of essentially normal duration before reporting for their next duty period. Even so, daytime alertness was substantially compromised, with drowsiness tending to increase as waking periods progressed. A common strategy on the second day of the layover was for the pilot to take a nap before commencing the next leg of the flight itinerary, particularly when that flight was scheduled to occur at nighttime. This practice was endorsed by the researchers as a means of reducing drowsiness and performance decrement

---

*This test requires subjects to interrupt their activities, lie down in a darkened room, and close their eyes; the speed with which they fall asleep, if they do so at all, is taken as a measure of daytime sleepiness and, by implication, of the quality of sleep previously obtained.

during the flight, and has also been supported by other studies of layover naps.[26,27,31] A second recommendation for westbound flights concerned the scheduling of the subsequent flight after the layover: the latter part of the flight, it was suggested, should be timed to coincide with the increase in alertness associated with the early morning rise in body temperature.

Eastbound flights presented a more complex set of problems, it was found: humans apparently find it more difficult to adjust to a shortening of their day than to a lengthening. Layover sleep following such flights was shorter, more fragmented and, in subjective terms, of poorer quality than normal sleep at home. The scheduling of sleep within the layover period was also less predictable than after westbound flights. One common pattern was for the pilot to go to bed upon arriving at the layover destination but to wake up within a relatively short period; subsequent sleep episodes then varied considerably in their timing and duration. Some individuals attempted to manipulate their sleep by remaining awake until an hour corresponding to their customary bedtime at home, while others apparently slept whenever they felt the need to do so.

Many pilots expressed a belief that the final sleep obtained before the next duty period was the most important. The researchers, working from this premise, therefore recommended that the pilot arriving on layover resist the temptation to sleep, and wait until the local night before going to bed. This strategy, they suggested, while possibly increasing fatigue in the short term, would maximize sleepiness and enhance sleep quality during the *second* local night of the layover and ensure that the pilot was well rested immediately before the next flight.[19]

While it is true that sleep may be deeper following excessive fatigue and tends to last longer when it coincides with the local night,[15] there are several assumptions in evidence here which may not fully hold up under scrutiny. One appears to be that if deeper sleep can be encouraged by an extended period of forced wakefulness beforehand, not only will this prior sleep deprivation be fully compensated for, but the individual may experience a 'net gain', as it were, in restedness. Another apparent assumption is that a person who wakes up spontaneously after an extended period of sleep is necessarily fully rested.

In fact there is good evidence that aircrew performing multiple long haul flights often experience a substantial accumulation of fatigue. An acknowledged limitation of the NASA cooperative study is that it examined only the layover periods following a single long distance flight; in reality, of course, the initial layover in a pilot's duty week is followed by additional flights, additional layovers in yet other time zones, and, quite likely, further circadian desynchronization. Add to this the fact that some of these flights may occur overnight and require extended periods of wakefulness, and the potential for an accumulated sleep deficit is obvious. It may therefore be shortsighted to evaluate 'restedness' only in terms of the immediately preceding sleep episode. More recently some of the same investigators (again sponsored by Ames Research Center) have looked at aircrew sleep patterns over entire trip sequences, and they are now suggesting that postponing sleep to conform to local time may not be advisable if it has the effect of reducing the total amount of sleep obtained. This is particularly true in the latter part of the duty week.[15]

Successive layovers

Existing models of aircrew rest requirements have proceeded from a general supposition that layover sleep is a fixed entity affected by the same kinds of factors at any given time. This assumption allows a single formula to be applied to all segments of a flight itinerary. In reality, of course, it is possible that considerable changes may be occurring in successive legs of an itinerary, where pilots are undergoing not one but repeated shifts in time zone and, presumably, continued and augmented circadian desynchronization. Cumulative sleep deficit is also a distinct possibility under such circumstances. The subject of sleep differences in successive layovers is obviously not a simple one and has yet to receive detailed research attention; however, recent research (again sponsored by NASA) has yielded some interesting data concerning sleep variations within the course of a single layover. Specifically, it appears that where two sleep episodes occur within one layover, the second of these is governed by different factors than the first -- a finding that may have important theoretical implications for future research on many aspects of aircrew rest requirements.

The study in which this discovery was made monitored aircrew sleep patterns during successive layovers within a variety of international flight itineraries.[15] Duty periods averaged approximately ten hours in length and alternated with layovers of about twenty-four hours. Pilots typically had two major sleep episodes within the span of one layover, and a wake episode in between amounting to an average of seven and a half hours (not including time spent napping). The data collected included continuous monitoring of circadian phase (via rectal temperature, heart rate, and activity of the nondominant wrist), as well as records of sleep onset and wake times, and pilots' subjective evaluations of the quality of that sleep. This information was incorporated into quantitative analyses of the various factors influencing layover sleep, including circadian rhythm phase, local time, level of fatigue (i.e., sleep debt), and duty requirements.

The timing of the initial sleep episode was influenced most markedly by circadian phase: sleep onset was most likely to occur shortly before the daily temperature minimum, just as it does normally. Other influences on the timing of initial sleep onset included local time (there was a strong preference for sleeping during the local night or, secondarily, early in the local afternoon), and the presence of sleep debt.

Circadian phase was less of a factor, however, in determining when the pilot *awoke* from this first sleep period. This is not to say that it was entirely irrelevant -- the sooner before the daily temperature minimum sleep commenced, the longer it was likely to last -- but the most important variable governing awakening proved to be local time. One pattern commonly observed following eastbound flights, for example, was for a pilot to arrive during the afternoon, sleep for a few hours, and awaken in the early evening. Since naps of this sort occurred during various phases of the circadian temperature cycle they were assumed to arise from an accumulated sleep debt that overrode existing internal rhythms; therefore, the fact that the sleep terminated after a few hours indicated not a state of full restedness but more likely a response to social conditions (for example, dinnertime). This interpretation of the data is supported by the observation that when initial sleep was postponed until the local night it was typically substantially longer. No positive relationship was recorded between the duration of the initial sleep episode and the length of time the individual had previously been awake, a finding which may seem counterintuitive but which is well corroborated in the sleep research literature.[5]

The second sleep episode within a layover was, as noted, subject to somewhat different influences than the first. The time of onset, for example, bore little relationship to circadian phase: rather, the most important factor governing the onset of the second sleep episode was the length of the preceding one, that is, the amount of sleep already obtained. There was also a marked preference for sleeping during the local night, which suggests that the pilots were beginning to synchronize to local time. The *duration* of the second sleep period, however, was most strongly constrained by upcoming duty requirements and the desire to get as much rest as possible before the next leg of the flight itinerary: the primary controlling variable was the amount of time remaining until the next flight, and pilots typically awoke within a few hours of reporting for duty. (The study did not consider layovers lasting longer than twenty-four hours.) A secondary influence on second-sleep duration was circadian phase (as with the first sleep); since the rise in temperature following the daily minimum was likely to trigger awakening, sleep lasted longer if it began earlier in relation to this minimum. (It may be presumed that if the layover were longer and duty obligations not imminent, circadian phase would play a more prominent role in determining second-sleep duration, as would local time.)

To summarize, then, falling asleep and waking up were governed by somewhat different factors, both in the first and second sleep episodes. A third dimension to consider, however, is that of sleep quality. In this study, as in the majority of research on aircrew rest patterns, the quality of sleep was rated by means of subjective assessments provided by the pilots, with answers to questions concerning ease in falling asleep, depth of sleep, ease in arising, and feelings of 'restedness'. In general, the first sleep episode was felt to be more restful than the second, and correlated with the length of the preceding wake duration (which sometimes exceeded twenty-four hours).

This finding is quite consistent with the general observation that sleep following extended wakefulness tends to be deeper than normal.[5] Also, as noted earlier, the initial sleep episode was more closely linked to circadian phase, and was consequently less likely to be disrupted by rises in temperature and other physiological phenomena normally associated with awakening. For both sleep episodes, however, the factor most strongly correlated with high quality, restful sleep was the duration of that sleep. The operational implications of this finding are clear: as the authors of the study[15] put it, "this reinforces the importance of ensuring that adequate time is available for sleep" (p. 31).

Strategies for aircrew rest management

Timing of sleep episodes

One question confronting pilots when they come off a duty period is when to schedule their sleep during the layover. For travellers who plan to remain at the new destination for an extended period, the usual strategy is to try to resynchronize their sleep/wake cycles to the local time zone as quickly as possible, even if this means incurring some sleep deficit in the short term. Aircrew, however, have somewhat different needs. Since they will typically be flying on to yet another time zone within the next few days, their interest is less in going out of their way to adapt to the current environment than in obtaining adequate rest before the next duty period.

Arguments can be presented to support a variety of strategies. For example, there is a widespread preference among pilots in favor of sleeping during the local night, which is presumably related to conditions of light, noise, and social circumstances such as meal availability. On the other hand, there is also evidence that sleep is likely to occur more readily, be of better quality, and last longer when it is in harmony with the individual's internal time, or 'circadian phase'. This fact would appear to argue in favour of timing sleep to coincide with nighttime at the home base, when the pilot is most likely to feel naturally sleepy. However, another possibility is suggested by Dement, who points out that drowsiness, or the propensity to fall asleep peaks not once but twice in each twenty-four-hour period -- at bedtime and also during the early part of the afternoon (the so-called 'post-lunch decrement').[6] Pilots can therefore take advantage of this period as well when planning sleep times.

There is, however, a potential complication attendant upon scheduling sleep in accordance with physiological rhythms. It may be relatively easy to determine circadian phase after a single transmeridian flight, but the pilot who makes successive changes in time zone over the course of a week may find it increasingly difficult to know where in the circadian cycle he is at any given moment. One approach to this difficulty has been proposed by Sasaki, who suggests that pilots could identify their circadian phase with the help of the Multiple Sleep Latency Test.[37] While the logistics of the test might require that a sleep laboratory be added to the hotel facilities where pilots stay, it could be, at least in theory, one way to help aircrew make the most effective use of their layover time.

It might also be possible for pilots to determine circadian phase by monitoring changes in body temperature. This method has the obvious advantage of requiring neither special equipment nor trained personnel. However, it may be less than reliable, as temperature is affected by the level of physical activity as well as by circadian rhythms; also, if taken orally, readings can also be corrupted by the temperature of the ambient air or of recently consumed food and drink.

The actual schedule adopted will be affected by several factors. One of these is direction of travel. Flights from east to west place the traveller in a situation where his circadian phase is ahead of the local time. This is termed *phase delay:* internal time must slow down, in effect, in order to synchronize itself to local time. When the flight is from west to east, in contrast, circadian rhythms must speed up for the individual to become entrained to the new environment; this type of shift is referred to as a *phase advance.* In general, westbound flights are associated with fewer sleep difficulties. Another factor which often interacts with direction of flight is the time of arrival at the layover destination. For example, a pilot arriving in the evening after a daytime, westbound flight is likely to have relatively little difficulty falling asleep at the local bedtime. He will, in effect, merely have had an unusually long day, although his more advanced circadian rhythms may cause some wakefulness as morning approaches.[19] On the other hand, a pilot arriving in the morning after an overnight east-bound flight will most likely be experiencing not only task related fatigue but a substantial sleep deficit, and unlike the westbound pilot will find his need for sleep to be considerably at odds with that of the local population. With an extended period of wakefulness behind him and many hours of daylight still ahead, he would probably find it impractical if not impossible to wait until the local bedtime before sleeping. One response might be to sleep at the time corresponding to afternoon of the individual's home time. Another might be to nap for a few hours upon arrival and then remain awake until the local evening.

Naps

Layover naps. Naps -- that is, brief episodes of sleep in addition to the longer 'primary' sleep periods -- have also been the object of some study. Many pilots resist the urge to nap during layovers, even if they may feel the need. This apparently stems from a belief that drowsiness during flight can best be prevented by obtaining as much sleep as possible immediately before reporting for duty.[15] Some aircrew members even go so far as to deliberately incur sleep deficit early in the layover period so as to maxi-mize sleep at the end of it.[6] To some extent this strategy has even been endorsed by researchers.[19] However, it has also been pointed out that this recommendation is based only on observations of pilots on the initial layover of a duty week; monitoring of pilot sleeping patterns on successive layovers indicates that sleep deficit can accumulate significantly as the week progresses. Given this circumstance, it would appear to be more important to concentrate on maximizing the total amount of sleep obtained over the course of a layover.

A different type of napping strategy involves taking *only* naps. Dement has suggested, for example, that if short sleeps of two to six hours are scheduled for each of the two daily lows in alertness (afternoon and nighttime), the total amount of sleep obtained may be adequate for each twenty-four-hour period.[6] This type of practice has been the object of some investigation within the context of various kinds of prolonged operations.[9,10,11,28] These studies suggest that alertness and overall performance can be maintained for quite extended periods of time (for example, as long as nine days) on a sleep regime consisting exclusively of naps. However, it should be noted that these studies have been conducted in settings where longer periods of sleep are impracticable -- for example, in military maneuvers of various kinds -- and to implement this type of schedule in commercial aviation would entail a radical restructuring of duty-rest cycles as they currently exist. Such a restructuring is unlikely to happen in the absence of compelling need, since there is no evidence to suggest that brief, frequent naps are inherently better than, or even as good as, more traditional sleep habits.

Flight deck naps. Napping can take place not only in off-duty periods but during flight. While doing so has often been officially prohibited, there is numerous anecdotal evidence to indicate that it is not an uncommon occurrence. Because of this, many researchers are now arguing that it may be better to schedule nap periods deliberately than to allow sleep to occur spontaneously and unpredictably. Research indicates that cockpit naps can have a beneficial effect upon subsequent flying performance. Several recent studies have demonstrated that brief scheduled naps (of forty minutes' duration) have improved aircrew alertness, as measured by reaction time as well as by brainwave and eye movement activity.[8,34,35]

A study of cockpit napping supported by NASA Ames Research Center offers the following guidelines: naps should be planned rather than spontaneous, allowing them to be integrated into the flight operation as a whole; there should be an established rotation schedule so that only one crew member sleeps at any given time; naps should be scheduled during low workload portions of the trip and terminate well before descent; naps should be preceded and followed by formal briefing and transfer of responsibilities. Also, to avoid sleep inertia (grogginess upon awakening), naps should be limited to forty-five minutes or less, and a post-nap recovery period should occur before the crew member is briefed and resumes his duties.[34]

Pharmacological interventions

Prescription and nonprescription medications may also be used in meeting the demands of duty and rest schedules. *Stimulants* may work either preventively, with the goal of maintaining alertness for long periods of time, or as a recovery aid, intended to ameliorate effects of sleep deprivation.[1] On the nonprescription side, caffeine is course a well-known stimulant, and can enhance alertness both on the flight deck and during off-duty periods when the individual is attempting to postpone sleep. However, for transmeridian travellers caffeine has another use as well. It functions as a 'zeitgeber enhancer' -- that is, it increases sensitivity to time cues in the new environment. As such it speeds up the rate at which the individual is able to adapt to the change in time zone, and can be useful in manipulating the sleep/wake cycle and other circadian rhythms. *Relaxants* such as alcohol, on the other hand, may serve as an appropriate 'sleep aid' when consumed in moderate amounts, especially given that many pilots express a need to 'unwind' after completing a flight.[6] There may even be a role for the occasional administration of short-life benzodiazepines.

Pilot education

It has been observed that although the traditional approach to minimizing the effects of pilot fatigue and circadian desynchronization has been via the scheduling of rest periods, a strong case could also be made for pilot education.[15] Pilots naturally utilize a range of strategies for making optimal use of alloted rest periods. Some of these are implicit in the preceding discussion: for example, a pilot can decide whether to sleep at will or to schedule sleep periods; if the latter, a further decision is whether to conform to the home time zone or the present one. Supplementary naps may or may not be taken; the timing of sleep may also be manipulated via the use of stimulants such as caffeine or depressants such as alcohol and sleep remedies. An additional role may be played by dietary factors, i.e., the timing and content of meals; this subject has received some attention from chronobiologists but rather less in the world of aviation medicine.

In short, physiological adjustment to the demands of long distance transmeridian flight is influenced not only by external scheduling conditions but by various aspects of pilots' own behaviour. At present decisions concerning this behaviour tend to be reached according to individual experience and inclination, often with the aid of informal heuristics and 'rules of thumb' that may be shared among fellow crew members. Certainly the more information aircrew have about sleep and circadian rhythms, however, the better use they will be able to make of layover time and the more they will be able to tailor it to specific circumstances.

References

1. Babkoff, H., and Krueger, G.P. (1992), 'Use of stimulants to ameliorate the effects of sleep loss during sustained performance', *Military Psychology,* vol. 4, no. 4.

2. Beh, H.C., and McLaughlin, P.J. (1991), 'Mental performance of air crew following layovers on transzonal flights', *Ergonomics,* vol. 34, pp. 123-35.

3. Buley, L.E. (1970), 'Experience of a physiologically-based formula for determining rest periods on long-distance air travel', *Aerospace Medicine,* vol. 41, pp. 680-3.

4. Czeisler, C.A., Weitzman, E.D., Moore-Ede, M.C., Zimmer, J.C., and Knauer, R.S. (1980), 'Human sleep: its duration and organization depend on its circadian phase', *Science,* vol. 210, pp. 1264-7.

5. Daan, S., Beersma, D., and Borbely, A.A. (1984), 'Timing of human sleep: recovery process gated by a circadian pacemaker', *American Journal of Physiology,* vol. 246, pp. R161-78.

6. Dement, W.C., Seidel, W.F., Cohen, S.A., Bliwise, N.G., and Carskadon, M.A. (1986), 'Sleep and wakefulness in aircrew before and after transoceanic flights', *Aviation, Space, and Environmental Medicine,* vol. 57, pp. B14-28.

7. Dinges, D.F. (1990), *Crew Rest and Sleep Deprivation,* Flight Safety Foundation, 35th CASS, Montreal.

8. Dinges, D.F., Graeber, R.C., Connell, L.J., Rosekind, M.R., and Powell, J.W. (1990), 'Fatigue-related reaction time performance in long-haul flight crews', *Sleep Research,* vol. 19, p. 117.

9. Dinges, D.F., Orne, E.C., Evans, F.J., and Orne, M.T. (1981), 'Performance After Naps in Sleep-Conducive and Alerting Environments', in Johnson, L.C., Tepas, D.I., Colquhoun, W.P., and Colligan, M.J. (eds.), *Advances in Sleep Research, vol. 7: Biological Rhythms, Sleep, and Shift Work,* Spectrum Publications, New York.

10. Dinges, D.F., Orne, M.T., and Orne, E.C. (1985), 'Assessing performance upon abrupt awakening from naps during quasi-continuous operations', *Behavior Research Methods, Instruments, and Computers,* vol. 17, pp. 37-45.

11. Dinges, D.F., Orne, M.T., Orne, E.C., and Whitehouse, W.G. (1986), 'Napping to Sustain Performance and Mood: Effects of Circadian Phase and Sleep Loss', in Haider, M., Kollar, M., and Cervinka, R. (eds.), *Studies in Industrial and Organizational Psychology: Vol. 3. Night- and Shiftwork: Long Term Effects and Their Prevention.* Proceedings of the VII International Symposium on Night- and Shiftwork, Peter Long, New York, pp. 23-30.

12. Dodge, R. (1982), 'Circadian rhythms and fatigue: a discrimination of their effects on performance', *Aviation, Space, and Environmental Medicine,* vol. 53, pp. 1131-6.

13. Endo, S., Yamamoto, T., and Sasaki, M. (1981), 'Effects of Time Zone Changes on Sleep', in Johnson, L.C., Tepas, D.I., Colquhoun, W.P., and Colligan, M.J. (eds.), *Advances in Sleep Research, vol. 7: Biological Rhythms, Sleep, and Shift Work,* Spectrum Publications, New York.

14. Evans, J.I., Christie, G.A., Lewis, S.A., Daly, J., and Moore-Robinson, M. (1972), 'Sleep in time zone changes: a study in acute sleep reversal', *Archives of Neurology,* vol. 26, pp. 36-48.

15. Gander, P.H., Graeber, R.C., Connell, L.J., and Gregory, K.B. (1991), *Crew Factors in Flight Operations: VIII. Factors Influencing Sleep Timing and Subjective Sleep Quality in Commercial Long-Haul Flight Crews,* NASA Technical Memorandum 103852, Ames Research Center, Moffett Field, California.

16. Gander, P.H., Myhre, G., Graeber, R.C., Anderson, H.T., and Lauber, J.K. (1989), 'Adjustment of sleep and circadian temperature rhythm after flights across nine time zones', *Aviation, Space, and Environmental Medicine,* vol. 60, pp. 733-43.

17. Gerathewohl, S.J. (1974). 'Simple calculator for determining the physiological rest period after jet flights involving time zone shifts', *Aerospace Medicine,* vol. 45, pp. 449-50.

18. Graeber, R.C. (1988), 'Aircrew Fatigue and Circadian Rhythmicity', in Wiener, E.L. and Nagel, D.C. (eds.), *Human Factors in Aviation,* Academic Press, Inc., San Diego, London.

19. Graeber, R.C., Dement, W.C., Nicholson, A.N., Sasaki, M., and Wegmann, H.M. (1986), 'International cooperative study of aircrew layover sleep: operational summary', *Aviation, Space, and Environmental Medicine,* vol. 57 (Suppl.), pp. B10-B13.

20. Graeber, R.C., Lauber, J.K., Connell, L.J., and Gander, P.H. (1986), 'International aircrew sleep and wakefulness after multiple time-zone flights: a cooperative study', *Aviation, Space, and Environmental Medicine,* vol. 57 (Suppl.), pp. B3-B9.

21. Klein, K.E., and Wegmann, H.M. (1979), 'Circadian Rhythms of Human Performance and Resistance: Operational Aspects', in AGARD Lecture Series No. 105, *Sleep, Wakefulness, and Circadian Rhythms,* NATO, Neuilly-sur-Seine.

22. Klein, K.E., Wegmann, H.M., Athanassenas, G., Hohlweck, H., and Kuklinski, P. (1976), 'Air operations and circadian performance rhythms', *Aviation, Space, and Environmental Medicine,* vol. 47, pp. 221-30.

23. Mills, N.H., and Nicholson, A.N. (1974), 'Long Range Air-to-Air Refuelling. A Study of Duty and Sleep Patterns', in Nicholson, A.N. (ed.), *Simulation and Study of High Workload Operations,* AGARD-CP-146, NATO-AGARD, Neuilly-sur-Seine.

24. Mohler, S.R. (1976), 'Physiological index as an aid in developing airline pilot scheduling patterns', *Aviation, Space, and Environmental Medicine*, vol. 47, pp. 238-47.

25. Monk, T.H., Moline, M.L., and Graeber, R.C. (1988), *Inducing Jet Lag in the Laboratory: Patterns of Adjustment to an Acute Shift in Routine*, Aerospace Medical Association, Washington, DC.

26. Mullaney, D.J., Kripke, D.F., Fleck, P.A., and Johnson, L.C. (1983), 'Sleep loss and nap effects on sustained continuous performance', *Psychophysiology*, vol. 20, pp. 643-51.

27. Naitoh, P. (1981), 'Circadian Cycles and Restorative Power of Naps', in Johnson, L.C., Tepas, D.I., Colquhoun, W.P., and Colligan, M.J. (eds.), *Advances in Sleep Research, vol. 7: Biological Rhythms, Sleep, and Shift Work*, Spectrum Publications, New York.

28. Naitoh, P., and Angus, R.G. (1989), 'Napping and Human Function During Prolonged Work', in Dinges, D.F. and Broughton, R.J. (eds.), *Sleep and Alertness: Chronobiological, Behavioral and Medical Apsects of napping*, Raven, New York, pp. 221-46.

29. Nicholson, A.N. (1970), 'Sleep patterns of an airline pilot operating world-wide east-west routes', *Aerospace Medicine*, vol. 41, pp. 626-32.

30. Nicholson, A.N. (1972), 'Duty hours and sleep patterns in aircrew operating world-wide routes', *Aerospace Medicine*, vol. 43, pp. 138-41.

31. Nicholson, A.N., Pascoe, P.A., Roehrs, T., Roth, T., Spencer, M.B., Stone, B.M., and Zorick, F. (1985), 'Sustained performance with short evening and morning sleeps', *Aviation, Space, and Environmental Medicine*, vol. 56, pp. 105-14.

32. Preston, F.S. (1973), 'Further sleep problems in airline pilots on world-wide schedules', *Aerospace Medicine*, vol. 44, pp. 775-82.

33. Preston, F.S., and Bateman, S.C. (1970), 'Effect of time zone changes on the sleep patterns of BOAC B-707 crews on world-wide schedules', *Aerospace Medicine,* vol. 41, pp. 1409-15.

34. Rosekind, M.R., Connell, L.J., Dinges, D.F., Graeber, R.C., Rountree, M.S., and Gillen, K.A. (1992), *Crew Factors in Flight Operations: IX. Effects of Planned Cockpit Rest on Crew Performance and Alertness in Long-Haul Operations,* NASA Technical Memorandum 103884, Ames Research Center, Moffett Field, California.

35. Rosekind, M.R., Connell, L.J., Dinges, D.F., Rountree, M.S., and Graeber, R.C. (1991), 'Preplanned cockpit rest: EEG sleep and effects on physiological alertness', *Sleep Research,* vol. 20.

36. Sasaki, M., Endo, S., Nakagawa, S., Kitahara, T., and Mori, A. (1985), 'A chronobiological study on the relation between time zone changes and sleep', *Jikeikai Medical Journal,* vol. 32, pp. 83-100.

37. Sasaki, M., Kurosaki, Y., Mori, A., and Endo, S. (1986), 'Patterns of sleep-wakefulness before and after transmeridian flight in commercial airline pilots', *Aviation, Space, and Environmental Medicine,* vol. 57, pp. B29-42.

38. Wegmann, H.M., Conrad, B., and Klein, K.E. (1983), 'Flight, flight duty, and rest times: a comparison between the regulations of different countries', *Aviation, Space, and Environmental Medicine,* vol. 54, pp. 212-7.

39. Wegmann, H.M., Hasenclever, S., Michel, C., and Trumbach, S. (1985), 'Models to predict operational loads of flight schedules', *Aviation, Space, and Environmental Medicine,* vol. 56, no. 1, pp. 27-32.

40. Winget, C.M., DeRoshia, C.W., Markley, C.L., and Holley, D.C. (1984), 'A review of human physiological and performance changes associated with desynchronosis of biological rhythms', *Aviation, Space, and Environmental Medicine,* vol 55, pp. 1085-96.

10 Stress in air traffic control

It is ... inappropriate to describe ATC work as unusually stressful.
-- Melton, *Physiological Stress in Air Traffic Controllers*

Air traffic control seems to be an extreme task.
-- Luczak, *Work under Extreme Conditions*

The work of the air traffic controller

Air traffic control (ATC) personnel carry out a broad range of functions in many locations within a sometimes vast network. Their duties include tower control, terminal radar control, en route flight monitoring, weather obervation, and much more. However, the basic objective is always the same -- to keep aircraft separated and to ensure a smooth, efficient flow of traffic. The air traffic control network is a complex one with many components: Figure 10.1 (overleaf) shows a schematic representation of the ATC system as it exists in the United States.

The most visible ATC location is, of course, the control tower: behind the familiar sloping glass of the tower's 'cab', controllers coordinate the movements of aircraft within the immediate airspace as well as on the taxiways and runways; they also coordinate the movements of surface vehicles in these areas. The ground controllers and the tower controllers must communicate with the aircraft and with each other to ensure the even flow of traffic in and out of the airport. They must be able to recall aircraft types, registration numbers, positions, speeds, and many other pertinent details; they also need to be able to remember which set of flight rules (visual or instrument) each pilot is operating within. In addition to briefing pilots, tower staff also make regular weather observations and relay their instrument readings to distant weather facilities. They must also communicate and coordinate with their colleagues in the dark of the radar room below them.

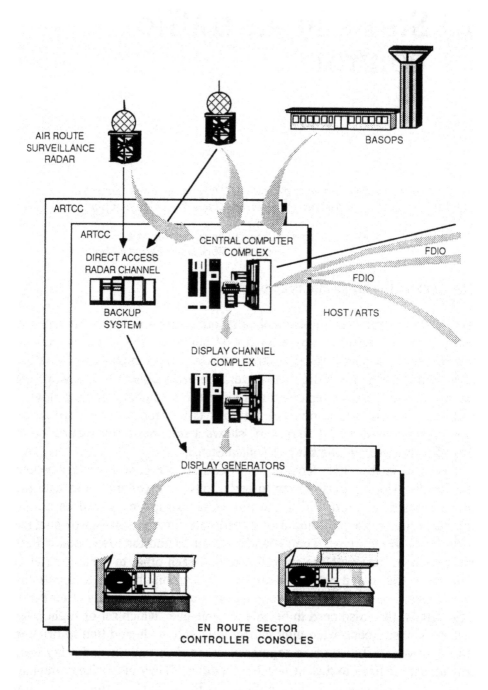

Figure 10.1 Operational elements of ATC system *(Alexander et al.[1])*

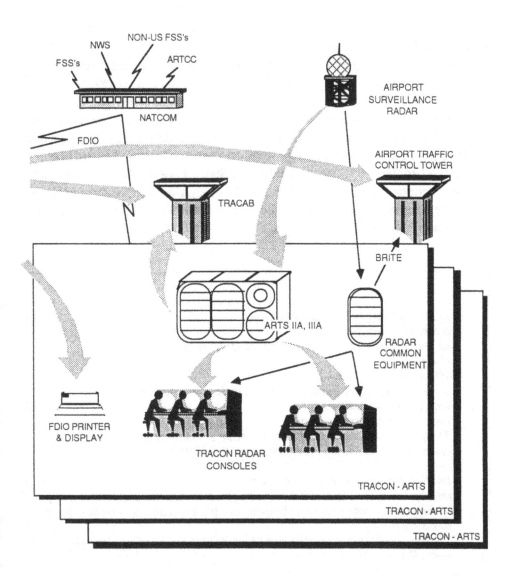

Figure 10.1 *(Continued)*

Controllers in the radar room monitor large screens (see sidebar below). They communicate with aircraft approaching or departing from the terminal area and maintain liaison with other towers and with En Route ATC centres. These centres keep aircraft separated as flights move along and across the crowded airways between terminal areas, providing clearances, advice, and if necessary, search and rescue services. En Route centres may be large and busy installations, equipped with scores of radar screens and staffed by hundreds of controllers.

Even this necessarily impoverished 'thumbnail' representation of the controller's duties suggests that the potential for high workload can be considerable. Given that air traffic control also involves an element of risk, should it be assumed that it is an inherently stressful occupation? Certainly it is often perceived to be an unusually challenging vocation that carries with it an above average level of responsibility. According to a recruiting brochure put out by the United States Federal Aviation Administration,[16] controllers are "a special breed -- tough-minded, alert, not-quite-ordinary people". The brochure goes on to add, "Which figures. It's not an ordinary job" (p. 2).

In the cool dark of the radar room
a controller watches
as the radar beam swings its way around the radius of the screen's
circle.
Within the circle, green blips --
some moving, some stationary; some single, some double; some important, some irrelevant --
compose a pale green galaxy.
This pattern, made up of light and the beam's regular rhythm,
could lull an unknowing eye to the restfulness of sleep.

But in the mind's eye of the controller,
the blips compose a constantly changing three-dimensional picture
of the planes moving through the area, at different altitudes, speeds and
directions.
The ability to carry mental pictures is vital to the work of an air traffic
controller.

-- Federal Aviation Administration,[16] p. 1

The FAA is not alone in expecting a lot from ATC personnel. Many members of the general public are understandably not fully aware of the complex web of responsibilities distributed between controllers, pilots, dispatchers, and others in the network. To many it probably appears that a controller's responsibility is self evidently to 'control' air traffic in a simple, directive, centralized, and perhaps even authoritarian sense. Within this conception events are in the controllers' hands, and it is only natural, if a situation gets out of control, for the layman's (or reporter's) thoughts to turn first to ATC to account for the ensuing incident or mishap. The assumption is often that if an aircraft has (for example) made a navigational error or flown into dangerous weather, it was probably not 'controlled' properly from the ground.

Of course, when all goes well (that is, almost all of the time), the role of ATC has little public visibility. There are few ATC heroes: as with diplomats and anaesthetists, the work of air traffic controllers is very largely taken for granted. Only the errors are noticed. Accidents, incidents, and disputes in aviation stir intense public and media interest, and regrettably it is almost exclusively within these contexts that the role of ATC personnel comes to the public's attention. Given this balance of workload, responsibility, and recognition, then, it could be argued or assumed that the air traffic controller's job has an inherent potential for stress. Certainly the popular press has made this assumption.[46]

In the United States public attention was first directed toward this issue in the late 1960s, when disputes began to develop between air traffic controllers and their managers within the Federal Aviation Administration.[61] Later, more massive publicity was engendered throughout the western world by the American controllers' strike of 1981, which ended with the dismissal of over 11,000 controllers by President Reagan. One aspect of the dispute concerned claims by the Professional Air Traffic Controllers Organization (PATCO) that controllers suffered from high levels of workplace stress -- high enough, they asserted, to be responsible for a variety of adverse health effects.[47]

This chapter evaluates the evidence for and against the presence of unusually high levels of stress in ATC work, and its implications for controllers' health, well-being, and performance. In keeping with the book's transactional and appraisal based approach to stress (and also with claims by the FAA that the striking controllers were somehow unusual in their perception of high workplace stress), we will first consider the issue of personality traits commonly observed in air traffic controllers.

Personality issues

A 1980 report by the FAA Civil Aeromedical Institute asserted that "the problem is to discern to what extent the incidence of hypertension or other physical or psychological problems results from the work, not the person" (Smith,[61] p. 11). This is, of course, a rather revealing 'nontransactional' statement, which, at a time of rock-bottom management relations between American controllers and the FAA, sought to 'blame' workplace stress on the controllers themselves rather on any job related circumstances. What the FAA was suggesting was that personality features specific to air traffic controllers were an important source of the physiological and psychological responses observed in ATC work, and would be so in any work circumstance.

It is not entirely clear how this suggestion squares with the assertion cited earlier that ATC personnel are a "special breed" of "not-quite-ordinary" individuals (a statement that seems suspiciously reminiscent of the folklore surrounding pilots' personalities discussed in Chapter 6). While far fewer studies have been conducted on the personalities of air traffic controllers than on those of pilots, available research does not suggest that air traffic controllers are a highly unusual group of people. For example, a study using the California Personality Inventory showed no significant differences between air traffic controllers and the general male population.[50,70] Another personality test, the Strong Vocational Inventory Blank,[5] similarly failed to demonstrate that air traffic controllers form a unique occupational group.[60]

Other studies have identified differences between air traffic controllers and population norms, but they have tended to be neither large nor consistent. For example, on the Cattell 16 Personality Factor (16PF) inventory,[8] controllers have obtained higher than average scores on four factors: intelligence, group conformity, 'tough mindedness', and compulsivity.[33,50,59] Also, a 1990 study of over six hundred British air traffic controllers found that controllers tended to be less aggressive, ambitious, and competitive than several comparison occupational groups. They were also higher than average in behavioural control.[15,68]

However, these findings do not by themselves throw much light on the *stress reactions* of air traffic controllers. The relationship between personality traits and stress was, of course, discussed at some length in Chapter 6, and several factors were identified that appear to have some bearing on individual reactions to external circumstances. One of the most general stress related personality constructs identified was that of trait anxiety (see also Chapter 1), and we will focus on this particular measure here because it has been studied in several populations of air traffic controllers. Certainly if controllers as a group were found to be unusually trait anxious, this might help to explain the high stress levels that they have sometimes reported. In fact, however, there is no evidence to suggest that controllers are particularly anxiety prone. If anything, the opposite is true. For example, one broad based survey conducted for the US Department of Health, Education, and Welfare found that relative to members of other occupations, ATC personnel tend to exhibit low trait anxiety scores.[6] Further evidence that air traffic controllers are not a particularly nervous population comes from another study[50] which reported low scores in a substantial majority of ATC personnel taking the Tension Anxiety Scale of the Profile of Mood States.[38] The British study referred to on the previous page also found that, in terms of trait anxiety, UK controllers closely resembled established population norms.[15]

Low trait anxiety scores have also been identified in FAA studies of air traffic controllers.[42,44,45,46,63] However, FAA researchers[64] have suggested a possible confounding variable. Anxiety research dating back to the early 1960s suggests that individuals tend to report lower anxiety levels as they get older,[7] and the normative group to which controllers in the FAA studies were compared consisted of college students. Therefore, the low trait anxiety scores sometimes reported for air traffic controllers might, it has been suggested, simply reflect the fact that they are older. That age is not the only factor, however, is suggested by one small study which assessed anxiety levels in student pilots, some of whom also happened to be air traffic controllers: this 'dual qualified' subgroup did exhibit lower trait anxiety scores than the noncontrollers in the study.[64] The small number of subjects (n = 15) precluded any definitive conclusions; however, similar results were obtained in a much larger study, which collected normative data from over 1,800 adults in the same age range as the population of controllers studied.[61] Average anxiety scores for this older sample were indeed lower than those that had been previously established for college undergraduates,[66] but still significantly higher than those that had been previously obtained for US air traffic controllers.

Trait anxiety may also influence the performance of controllers while they are in training. A recent American study examined the relationship between training success and trait anxiety levels of 1,790 ATC trainees.[10] First, it was found that entrants to the FAA Academy had relatively low trait anxiety scores compared to norms for college students and Navy recruits. This would seem to indicate a certain degree of self selection on the part of individuals who choose to become controllers. However, trait anxiety also proved to be a predictor of training success for those students already enrolled: higher scores tended to be associated with greater dropout and failure rates as well as higher field attrition.

Stress reactions in air traffic controllers

In the early 1970s the Federal Aviation Administration began a ten year program of research into the stress experienced by air traffic controllers. Stdies were, in general short term in nature and consisted primarily of physiological and biochemical assessments of ATC crew members going about their work, along with a few psychological evaluations. Physiological functions measured included galvanic skin response, blood pressure, and body temperature; ambulatory electrocardiograms were also taken. Biochemical measurements initially included plasma fibrinogen and phospholipids, as well as urinary 17-OH corticosteroids, epinephrine, norepinephrine, sodium, phosphorus, potassium, urea, and creatinine.* This heavily physiological approach to stress does, of course, have important limitations with respect to the more cognitively oriented models discussed in this book; some implications of the FAA's response based orientation will be addressed subsequently.

The first pair of studies assessed physiological arousal and anxiety levels in controllers at O'Hare International Airport in Chicago. Arousal, as measured by heart rate and phospholipid concentrations, was found to be elevated;[21] in some instances, in fact, phospholipid excretion exceeded that found in Vietnam fighter pilots.[41] (Blood pressure and galvanic skin response did not differ from that of controls, however.) A concurrent study[65] recorded the same individuals' stress and anxiety levels, as assessed by self report: test instruments used included Malstrom's Composite Mood Adjective Check List (CMACL),[35] the Nowlis Anxiety Scale,[49] and the Zuckerman Affect Adjective Check List.[73] Not surprisingly, feelings of

---

*For purposes of comparison across studies, it should be noted that blood sampling was eventually discontinued as it appeared to discourage subject participation and for various reasons of feasibility. The sodium, phosphorus, potassium, and urea tests were not found to be useful in measuring 'stress' and were eliminated as well. Galvanic skin response measurement was also discarded on the grounds that it hindered subjects' activities.[39]

> *On 10 September 1976 Gradimir Tasic was on duty at the understaffed Zagreb Air Traffic Control Centre, the second busiest in Europe. It was his third twelve hour shift in three days, and although officially an assistant in a two man team he was on his own, controlling eleven aircraft. The newly installed radar was still unreliable, and showed a British Trident aircraft at Flight Level 335 (33,500'). In fact it was at FL330. When a Yugoslavian DC-9 was cleared up to FL350 into Tasic's sector (without a squawk code -- the electronic label that gives altitude information), he was too busy to give it his full attention. And when his colleague finally arrived Tasic's workload actually increased, since he now had to provide a briefing. Only when the DC-9 reported climbing through FL327 did Tasic notice the danger: the two aircraft were closing at over 1000 mph. The DC-9 complied with an immediate instruction to level off, but inertia carried it the 300 feet to FL350, the Trident's actual altitude. In the resulting collision all 176 persons on the two aircraft perished. Tasic was found guilty of criminal misconduct under Yugoslavian law and was sentenced to seven years in prison. Due to the efforts of the International Federation of Air Traffic Controllers' Associations he was released in 1978. Subsequently the investigative inquiry was reopened and in 1982 reported that Tasic had become overloaded due to factors outside his control.*
>
> -- Condensed from Stanley Stewart's account in *Air Disasters*

fatigue were found to increase as the work shift progressed and were higher in night shift than in evening shift workers. Anxiety levels, however, were quite low, although they tended to be higher after a work shift than before. In general, significant psychological stress reactions were not found, although it is worth noting that little normative data for the CMACL existed, and conclusions were therefore necessarily limited.

This problem was addressed in a subsequent study conducted at Houston Intercontinental Airport,[42] which employed the State-Trait Anxiety Inventory[66] in addition to the CMACL. Both scales showed a pattern of responses similar to that in the O'Hare study, with fatigue and anxiety indicators higher at the end of a shift than at the beginning, and higher for night shift than for day shift workers. Use of the STAI also made possible comparison with established norms: these indicated that state anxiety was no higher than that of any normative groups. (As in other studies, trait anxiety was fairly low, in the 24th percentile). Physiological and biochemical measures of arousal (heart rate, urinary epinephrine and norepinephrine, and plasma phospholipid concentrations) correlated with activity levels in a given shift, tending to be higher during the day shift than at night, and higher at O'Hare than at the less busy Houston airport. These results are consistent with those found in an early Swiss study, in which catecholamine levels were found to be elevated when controllers were actively performing ATC duties, but not when they were performing clerical or supervisory duties.[53] In summary, then, the researchers were unable to infer remarkable levels of 'stress' on the basis of the physiological and biochemical data.

This general finding continued to be replicated in subsequent FAA research. A 1975 study, for example, evaluated ATC personnel at two additional sites: a general aviation airport with very high traffic and workload, and a radar facility with comparatively low workload. As in the previous study, controllers answered questions from the State-Trait Anxiety Inventory before and after each shift; a new feature was that they also provided a rating of the shift's level of difficulty. State anxiety was again found to be higher after a work shift than before, but it was also found that at both facilities the score for state anxiety increased more than twice as much during shifts that were rated as 'difficult'.[63] The finding that state anxiety increased more during difficult or demanding work periods was also replicated in a subsequent study of military air traffic controllers.[26]

A similar study was conducted at a number of small facilities with low traffic density and, presumably, a lower level of workload than that found in busier towers.[46] The finding that state anxiety increased over the course of a work shift was again replicated, as was the observation that air traffic controllers as a group had low scores for both state and trait anxiety relative to STAI norms. Anxiety ratings of the controllers working in these smaller facilities were in fact no different from those obtained in larger and busier airports. The level of epinephrine excretion was lower, however, and upon analysis was found to correlate very closely (0.96) with the level of traffic volume. No such correlation was found for norepinephrine and steroid levels. It was concluded that epinephrine excretion should be regarded merely as an indicator of ATC workload and not of the emotional state of air traffic controllers.*

---

*Similarly, in pilots heart rate has been reported to be an index of workload but not of emotional stress per se (see Chapter 2, p. 36).

Outside the United States there have been several studies of stress in ATC personnel which have not adopted the heavily physiological and biochemical approach favored by the FAA. For example, in 1988 researchers from Massey University in New Zealand reported a study of 164 controllers from four ATC centres in that country.[54] The study was designed in such a way as to facilitate comparison of results with those obtained in an earlier study of 207 Canadian controllers.[37] Perceived stress from a variety of sources was rated by controllers, and the following five main sources of stress emerged from the study (in order of importance):

(1) equipment limitations

(2) peak traffic

(3) requirement to report colleagues' errors

(4) poor work environment in general

(5) fear of causing an accident.

The mean values found for the two nationalities were very similar. Canadian controllers differed slightly, ranking fear of causing accidents third, bad weather fourth, and work environment and reporting of errors fifth and sixth, respectively. These similarities are notable, bearing in mind that the ATC systems in Canada and New Zealand have appreciable differences in size, organization, and climatalogical conditions. (One 'sore point' for Canadian controllers concerned the use of French; naturally, this was not identified as a stressor by the New Zealand controllers.)

Factor analysis of the stress ratings yielded the conclusion that "the air traffic controller's job produces high task stress" (p. 269), and that this emerged equally from overload and underload. It was also concluded that problems of organization and supervision were very important sources of occupational stress in air traffic control. The finding that "stress is endemic in this occupation" (p. 263) is at marked variance with the conclusions drawn by the FAA.

A 1990 study of British air traffic controllers also attempted to identify sources of workplace stress. In addition, however, the researchers set out to evaluate the effects of stress on health and well-being, and to identify relevant mediators in the form of personality variables and coping strategies.[15,68] As such the study adopted a relatively transactional approach. Two questionnaires were sent out to over 1100 controllers in twenty-five National Air Traffic Services (NATS) units.

The first questionnaire was a general non-domain specific test instrument, the Occupational Stress Indicator.[11] The second collected data relating specifically to air traffic control and also incorporated biographical questions. In addition to these questionnaires, workload was rated using the NASA Task Load Index (TLX),[24] and mood was evaluated via an adjective checklist that assessed depression, anxiety, and fatigue. The Cattell 16PF[8] was also administered.

Just over half the questionnaires were returned completed. As with other research reported earlier in this chapter, trait anxiety was not found to be particularly high. The most important general source of stress reported by the controllers concerned organizational structure and 'climate'. In particular, controllers tended to cite inadequate staffing and training, poor consultation, low morale, and a relative lack of autonomous control (an important stressor, as noted elsewhere).

In addition, three areas of concern were identifed that were specific to air traffic control. These included problems relating to workload, to equipment (its unreliability, positioning, and the like), and to 'external' factors (e.g., public comment). The workload factor comprised demand variables such as shiftwork, hours on duty, and traffic levels. Duty shifts without breaks or additional assistance were particularly stressful, as were traffic load peaks (a stressor also noted by other researchers[30]), extended periods at peak load, and 'extraneous' traffic.

These data were then used to create models of stress among controllers. Interestingly, the predominant effect of workload was a negative influence on perceptions of organizational structure and 'climate'. This, in turn, reduced the quality of sleep in controllers. Stress from workload was also associated with lowered job satisfaction, reduced physical and mental health, together with increases in depression and fatigue. The combination of workload and 'external' factors affected both physical and emotional well-being (as measured by state anxiety).

These results are consistent with, and expand upon, those of the New Zealand researchers. The British investigators conclude that stress is present in controllers, but stop short of stating that stress is, therefore, endemic to ATC work (in the sense of being an integral and inevitable component of the job). Rather, they suggest that many of the organizational and supervisory difficulties (for example, the shiftwork problems discussed later) could be 'fixed' -- in other words, programmed out of the system by relatively modest organizational changes. Where they cannot, appropriate countermeasures and adjustments in training could help air traffic controllers to accept and cope with a less than optimal working environment.

Health problems

As noted at the beginning of this chapter, the American air traffic controllers who walked off the job in 1981 claimed, among other things, that the stress they were experiencing in the workplace was sufficiently severe as to cause adverse health effects.[47] A number of researchers have examined the health status of ATC personnel; however, no definitive trends have been identified, and comparison of data across different studies yields an inconclusive picture. Some early studies, for example, associated air traffic work with gastrointestinal problems.[14,25] Additional research suggested that air traffic controllers suffered from both hypertension and peptic ulcers at a rate four times higher than that found in the overall male population;[9] similar findings were reported in an extensive study that followed nearly 400 controllers over a period of three years.[50]

On the other hand, a review of the medical records of 25,000 ATC personnel found a lower than average incidence of hypertension, and no unusual rate of gastrointestinal complaints.[2] Similarly, a small scale study of controllers working at O'Hare International Airport reported no exceptional incidence of ulcers.[55]

A study of blood pressure levels in both airline pilots and air traffic controllers reported that one-fifth of the controllers suffered from borderline hypertension, fully twice the rate observed in pilots.[3] This is consistent with the findings of a study from the 1960s, which also reported a higher incidence of hypertension in controllers than in a matched pilot population.[13] This may not, however, indicate that ATC work is inherently more 'stressful' than piloting, as these data may at least in part be explained by the more liberal medical waivers available to air traffic controllers.[3]

Smith of the FAA has pointed out that epidemiological comparisons of air traffic controllers with members of other occupations do not, as a rule, control for the effects of rotating and night shift work. He suggests that the high rate of health problems that some studies have reported for air traffic controllers may be due in part to the lower proportion of shift workers in the comparison populations, rather than to factors specific to ATC work itself.[61] However, there does appear to be good evidence from both US and British studies that there is some relationship between controllers' dissatisfaction with management and the development of adverse health effects.[50,68] This would seem to suggest that health problems among ATC personnel may have less to do with the work that they perform than with the social circumstances surrounding that work.

Emotional problems

One review of medical disqualifications in air traffic controllers revealed that of seventy-nine individuals permanently disqualified between 1972 and 1977, sixty-one were removed because of psychological problems.[57] Along similar lines a three year assessment of air traffic controller health, reported that fully one-half of the subjects studied suffered from at least one psychiatric problem. The most common of these was disturbance of impulse control, which was observed in 30 percent of the controllers. In addition, 20 percent developed significant marital problems, and 13 percent experienced depression and anxiety during the course of the study. Also, while only 8 percent were found to be alcohol abusers, over 50 percent were heavy drinkers, which suggests the possibility that additional subjects might develop alcohol problems over time.[50] The survey of ATC medical records cited earlier also identified a high incidence of psychological problems.[2] In another study, over 40 percent of a group of more than 650 air traffic controllers reported severe distress within a six month period, as measured by the Goldberg General Health Questionnaire.[36]

Overall, this would appear to be a rather high rate of psychopathology, although in the absence of comparable norms or a matched control group this is difficult to verify. Certainly it remains to be determined whether or not any of these problems manifest themselves in terms of workplace stress and a concommitant performance impairment on the job. It is also unclear to what extent the presence of psychiatric disorders might be an effect of preexisting personality factors rather than of the work itself. One researcher suggests that controllers could benefit from instruction in meditation and other relaxation techniques, as well as from counselling in strategies for stress reduction. Another has recommended that programs for the treatment of alcohol abuse be instituted in such a way that controllers are not penalized for seeking treatment.[31]

Job attitudes

Another indication of job stress is provided by measures of employee attitudes, which reflect general satisfaction or dissatisfaction in the workplace. Among air traffic controllers, these can be conveniently (if simplistically) divided into attitudes toward controlling aircraft as a job, and attitudes to ATC management and organization. For example, one survey of over 600 individuals reported that the majority of air traffic controllers actually enjoyed the fast pace and high demands of their work. However, many controllers expressed less positive feelings about certain other aspects of their jobs: areas of dissatisfaction included scheduling, relations with management, and the quality of equipment available.[62]

Similar findings were reported in another survey of nearly 800 controllers: dislikes tended to centre around management and working conditions (for example, night shifts), but the challenging nature of the work itself was regarded as a positive feature of the job. In fact, more than 92 percent of the controllers surveyed in this study expressed satisfaction with their work (as compared to an average of 80 percent for other occupations). Moreover, moderate and heavy air traffic was rated as being more enjoyable to monitor than light traffic, which, it was suggested, did not support the idea that air traffic control work was unusually stressful.[58] Of course, this interpretation apparently did not consider the potential role of underload, monotony, and boredom as sources of stress (an issue discussed in Chapter 12). There is also an assumption that low traffic density is necessarily associated with low workload; however, since air traffic control work requires a high degree of vigilance irrespective of traffic density, frustration may result when the arousal needed to maintain this constant alertness is not associated with high levels of activity. Indeed, it has often been observed that too little work can be as stressful as too much, or, indeed, even more so (see also Chapter 12).[31,40]

Finally, passing reference was made earlier to the 1981 strike by PATCO (the Professional Air Traffic Controllers Organization). While this event was not, of course, a controlled scientific investigation, no discussion of job attitudes in ATC can fail to mention it. On August 3, 1981, 11,500 air traffic controllers, representing some 80 percent of the American ATC workforce, walked out of their jobs -- most of them, as it transpired, forever. On the face of it, the factors mitigating against such a large scale action seem overwhelming. The strike was a violation of federal law and strikers risked legal recriminations. The target of the strike was the controllers' only real potential employer, the Federal Aviation Administration. The ATC management within the FAA were known to have an elaborate contingency plan to cope with just such a strike. The agency was supported by a very popular president, Ronald Reagan, who ultimately authorized the dismissal of the strikers. In other words, whatever the forces were that brought the air traffic controllers and the FAA to this point, they must have been singularly potent. Indeed, the strike has

> *Virginia, November, 1990: Two aircraft were being vectored southwest, bound for runway 19 Left and 19 Right, respectively. The first aircraft, a wide bodied jet, was given instructions to descend in front of the second aircraft, a medium sized airliner which was also descending. Less than standard wake turbulence separation occurred as the wide bodied jet passed in front of and above the other aircraft. The occurrence was reported by the supervisor who was monitoring me. The incident occurred after a very tense discussion with the air traffic manager about my pending transfer to another facility as a supervisor. I should not have assumed the controller position due to my emotional state.*
>
> *-- NASA Aviation Safety Reporting System (Accession No. 163964)*

been described by one researcher[4] as "perhaps the greatest labor relations disaster in the history of modern public administration" (p. 5).*

The sources of the controllers' dissatisfaction appear to have lain less with their actual work than with the environment in which this work was performed -- a theme also detectable in research reviewed above. The controllers consistently reported that what they really found stressful was the quality of management and administration.[56,58] Smith has also reported management issues to be a major source of ATC job dissatisfaction.[58,62] One report to the FAA on management and employee relationships criticized FAA management of air traffic controllers as being insensitive, inflexible, and overly authoritarian.[31] Other investigators identified a number of additional complaints: journeymen controllers, for example, felt that management was uninterested in their contributions, and there was frustration at the perceived lack of recognition for exceptional work. A desire was also expressed for greater latitude in problem solving.[50]

Effects of shiftwork and shift rotation schedules

As discussed in Chapters 8 and 9, disruption of circadian rhythms can have negative effects on performance, which may in turn give rise to safety implications. As noted previously, alertness is generally at its lowest be-

*Further details from an organizational perspective may be found on pp. 355-7.

tween 3:00 and 7:00 a.m.; this period should, in theory, be associated with high rates of operator error. Certainly work shift rotation has been linked with adverse psychological and health effects for decades.[23,48] Melton, a researcher for the Federal Aviation Administration, used a com-bined subjective evaluation and response based methodology to examine the shiftwork issue with respect to air traffic controllers. The first study (subsequently replicated) compared psychological, biochemical, and physi-ological reactions to two different shift schedules, which were used sequen-tially at the same airport.[43,45]

The first of these was a five day schedule, consisting of one week (five days) on the day shift, one week on the evening shift, and one week on the night shift, with two days off between each change. This was then fol-lowed by the so-called 2-2-1 schedule (two day shifts, two evening shifts, and one night shift, repeated after a two day rest). Subjective feelings of fatigue, as measured by the Composite Mood Adjective Check List,[35] were slightly more pronounced with the 2-2-1 schedule, while other psychologi-cal dimensions such as anxiety (assessed by the State-Trait Anxiety Inven-tory) were unchanged. Physiological and biochemical measures of arousal were reportedly slightly lower in some instances with the 2-2-1 schedule, but the difference was not significant.

An Italian study examined twenty air traffic controllers working three shifts at the Regional Air Control Centre in Rome.[12] These controllers worked a six day shift cycle, which was set up as a 'fast rotation' schedule in the following manner:

first day: afternoon [1300-2000]
second day: morning [0700-1300]
third day: night [2000-0700]
fourth day: rest
fifth day: off
sixth day: off.

The researchers monitored the controllers' workload in terms of aircraft controlled per hour, and also examined a number of physiological and bio-chemical variables such as heart rate, temperature, and endocrine activity. Performance measures included visual reaction time and critical flicker fusion frequency. Mood, fatigue, and physical fitness were also recorded. It was found that whereas workload varied very appreciably, especially from night to day, the trends in heart rate showed a fairly uniform 'pro-file', being, on average, marginally greater in the afternoon shift than in the morning or night shift. Temperature showed fairly normal circadian changes. Workload did not predict levels of vanillyl mandelic acid, a 'stress' hormone product; levels of this were found to remain high even during the night shift, despite the very low workload associated with this period. Mood worsened toward the end of each shift, as did fatigue, an effect that was strongest during the night shift. The performance test scores were best in the afternoon, but did not deteriorate over the course of a shift. These results in fact simply reflect the usual circadian pattern. Overall, the six day 'rapid rotation' shift arrangement, with the days off following the night shift, hardly altered the controllers' normal circadian patterns.

It is particularly interesting to note that the researchers interpreted the night shift results to mean that the controllers, faced with a very light traffic load, were nonetheless maintaining a level of arousal and performance appropriate to the vigilance required for air traffic control. That is, they remained alert without the external stimulation of workload. This was attributed to compensatory behaviours and good work organization; however, it should be noted that alertness in underload situations is not 'free' -- it can require considerable effort (see the discussions of vigilance in Chapters 3 and 12). Moreover, it has been suggested (on the basis of Canadian data) that most air traffic control incidents and errors tend to occur in just such conditions of apparent light workload.[32] However, this interpretation is called into question by the findings of a follow-up study conducted by the same Italian research team, consisting of a review of 'near miss' incidents in the preceding two year period. Of fifteen such incidents, only one occurred at night; the majority (nine incidents) occured during peak traffic hours at Rome. This finding is also consistent with American data to the effect that the night shift period is not associated with high rates of error.[40]

In the British study cited earlier, duty periods without breaks or additional assistance were found to be particularly stressful, as were traffic load peaks, extended times at peak load, and 'extraneous' traffic. However, shiftwork per se was not found to be a particularly important source of stress, although such problems as did occur were traceable to violations of certain basic principles of scheduling such as those discussed in Chapter 9. For example, it is now maintained that rotating shift schedules ideally should delay the sleep/wake cycle rather than advance it. In other words, human physiology can adjust more easily to an unnaturally lengthened 'day' (as with a shift rotation running from day to evening to night) than to a shortened one that requires the individual to try to sleep before he actually feels tired (as with a schedule involving night shifts, followed by evening shifts, followed by day shifts).

Some methodological problems may be noted in the collection and interpretation of work shift data as they relate to controllers. First, airports experience heavier traffic at certain times of the day; also, smaller airports that do not provide round-the-clock tower support are also likely to be less busy overall.[61] Circadian rhythm effects may be confounded with workload effects in another respect as well: as the night shift is the only shift associated with circadian rhythm disruption, and is typically associated with low workload, reduced arousal may actually exacerbate fatigue.[40]

Perhaps the most dramatic performance impairment associated with night shift work is a complete paralysis in which the person is conscious but 'frozen', that is, rendered immobile. The condition, which can last seconds or minutes, has been known for some decades having been reported shortly after the Second World War.[51,52] In a 1984 study of night nurses it was found that 'night shift paralysis', as it is called, had at one time or another afflicted 12 percent of the nurses surveyed.[20] In 1987 the same researchers conducted a survey of 435 air traffic controllers from seventeen different countries and found a much lower, but nevertheless appreciable, incidence of about 6 percent.[19] There is evidence that the sleep deprivation which contributes to night shift paralysis is cumulative and, therefore, that successive night shifts should be avoided, as should morning and night shifts occurring on the same day. Any level of controller incapacitation is clearly dangerous, and even the prospect of such incapacitation could, because of its potential consequences, represent a source of psychological stress.

That night shift paralysis is not more dangerous or stressful than it is may be due to the team nature of most air traffic control work: should any incapacitation occur it can, in theory, be spotted and compensated for. We say 'in theory' because the history of flight crews failing to detect or to intervene during subtle incapacitation in their colleagues is not encouraging. Nevertheless, in air traffic control as it currently exists humans do monitor humans (at least, potentially). However, as we will discuss in the following section, advanced automation may radically curtail the team aspect of air traffic control. In the future, human-machine dialogue may well predominate rather than human to human dialogue; in such systems, the controller will monitor the machines, but who (or what) will monitor the controller?

Automation

> Automation must provide information (whether on past, present, or future states of the system) which synchronizes well with the controller's flow ... If it does not synchronize, it may well place the controller outside the 'optimal experience' zone and become a significant stressor. (Westrum,[71] p. 369)

Air traffic control used to be, as it were, manual labour. In the absence of radar and computers the system depended entirely on procedural control -- time and distance calculations, position reporting, and the writing of flight progress strips which were physically passed from controller to controller. In the 1950s, however, the expansion of the air carrier system brought with it some early attempts at automating part of the ATC system. In the 1970s computer systems were introduced into air traffic control, albeit at different rates in different parts of the world. In the United States, for example, the ubiquitous IBM 360 (modified as the IBM 9020) was installed in all twenty En Route centres, followed by Univac's ARTS III and ARTS II (minicomputer) systems for services at terminal facilities.

The functioning of this system has been described in terms of closed loop control theory.[29] The configuration of the system at future points forms a set of objectives for a planning function. The desired system state involves maintenance of certain parameters that bear on the safety and efficiency of the system (for example, separation criteria). Excursions or deviations from this state are recognized and arrested by a controlling function which attempts to maintain a sort of system homeostasis. Communication with system elements (e.g., aircraft, other ATC units, ground vehicles) is a key part of this function, as is data management.

It has been pointed out, however, that there is an additional 'metafunction' which is affected by external forces such as weather variables and the unreliability both of human and nonhuman system components.[67] These factors can be difficult to predict. As we will discuss in Chapter 12, an important issue in human-machine system design concerns which tasks are best assigned to the machines (in this case, computers), and which to the human components of the system.[18] In practice, policies in this area have been largely technology driven. Thus, the early automated ATC systems simply collected data, stored it, and presented it for human interpretation and decision making. More recently, advances in data processing and display technology have allowed data to be transformed and labelled in various ways, and predictions to be made from present to future situations (for example, track deviations and conflict alerts).[28] At this stage humans, generally acting in teams, still retain overall planning, problem solving, and decision making control. It is at this level of automation, a level we might term 'automated support', that existing studies of automation and stress have been conducted (and there are few).

Melton and colleagues,[44] for example, performed both psychological and biochemical stress assessments of ATC personnel in two American facilities, before and after installation of ARTS III (Automated Radar Terminal Systems III). This system provides aircraft identity information together with height, position, and movement information. ARTS III is designed to reduce the amount of controller coordination needed; human-machine interaction time is increased (largely in keyboard entry tasks), but overall workload is said to be reduced. It was hypothesized that the introduction of the system might measurably reduce stress, at least as indexed by physiological measures and questionnaire results. In fact, total stress increased, these researchers concluded. No psychological changes (as measured by the State-Trait Anxiety Inventory) were observed either way; that is, work related anxiety seemed to be neither ameliorated nor exacerbated by ARTS III. Heart rate was also unaffected. However, catecholamine excretion increased rather than decreased with ARTS III, although baseline levels also increased.

In the United Kingdom, a 1980 study of computer aiding was undertaken by the University of Aston working with the Royal Signal and Radar Establishment.[72] This study examined an ATC simulation using computer assisted approach sequencing (CAAS), designed to assist in the regulation of inbound traffic to London Heathrow, and interactive conflict resolution (ICR), intended to aid in the detection and resolution of en route traffic conflicts. The results were generally favourable and included an unanticipated phenomenon: one controller team reallocated tasks between controllers such that inbound and outbound traffic was handled independently, although a single controller undertook all communication with the aircraft. This reorganization achieved rather better utilization of the ICR system. Workload with the computer assisted systems was judged to be generally acceptable, but low enough at times that concern was expressed that "computer aid might reduce demand on the controller below an optimum level" (p. 576).

The results of these two studies do not provide strong evidence that automation will be either a source of increased controller stress or, via its workload reducing effect, a net benefit to controller stress levels. However, the studies suffered from some important limitations. First, in the US study the ARTS III systems had only been in place for five months at the time of the experiment, and controllers were still not fully familiar with the new equipment. Second, both experiments were of short duration (a matter of days rather than of months), and it is possible, in unusual or nonroutine circumstances (requiring much longer periods to realistically sample effectively), that automation influences stress for better or for worse. Similarly, stress increases or decreases associated with the introduction of automation could be subtle, chronic, or cumulative, with predominant influences on cognition (for example, in the reinterpretation and reevaluation of the controller's role and importance). This would in any case be difficult to pin down with biochemical or physiological measures sensitive only to variations in arousal and difficult to evaluate with the 'blunt instrument' of a standardized questionnaire.

For our purposes, however, the most important (and to be fair to the researchers, inevitable) limitation of the studies discussed here lies in the restricted degree to which results can be extrapolated to more advanced automation. The studies examined an incremental change within a known system -- the provision of automated support for traditional controller functions. It did not involve the radical reformulation of the controller's role that could be entailed by very advanced and comprehensive automation. After all, the carpenter who happily sets aside his handsaw for an electric machine tool might balk at the introduction of a robot-carpenter. Even within the confines of the UK experiment, most of the controllers reported some unease at being 'driven' by the computer, propelled from problem to problem without being fully in charge of the situation. Some concern was also expressed over whether a 'mental picture' of the traffic situation would long survive failure of the computer equipment. Moreover, the unexpected and unilateral reorganization of one of the subject teams in the UK experiment is a telltale reminder of the need for humility in projections to the future performance of a large scale highly automated human-machine system based upon extrapolations from current equipment and practices. Radically new systems are likely to stimulate the evolution of radically new practices, for better or for worse. However, the adaptive changes in human response and team performance are among the most difficult variables to model beforehand. This emphasizes the desirability of realistic preservice testing of advanced automated ATC networks and raises the 'Star Wars' question -- how can a vast and intricate system be adequately tested before irrevocable commitment to the development and deployment of all of its interlocking parts?

In 1985 Field[17] asserted that "the computer is there to *assist* [the controller] in his task of the safe and orderly flow of air traffic, and must in no way go beyond the capability of the human being to retain control of decision-making" (p. 102). Today, nine years later, the air traffic controller still retains planning, analysis, and control functions while the computers play a supporting role, processing and presenting data to the controllers. This is a very significant role, to be sure, so much so that independent computerized backup systems such as the US Direct Access Radar Channel (DARC) may be integral parts of the system. Nevertheless, humans still 'retain control of decision making'. This is because in the present system controllers are able to maintain a mental model or picture of the airspace and are aware of the system state -- the positions, tracks, and intentions of aircraft within the airspace. Controllers can step in at any time should a computer failure occur. As a matter of fact, in many places the old 'manual' methods still largely coexist with the modern and form the ultimate 'last trench' backup should automated assistance fail. However, it is by no means clear to what extent this will be the case in the not-too-distant future:

> It seems highly probable that as we enter the 21st century we will see the black boxes in unmanned aircraft communicating and exchanging flight data with black boxes on the ground and receiving in return, from unmanned (at least by air traffic controllers) ATC centre's required instructions and clearances. Where or how will the future pilot and controller fit in? (p. 244)

This prediction is no journalist's flight of fancy but comes from Michael Tonner,[69] a Canadian air traffic controller and a senior official in CATCA, the Canadian Air Traffic Control Association. It is not clear that the system described is *probable* by the twenty-first century, but it is rapidly becoming possible. Advances in technology are now such that in a highly automated ATC system, the overall planning, analysis, and control functions could already be assigned to machines rather than to humans. Other informed commentators anticipate just this in ATC systems before the turn of the century.[29] Moreover, instead of monitoring flights along well-travelled airways, a fully automated system could clear myriad aircraft along individualized pilot requested routes, 'customized' in real time according to weather, traffic flow, and other exigencies. Computers would both generate and transmit the clearances that aircrew would act upon.

In such a system it would be much more difficult for a human controller to maintain in her 'mind's eye' a situational model that would permit rapid manual intervention in the event of computer failure. Nevertheless, the challenge is being taken up. In the United States, for example, the FAA's plan for a distributed "Advanced Automation System" (AAS) calls for a single integrated En Route and terminal system that will be monitored by controllers in tower cabs, TRACON rooms, and En Route centres. Gone will be the old flight progress strips, display consoles and, indeed, most of today's ATC paraphernalia. Instead of the system providing information for the controller to use, the controller will provide information for the system to use. The controller "will be responsible for determining the general health of the automated system" and for handling exceptions and failures (Hunt and Zellweger,[29] p. 27).

It is possible that in such a system ATC controllers could perceive their role to have deteriorated to the status of data entry clerks and machine minders -- clerks who nevertheless would be expected to work miracles on the rare occasions when the machines failed. While we are hopeful that this stark view of the matter presents too bleak a picture, it nevertheless cannot be shrugged off. The problem of boredom, for example, has been acknowledged even in the present system, although the relationship of monotony to safety is not particularly well researched or understood.[27,28] Moreover, the supportive, collegial, and professional atmosphere of team work may not survive intact in a system where team functions are largely replaced by one-on-one human-machine dialogue.[28]

If the management and supervisory milieu is somewhat suspect, as seems to be evidenced in some of the research findings, will reduced team interaction ameliorate or exacerbate discontent? There is clearly a future potential for stress from reduced job satisfaction and from the frustrations of responsibility without (or with reduced) power. It seems likely that the general public, controllers' employers, and controllers themselves will feel that the awesome responsibilities of ATC personnel are undiminished by automation (and perhaps increased), while controllers may perceive themselves to be servants of an opaque and impersonal system that makes the real decisions. This could lead to some dissonance. Perception of control, as we have discussed elsewhere, can have a powerful influence upon the level of stress perceived by an individual. An individual who feels that she can exercise meaningful authority over her environment will, other things being equal, tend to perceive her situation as being less stressful than one who feels that she has little control. Automation by its very nature takes some of that control away from the human in the system. On the other side of the equation, however, automation may reduce workload and free up attention required for other matters (we say *may*, because this is subject to management decisions, and historically, advanced technology, from radar to laptop computers, has been used to increase 'productivity' -- e.g., output, traffic flow -- rather than to create more slack time). Whether, on balance, automation is likely to be stress reducing or stress increasing, for whom, and in what circumstances, is obviously a complex question that is difficult to address simply as a 'thought experiment'. The answer is likely to be very sensitive to the precise details of the particular system in question, the technical and managerial structures within the system, and the indoctrination and training of personnel. These same difficulties are likely to beset empirical researchers intent upon obtaining a 'heads-up' on the problem and, in fact, little research of this nature is available.

Summary and conclusions

We are now in a better position to expand upon and reconsider the epigraphs that open this chapter. In 1982 Melton[39] of the FAA felt able to assert (on the basis of the previous ten years of US research) that "it is clearly inappropriate to describe ATC work, as is commonly done in the popular press, as an unusually stressful occupation. Popularized accounts deal with the exceptional rather than the typical..." (p. 47). Recently, however, Luczak,[34] a European specialist in work under extreme conditions, felt equally justified in stating nearly the opposite:

> Air traffic control seems to be an extreme task in terms of mental load: complaints and strikes are numerous and frequent ... comparable mean values of heart rate and deviations from conditions of rest are found only in working conditions that combine a high density of information flow with a high degree of 'danger' or 'responsibility', as is the case, for instance, with test pilots ... parachute jumping, ... automobile racing, ... stage plays, and examinations. (p. 709)

The difference in the two views is, in part, a reflection of differences in European and American research data and in its interpretation, as well as of different notions of workplace stress and, possibly, differences in the history of ATC employee-management relations. Although these views cannot be easily reconciled, a synthesis of the research discussed earlier does at least enable the differing outlooks to be understood.

In terms of personality, air traffic controllers do not appear to differ substantially from many other occupational groups. They may have above average intelligence, and tend toward conformity and self control. More significantly, however, from the standpoint of vulnerability to stress, multiple studies have demonstrated that air traffic controllers are, as a group, low in trait anxiety. State-trait theory suggests that they should be relatively well equipped to cope with stressful situations.

A number of American field studies show physiological and biochemical evidence of arousal in controllers, particularly in association with heavy traffic. However, the discussion of arousal and stress in Chapter 2 makes the point that arousal is not a unidimensional variable, much less a synonym for stress. In the case of the US controllers, arousal has not been shown to correlate with negative affect (the feeling of being overstressed). Other, less physiologically oriented studies from other countries indicate that workload may not be a significant source of stress in air traffic controllers unless it is particularly heavy, as at times of peak traffic load. In general, controllers enjoy their work and derive satisfaction from meeting the challenges that it imposes. Indeed, they may become frustrated when there is not enough for them to do. Even shiftwork does not appear to be a major source of subjectively experienced stress in ATC personnel, unless poor scheduling violates basic principles of human circadian rhythm adjustment. A rare but serious phenomenon, however, is night shift paralysis (which has also been observed in other night workers).

The picture is rather less clear when evidence from studies of controllers' physical and mental health is considered. Many studies have reported a variety of (possibly stress related) health problems in air traffic controllers, but it is unclear whether controllers differ from the general population in this respect. Rotating schedules and night shift work are typically associated with adverse health effects in all occupations and may account for some of the problems reported; problems experienced with supervisors and managers have also been correlated with the emergence of health problems. Such research as exists on psychological problems in air traffic controllers has reported what appears to be an unusually high incidence of psychiatric conditions, although it is difficult to be certain of this owing to the absence of control populations in the studies concerned. A variety of treatment programs have been suggested. Life events and (non-ATC related) daily 'hassles' are seldom controlled out of (or factored into) studies of air traffic controllers, and the interaction of emotional problems with other influences on job stress and performance remains to be determined.

Where job dissatisfaction is expressed by air traffic controllers, it is more likely to concern aspects of working conditions, relations with supervisors, or poor management than workload or shiftwork per se. Desires for a more collegial and less authoritarian environment are often expressed. Field studies confirm that the major stress factors tend to be organizational and managerial problems, equipment deficiencies, lack of control or consultation, and poor shift scheduling.

It is an oversimplification, but not an egregious one, to suggest that controllers are stressed not by ATC work itself as much as by factors that, as they perceive it, hinder them from doing their jobs well. These largely institutional factors are seen as impairing both 'climate' and efficiency in the workplace. It should be noted, however, that similar concerns have been expressed by controllers in many different countries, working in various ATC systems. It may be the case that the type of person who chooses to become an air traffic controller shares some characteristics with pilots -- self reliant, self confident, controlling individuals taking pride in their own technical abilities. Traditional hierarchical and nonconsultative organizational structures may be too stifling and regimented for these types of workers.

Pilots, of course, largely do their work independently, free of the direct supervision and 'office politics' of their parent companies. ATC personnel are not so fortunate. Similarly, there may be tasks or occupations in which standard hierarchical structures are less than optimal.[22] These may include certain tightly coupled nonlinear organizations (see Chapter 11) which feature high individual responsibility and technical competence, which place a premium on communications efficiency, and in which the 'stakes' are high (in lives and money). Perhaps greater attention to organizational and supervisory issues could benefit controllers worldwide. A reconsideration of the controller's role in the ATC organization and in the ATC system is timely, given the imminence of advanced automation.

It has sometimes been assumed that automated support systems should reduce controller workload (and hence stress, on the supposition that workload is the controllers' main stressor). However, such research as exists (and surprisingly little exists) does not particularly indicate that automation reduces stress. As far as can be determined, the levels of automation examined so far appear to have a more or less neutral effect on controllers' emotional state, while physiological arousal may if anything increase under conditions of automation. The latter phenomenon, however, is possibly a temporary effect of the learning curve associated with new equipment and new procedures. Whether there are also more chronic or cumulative sequelae has yet to be determined.

References

1. Alexander, J.R., Ammerman, H.L., Fairhurst, W.S., Green, R., Hostetler, C.M., and Jones, G.W. (1991), *FAA Air Traffic Control Operations Concepts. Volume I: ATC Background and Analysis Methodology (Change 2)*, CTA Incorporated, Colorado Springs.

2. Booze, C.F. (1978), *The Morbidity Experience of Air Traffic Control Personnel*, FAA Office of Aviation Medicine Report No. AM-78-21.

3. Booze, C.F. (1982), 'Blood pressures of active pilots compared with those of air traffic controllers', preprints *Aerospace Medical Association.*

4. Bowers, D.C. (1983), 'What would make 11,500 people quit their jobs?', *Organizational Dynamics*, Winter, pp. 5-19.

5. Campbell, D.P. (1966), *Manual for the Strong Vocational Interest Blank*, Stanford University Press, Stanford, California.

6. Caplan, R.D., Cobb, S., French, J.R.P., Harrison, R.V., and Pinneau, S.R. (1975), *Job Demands and Worker Health*, Department of Health, Education, and Welfare, National Institute for Occupational Safety and Health Report No. NIOSH 75-160.

7. Cattell, R.B. (1962), *Manual for the Sixteen Personality Factor Questionnaire (Forms A and B)*, Institute for Personality and Ability Testing, Champaign, Illinois.

8. Cattell, R.B., Eber, H.W., and Tatsuoka, M.M. (1970), *The 16PF Test*, Institute for Personality and Ability Testing, Champaign, Illinois.

9. Cobb, S., and Rose, R.M. (1973), 'Hypertension, peptic ulcer and diabetes in air traffic controllers', *Journal of the American Medical Association*, vol. 224, pp. 489-92.

10. Collins, W.E., Schroeder, D.J., and Nye, L.G. (1991), 'Relationships of anxiety scores to screening and training status of air traffic control-

lers', *Aviation, Space, and Environmental Medicine,* vol. 62, pp. 236-40.

11. Cooper, C.L., Sloan, S.J., and Williams, S. (1988), *Occupational Stress Indicator,* NFER-Nelson, Windsor.

12. Costa, G., Pinchera, E., Pistilli, M., Battistic, S., and Munafo, E. (1989), 'Stress and performance of air traffic controllers', *Ergonomia,* vol. 12, pp. 93-100.

13. Dougherty, J.D. (1967), Cardiovascular findings in air traffic controllers, *Aerospace Medicine,* vol. 38, pp. 26-30.

14. Dougherty, J.D., Trites, D.K., and Dille, J.R. (1965), 'Self-reported stress-related symptoms among air traffic control specialists (ATCS) and non-ACTS personnel', *Aerospace Medicine,* vol. 36, pp. 956-60.

15. Farmer, E.W., Belyavin, A.J., Berry, A., Tattersall, A.J., and Hockey, G.R.J. (1990), *Stress in Air Traffic Control I: Survey of NATS Controllers,* RAF Institute of Aviation Medicine Report No. 689.

16. Federal Aviation Administration (1988), *Air Traffic Control Specialist,* Announcement No. FAA/ATC-008 Revised 3-88, Mike Monroney Aeronautical Center, Oklahoma City, Oklahoma.

17. Field, A. (1985), *International Air Traffic Control: Management of the World's Airspace,* Pergamon Press, Oxford.

18. Fitts, P.M. (ed.) (1951), *Human Engineering for an Effective Air-Navigation and Traffic Control System,* National Research Council, Washington, DC.

19. Folkard, S., and Condon, R. (1987), 'Night shift paralysis in air traffic control officers', *Ergonomics,* vol. 30, pp. 1353-63.

20. Folkard, S., Condon, R., and Herbert, M. (1984), 'Night shift paralysis, *Experientia,* vol. 40, pp. 510-2.

21. Hale, H.B., Williams, E.W., Smith, B.N., and Melton, C.E., Jr. (1971), 'Excretion patterns of air traffic controllers', *Aerospace Medicine,* vol. 42, pp. 127-38.

22. Hancock, P.A. (1989), 'Stress, Information-Flow, and Adaptibility in Individuals and Collective Organizational Systems', in Hendrick, H.E. and Brown, O. (eds.), *Proceedings of the Second International Symposium on Organizational Design and Management,* North Holland, Amsterdam.

23. Harrington, J.M. (1978), *Shift Work and Health,* University of London, London School of Hygiene and Tropical Medicine, London.

24. Hart, S.G., and Staveland, L.E. (1989), 'Development of a NASA TLX (Task Load Index): Results of Empirical and Theoretical Research', in Hancock, P., and Meshkati, N. (eds.), *Human Mental Workload,* Elsevier, Amsterdam.

25. Hauty, G.T., Trites, D.K., and Berkley, W.J. (1965), *Biomedical Survey of ATC Facilities: 2. Experience and Age,* FAA Office of Aviation Medicine Report No. AM-65-6.

26. Hibler, N.S. (1978), *The Effects of Stress on State Anxiety in Air Traffic Controllers,* Doctoral dissertation, University of South Florida.

27. Hopkin V.D. (1980), 'Boredom', *The Controller,* vol. 19, pp. 6-9.

28. Hopkin V.D. (1991), 'The Impact of Automation on Air Traffic Control Systems', in Wise, J.A., Hopkin, V.D., and Smith, M.L. (eds.), *Automation and Systems Issues in Air Traffic Control,* NATO ASI series, Springer-Verlag, Berlin.

29. Hunt, V.R., and Zellweger, A. (1987), 'Strategies for future air traffic control systems', *Computer,* pp. 19-32.

30. Hurst, M.W., and Rose, R.M. (1978), 'Objective workload and behavioural response in airport radar control rooms', *Ergonomics,* vol. 21, pp. 559-655.

31. Jones, L. (1982), *Management and Employee Relationships Within the Federal Aviation Administration,* Contract DTFAO1-82-C-30006, Federal Aviation Administration, Washington, DC.

32. Jorna, P.G.A.M. (1990), 'Operator Workload as a Limiting Factor in Complex Systems', in Wise, J.A., Hopkin, V.D., and Smith (eds.), *Automation and Systems Issues in Air Traffic Control* (pp. 281-92), NATO ASI series, Springer-Verlag, Berlin.

33. Karson, S., and O'Dell, J.W. (1974), 'Personality makeup of the American air traffic controller', *Aerospace Medicine,* vol. 45, pp. 1001-7.

34. Luczak, H. (1991), 'Work under extreme conditions', *Ergonomics,* vol. 34, pp. 687-720.

35. Malstrom, E.J. (1968), *Composite Mood Adjective Check List,* Unpublished manuscript, Department of Psychology, University of California, Los Angeles.

36. McBride, A., Lancee, W., and Freeman, S.J., (1979, September 25-29), *Minimal Use of Professional Support Within a High Stress Occupation,* Paper presented to the Canadian Psychiatric Association, Vancouver, British Columbia.

37. McBride, A., Lancee, W., and Freeman, S. (1981), 'The psychosocial impacts of a labour dispute', *Occupational Psychology,* vol. 54, pp. 125-34.

38. McNair, D.M., Lorr, M., and Dropplman, L.F. (1971), *Profile of Mood States: Manual,* Educational and Testing Service, San Diego, California.

39. Melton, C.E. (1982), *Physiological Stress in Air Traffic Controllers: A Review,* FAA Office of Aviation Medicine Report No. AM-82-17.

40. Melton, C.E., and Bartanowicz, R. (1986), *Biological Rhythms and Rotating Shift Work: Some Considerations for Air Traffic Controllers and Managers,* FAA Office of Aviation Medicine Report AM-86-2.

41. Melton, C.E., McKenzie, J.M., Polis, B.D., Funkhouser, G.E., and Iampietro, P.F. (1971), *Physiological Responses in Air Traffic Control Personnel: O'Hare Tower*, FAA Office of Aviation Medicine Report No. AM-73-21.

42. Melton, C.E., McKenzie, J.M., Polis, B.D., Hoffmann, S.M., and Saldivar, J.T. (1973), *Physiological Responses in Air Traffic Control Personnel: Houston Intercontinental Tower*, FAA Office of Aviation Medicine Report No. AM-74-11.

43. Melton, C.E., McKenzie, J.M., Smith, R.C., Polis, B.D., Higgins, E.A., Hoffmann, S.M., Funkhouser, G.E., and Saldivar, J.T. (1973), *Physiological, Biochemical, and Psychological Responses in Air Traffic Control Personnel: Comparison of the 5-Day and 2-2-1 Shift Rotation Patterns*, FAA Office of Aviation Medicine Report No. AM-73-22.

44. Melton, C.E., Smith, R.C., McKenzie, J.M., Hoffmann, S.M., and Saldivar, J.T. (1976), 'Effects of ARTS-III', *Aviation, Space, and Environmental Medicine*, vol. 47, pp. 925-30.

45. Melton, C.E., Smith, R.C., McKenzie, J.M., Saldivar, J.T., Hoffmann, J.M., and Fowler, P.R. (1975), *Stress in Air Traffic Controllers: Comparison of Two Route Traffic Control Centers on Different Shift Rotation Patterns*, FAA Office of Aviation Medicine Report No. AM-75-7, 1975.

46. Melton, C.E., Smith, R.C., McKenzie, J.M., Wicks, S.M., and Saldivar, J.T. (1978), 'Stress in air traffic personnel: low-density towers and flight service stations', *Aviation, Space, and Environmental Medicine*, vol. 49, pp. 724-8.

47. Mohler, S.R. (1983), 'The human element in air traffic control: aeromedical aspects, problems, and prescriptions', *Aviation, Space, and Environmental Medicine*, vol. 54, pp. 511-6.

48. Mott, P.E., Mann, F.C., McCLoughlin, Q., and Warwick, D.P. (1965), *Shift Work*, University of Michigan Press, Ann Arbor, Michigan.

49. Nowlis, V. (1965), 'Research with the Mood Adjective Check List', in Tomkins, S.S., and Izard, C.E. (eds.), *Affect, Cognition and Personality*, Springer, New York.

50. Rose, R.M., Jenkins, C.D., and Hurst, M.W. (1978), *Air Traffic Controller Health Change Study*, FAA Office of Aviation Medicine Report No. AM-78-39.

51. Rudolph, G. deM. (1946a), 'Psychological aspects of a conscious temporary generalized paralysis', *Journal of Mental Sciences*, vol. 92, pp. 814-6.

52. Rudolph, G. deM. (1946b), 'Night nurse paralysis: a temporary tonic motor paralysis', *Bristol Med. Chir. J.*, vol. 43, pp. 132-5.

53. Schad, R., Gilgen, A., and Grandjean, E. (1969), 'Excretion of catecholamines in air traffic personnel', *Schweizerische Medizinische Wochensschrift*, vol. 99, pp. 889-92.

54. Shouksmith, G., and Burrough, S. (1988), 'Job stress factors for New Zealand and Canadian air traffic controllers', *Applied Psychology: An International Review*, vol. 37, pp. 263-70.

55. Singal, M., Smith, M.J., Hurrell, J.J., Bender, J., Kramkowski, R.S., and Salisbury, S.A. (1977), *Hazard Evaluation and Technical Assistance Report: O'Hare International Airport*, National Institute for Occupational Safety and Health, Report No. TA 77-67.

56. Singer, R., and Rutenfranz, J. (1971), 'Attitudes of air traffic controllers at Frankfurt Airport towards work and the working environment', *Ergonomics*, vol. 14, pp. 633-9.

57. Smith, G. (1978, June 2), *Communication Concerning Partial Summary of Medical Disqualifications at Level 5 Terminals -- 1972-1977*, FAA Aeromedical Services Division, Washington, DC.

58. Smith, R.C. (1973), 'Comparison of job attitudes of personnel in three air traffic control specialties', *Aerospace Medicine*, vol. 44, pp. 918-27.

59. Smith, R.C. (1974), *A Realistic View of the People in Air Traffic Control*, FAA Office of Aviation Medicine Report No. AM-74-12.

60. Smith, R.C. (1975), 'Vocational interests of air traffic control personnel', *Aerospace Medicine*, vol. 46, pp. 871-7.

61. Smith, R.C. (1980), *Stress, Anxiety and the Air Traffic Control Specialist: Some Conclusions From a Decade of Research*, FAA Office of Aviation Medicine Report No. FAA-AM-80-14.

62. Smith, R.C., Cobb, B.B., and Collins, W.E. (1972), 'Attitudes and motivations of air traffic controllers in terminal areas', *Aerospace Medicine*, vol. 43, pp. 1-5.

63. Smith, R.C., and Melton, C.E. (1975), 'Susceptibility to anxiety and shift difficulty as determinants of state anxiety in air traffic controllers', *Aerospace Medicine*, vol. 45, pp. 599-601.

64. Smith, R.C., and Melton, C.E. (1978), 'Effects of ground trainer use on the anxiety of students in private pilot training', *Aviation, Space, and Environmental Medicine*, vol. 49, pp. 406-8.

65. Smith, R.C., Melton, C.E., and McKenzie, J.M. (1971), 'Affect adjective check list assessment of mood variations in air traffic controllers', *Aerospace Medicine*, vol. 42, pp. 1060-4.

66. Spielberger, C.D., Gorsuch, R.L., and Lushene, R.F. (1970), *Manual for the State-Trait Anxiety Inventory*, Consulting Psychologists Press, Palo Alto, California.

67. Stein, E.S. (1987), 'Where Will All Our Air Traffic Controllers be in the Year 2001?', *Proceedings of the Fourth International Symposium on Aviation Psychology*, Ohio State University, Columbus.

68. Tattersall, A.J., Farmer, E.W., and Belyavin, A.J. (1990), 'Stress and Workload Management in Air Traffic Control', in Wise, J.A., Hopkin, V.D., and Smith (eds.), *Automation and Systems Issues in Air Traffic Control* (pp. 255-66), NATO ASI series, Springer-Verlag, Berlin.

69. Tonner, M. (1990), 'The Controller in Human Engineering', in Wise, J.A., Hopkin, V.D., and Smith (eds.), *Automation and Systems Issues in Air Traffic Control* (pp. 243-8), NATO ASI series, Springer-Verlag, Berlin.

70. Trites, D.K., Kurek, A., and Cobb, B.B. (1967), 'Personality and achievement of air traffic controllers', *Aerospace Medicine,* vol. 38, pp. 1145-50.

71. Westrum, R. (1990), 'Automation, Information and Consciousness in Air Traffic Control', in Wise, J.A., Hopkin, V.D., and Smith (eds.), *Automation and Systems Issues in Air Traffic Control* (pp. 367-80), NATO ASI series, Springer-Verlag, Berlin.

72. Whitfield, D., Ball, R.G., and Ord, G., (1980), 'Some human aspects of computer aiding concepts for air traffic controllers', *Human Factors,* vol. 22, pp. 569-80.

73. Zuckerman, M. (1960), 'The development of an affect adjective checklist for the measurement of anxiety', *Journal of Consulting Psychology,* vol. 24, pp. 457-62.

11 Organizations, stress, and accidents

The working of great institutions is mainly the result of a vast mass of routine, petty malice, self interest, carelessness, and sheer mistake. Only a residual fraction is thought.

-- Santayana, *The Crime of Galileo*

A lot of lip service is paid to the myth of command residing in the cockpit, to the fantasy of the captain of the ship as ultimate decision-maker. But today the commander must first consult with the accountant.

-- Stephan Wilkinson, *The November Oscar Incident*

On the evening of June 2, 1979, Downeast Flight 46, a de Havilland Twin Otter, crashed into a fog shrouded shoreline forest while on final approach to Rockland, Maine. Seventeen people were killed.[34] The immediate cause of the crash was the failure of the crew to arrest the descent of the aircraft at the MDA (minimum descent altitude) of 440 feet. This resulted from the failure of the captain and first officer to monitor the instruments, which were indicating an unusually high rate of descent. The descent rate, in turn, resulted from an earlier error, the captain's mis-setting of the landing flaps to 20 degrees instead of 10 degrees. Traditionally the discovery of such a mistake would have largely 'wrapped up' the accident investigation and it would have been diagnosed as a clear cut case of pilot error.

On this occasion, however, human performance specialists from the National Transportation Safety Board, tipped off about deeper problems within the airline, probed further. The captain of the Otter had been tired and working under some kind of stress, it was said, and the first officer had at times been only marginally proficient and was in need of additional inservice training. Moreover, the Otter had had engine serviceability problems, which may have added to crew anxiety and distraction.

As investigators continued to backtrack, it became increasingly apparent that these problems were not isolated and unrelated, but rather were the collective legacy of longstanding management policies within the airline. It was found that the management had fostered a corporate culture in which

330

short term revenue rather than safety had become the primary guiding principle for decisions. The results of this were far-reaching. For example, since training cost money, the airline provided little or none of the proficiency training from which the Otter's first officer would have benefited. Scrimping on maintenance costs decreased the serviceability of the airline's fleet, creating cynicism and nagging doubts in the minds of pilots. Stress and fatigue stemmed from management pressure to bring in revenue and minimize costs, even if this meant flying long duty days in poorly maintained aircraft and marginal weather. Most disturbing, there was pressure to 'bend' safety rules or to disregard them outright.[20] This pressure was sometimes quite overt, as, for example, when pilots who dissented with these policies were fired (or not promoted) on the grounds that they lacked what was institutionally regarded as a 'can do' attitude. It hardly needs pointing out that this alone could represent a potent source of stress.

The pressure placed on pilots did not end here, however. It also took subtler, more pervasive forms, and emerged from a pernicious company culture in which incentives and disincentives, praise and blame, were distributed by reference to the airline's uncompromising pursuit of short term profit. For example, the cautious were sneered at as overcautious, and their competence and even manhood were questioned. (John Nance records that the general manager of the airline had been known to call such pilots 'pantywaists'.[33]) Pilots had the invidious and distressing task of juggling their responsibilities to their employer (and to their families) with conflicting responsibilities to the Federal Aviation Administration and to the principles of safety and integrity drilled into them from their first training flight. As Nance also records, the National Transportation Safety Board found that it was in this corporate context that the pilots of Downeast Airlines were routinely expected to descend below the minimum descent altitude in bad weather simply to avoid an expensive diversion to a more distant airport -- a shocking revelation and one which casts the loss of Flight 46 in a very different light.

Organizations, accidents, and causes

The Downeast accident illustrates some ways in which organizational and management factors can affect both aircrew well-being and air safety. The social dimensions of human performance within complex, high risk systems such as aviation have received increasing research attention in recent years, in part because insights in this area may help to prevent future accidents, and also because they raise important issues of individual versus corporate responsibility when mishaps do occur. Perhaps for these reasons, this research has thus far tended to focus more on accident investigation (and prevention) than on operator stress per se. Even so, studies conducted from this perspective can potentially contribute much to our understanding of organizational precursors of stress in the cockpit. (Indeed, it has been suggested that research on high risk systems could itself benefit from closer links with organizational psychology, and future efforts in this area are likely to draw upon both disciplines.[32]) In order to set a context for evaluating the role and importance of organizational stress, as well as some aspects of its provenance and incubation, we therefore need to digress a little from the subject of stress and consider matters of organizational structure, as well as current views on the aetiology of accidents.

At the time of the Downeast Flight 46 accident in 1979, very little had been written about organizational precursors of accidents or about distal (nonproximate) factors in general. Since then, however, there has been a series of well-publicized disasters in which organizational factors have been shown to have had an important role. Examples include the escape of deadly methyl isocyanate from the Union Carbide plant in Bhopal, India; the destruction of the Piper Alpha oil rig in the North Sea; the Chernobyl and Three Mile Island nuclear power plant accidents; the railway accident at Clapham Junction, London; and the explosion of the space shuttle *Challenger*. In each case the immediate or proximate cause -- such as the failure of the rubber O-ring seals on Challenger's fuel tank or the shorted wire in the signal light at Clapham -- was found to be merely the last factor in a complex of circumstances embedded in the (often longstanding) politics and practices of the organization. Indeed, it has been argued that in many accidents organizational variables have been more important than individual operator errors.[31] One way of viewing the traditionally cited or proximate cause of an accident, therefore, is to regard it as merely the *occasioning* of the accident, the final, local, 'triggering' event.

This attention to distal factors represents a relatively new way of looking at accident causation. Traditionally, of course, standing conditions such as the structure or politics of an organization have tended to be regarded as 'givens', elements of the system beyond challenge. To consider otherwise, in explaining disasters or other untoward occurrences, is to raise the issue of defining how broad a framework of inquiry is necessary and legitimate.

It is a matter of specifying the 'causal field', a concept that has been likened to the field of view through a microscope at varying levels of magnification.[8,29] Organizations, concerned perhaps with 'damage control' in its political rather than physical sense, often prefer localized responsibility and favour a narrow focus and proximate causes. There may indeed be considerable institutional resistance to broadening of the causal field, since this may bring senior individuals and policies under scrutiny. (The Watergate and Iran Contra affairs are, perhaps, the most obvious and certainly the most political of examples.) For root causes, however, it is sometimes necessary to look at organizational issues of some complexity.

The structure of organizational systems

When the human factors specialist speaks of a system, she is usually referring to a human-machine system -- that is, a functional entity made up of several interacting components: some human and fallible, and some designed by fallible humans. Systems vary in complexity. The UK Meteorological Office, with its network of observer stations, high speed computers, and teams of technicians, analysts and forecasters, forms a system; so does a man on a bicycle. Both take inputs, pass data between components, and create outputs, all in interaction with the environment. An aircraft and its crew form a system, but an organization such as an airline is also a system -- one that is made up of subsystems including aircraft and crews, maintenance facilities, dispatch departments, and the like. Moreover, the airline is itself linked to, and in a sense is part of, a wider and more amorphous system -- the airspace and air traffic control system. These large and complex organizational systems can give rise to *system accidents* -- unforeseen outcomes of the interaction of many components of the system.

Linear and complex systems

Since all systems are by definition interactive, the possibility always exists that compenents will interact in unanticipated ways. However, this is more likely to occur in systems that are large and complicated. The rate or probability of unanticipated events is not simply a function of the number of components in the system, but also depends upon the way in which the system is organized. Many systems are largely *linear*: one operation or process tends to be linked to the next in an obvious and visible sequence.

An aircraft production line and an airline's salaries department, for example, are hardly simple systems, but the flow of information and materials through them is mostly, if rarely entirely, linear. Failures, when they occur, generally have predictable consequences 'downstream' of the error, outcomes which may be backtracked to the source of the problem fairly readily.[36]

More *complex* systems, in contrast, are characterized by a greater number of nonlinear interactions between their component parts. Many parts may operate in 'common mode': that is, they may serve multiple functions, some or all of which may be hidden. Components may also be interlinked in such tangled ways that the functioning of the whole is difficult to observe or understand (a problem touched upon in the discussion of automation in Chapter 12; see also Chapter 10). The human operators may work routinely with an inaccurate or oversimplified mental model of the system. Thus, failures, when they occur, may have surprising consequences which seem to 'pop up' in unanticipated or remote parts of the system. An irony of complexity is that the greater the number of safety gadgets, alarms, and warning devices, the more complex the interactions may be, and the more confused and inaccurate the operators' mental model may become in nonstandard situations (see sidebar).

Tightly and loosely coupled systems

A further important characteristic of systems has been referred to as *coupling*.[36] Loosely coupled systems have a certain amount of 'slack' built into them: that is, the components of the system have a degree of autonomy and independence that helps to contain and localize failures. Such systems tolerate local perturbations without overall system destabilization. Errors and breakdowns tend to be 'absorbed', that is, identified and corrected before they propagate. Tightly coupled systems, by contrast, are characterized by the proximity (in space and/or time) and interdependence of their components. In tightly coupled systems even small failures can propagate, multiply, and expand through the system before the problem is diagnosed properly or before individuals can react. Charles Perrow identifies aircraft and air traffic control as both complex and tightly coupled systems, and airlines and airways as moderate in both respects.

What, then, are the implications, if any, of complexity and tight coupling for workplace stress, anxiety, and individual cognitive performance? Very little research has actually addressed this problem, and we must

Too Few Resources?

The loss-of-coolant accident at the Three Mile Island nuclear plant is often cited as an example of confusion associated with multiple warning systems. The accident itself need not be detailed here as it has been fully explored in several books;[16,25,47] suffice it to say that the power plant's operators concluded that there was an excess of coolant in the reactor, shut off the emergency cooling system and were faced with an impending meltdown of the reactor core. For over two hours they were exposed to a barrage of audible alarms, visual warnings, and indicators, but nevertheless clung to an erroneous and almost catastrophic conception of the nature of the problem at hand until another operator came onto the shift and promptly recognized the true state of affairs.

Various explanations have been offered for the failure of the control room staff to adequately diagnose the nature of the problem. It has been suggested, for example, that the multiple alarms may have given rise to overarousal (i.e., excitement, fear, or stress) and consequent 'cognitive tunnel vision' on the part of the operators.[16] However, it may also be useful to consider Norman and Bobrow's distinction between resource limited and data limited cognitive processing.[35] The overarousal contention is a claim about limits placed upon cognitive resources, i.e., that the delay in recognizing the true state of affairs stemmed from constraints placed upon attention and memory by, in this case, acute reactive stress. However, it seems at least as likely that stress per se was not the primary source of the delayed diagnosis of the failure. It could be argued that the activation of all of a system's alarms is likely to provide little if any more diagnostic data than total inactivation of the alarms. In other words, the difficulty may well have resided primarily in the information 'white out' that effectively data limited the plant operators' diagnostic performance.

extrapolate what we can from first principles. First, complexity, as we have discussed, keeps processes hidden, and unsuspected problems can spring up in unanticipated places at unpredictable times. In short, complexity generates uncertainty and reduces perception of control -- both potent and notorious stress multipliers. Second, tight coupling tends to encourage the rapid 'snowballing' or propagation of problems, thereby restricting preemptive intervention. That is, it creates time pressure -- a second potent stressor and one that also interacts with uncertainty.

Perhaps, then, we need not concern ourselves about loosely coupled or moderately coupled systems of low or moderate complexity, such as airlines and airways? Such an assumption is based on a view of organizational systems as belonging to static categories, a view we regard as too rigid and structural. Organizations are staffed by inventive people, whose behaviour is not static but highly responsive to uncertainty and threat. A more organic view of organizations would acknowledge that coupling and complexity could vary continuously (within certain parameters) as a function of cultural 'climate'. Thus, moderately coupled and somewhat linear systems, such as airlines, may change temporarily, in whole or in (possibly critical) parts, to more complex, more tightly coupled systems when the organization is stressed. This could be brought about by bankruptcy, poor industrial relations, poor management, high staff turnover, and so forth.

For example, when an organization is under stress, uncertainty is high and hierarchies become more salient. Individuals defer to leaders, to formal authority, and so the system centralizes.[7,46] Decision making becomes less distributed, less rapid, and more dependent upon communications making their way up and down the hierarchy. It has been noted that this alone accounts for slow reactivity and poor adaptivity in stress.[15,38] However, as we noted in Chapter 4, actual communication content may be degraded too, with decisions becoming more prone to uncritical 'groupthink'. Threat, as Weick[46] has stated, "tightens couplings between formal authority and solutions that will be influential, even though the better solutions may be in the hands of those with less authority" (p. 129). Complexity also increases in part because resourceful humans adopt 'survival' tactics that may generate more system components than those that figure in the formal organizational diagrams, and more (undocumented and nonstandard) ways of doing things. This gives increased scope for surprise and unexpected interactions.[*]

A decision making Catch-22. An intriguing picture emerges from these discussions in the light of what is known about expert decision making in dynamic, risk prone environments. As discussed in Chapter 4, individuals

---

[*]A very literal example of an additional system component was the escape tunnel built by RAF POWs which was 'found' by a German prison camp guard (when the ground beneath him collapsed). However, the notion need not be taken this literally -- consider the complexity and unpredictability introduced by 'black market' activities in stressed economies, or the unofficial 'fixes' and creative record keeping observed in some overworked and underfunded flight maintenance shops.

who have become experts in a given endeavour (e.g., aviation, firefighting, or chess) do not necessarily have better memories or greater powers of diagnostic inference than nonexperts.[4,48] Rather, they make their superior decisions largely on the basis of experience, by matching situational cues with elements in long term memory.[24,44] This process has been termed recognition primed decision making,[23] and is very fast and effective, as well as using few attentional resources. Only when this mechanism fails do experts fall back upon much slower, less reliable, and more attention demanding cognitive skills involving computationally intensive processes of information integration and inference in working memory.[45]

Given this, it appears that system complexity and tight coupling may provide a 'Catch-22' for expert system operators. First, system complexity increases the probability that a brand new problem will emerge from some arcane conjunction of events, or that an old problem will manifest itself in some never-before-seen manner. In other words, complexity by its nature creates conditions liable to defeat recognition primed decision making and force a 'cognitive retreat' to a time consuming, less efficient analytical decision making process. These analytical processes, in turn, may be vulnerable if the system is also a tightly coupled one, as tight coupling increases the probability that malfunctions will ripple rapidly through the system, denying the operators the time needed to diagnose the

---

September, 1991: a rainy night in Syracuse, New York. The left bleed air fail light was on, but we decided to proceed: mistake #1. As we turned onto taxiway A, I turned the taxi light out. The first officer noticed that the attitude indicator rolled to 10 degrees of bank. I had my head down completing the 'final items' checklist when I heard a pop. The first officer had apparently taxied over a runway or taxiway light. We were already cleared for takeoff. Not thinking of propeller damage, and since the control tower didn't see us do anything wrong, we decided to take off: mistake #2. Upon landing at Rochester the first officer advised me that the left prop was badly damaged but it would be OK for the next leg to Albany. Taking into account how much we had already let slide, the company's Chapter 11 bankruptcy status, and the need for revenue, I decided to depart in the darkness for Albany: mistake #3 and the one that cost me my job. It was a bad decision, I'm just glad nobody was hurt.

-- NASA Aviation Safety Reporting System (Accession No. 190042)

problem before it reaches critical proportions and ensuring that their 'mental model' lags behind the actual system state.

In terms of cognitive performance there is considerable evidence that such processes may occur. In addition to the examples of Three Mile Island and the 1979 DC-10 crash at O'Hare (see p. 104), there have been several mishaps in highly automated (and thus, very complex, tightly coupled) aircraft such the Airbus 320. In two separate controlled-flight-into-terrain crashes in India and France, crews of the A320 became overly confident in the aircraft's (admittedly remarkable) flying qualities and were unaware, until too late, that they had strayed outside its normal flight envelope. They were highly expert crews (in one case, company test pilots), yet they failed to recognize the true state of affairs (see Chapter 12).

Appearances versus reality

The 'safety first' culture

Many systems, particularly complex, tightly coupled systems, are well defended by engineered safety devices (ESDs) such as interlocks, fire sensors, automatic shutoffs, multiple redundant components, and the like. More importantly, from an organizational perspective, they also tend to feature policy safeguards, a 'safety first' ethic, well-defined zones of responsibility, regulatory control, and, at the 'coal face' of operations, procedural safety nets, checklists, drills, and Standard Operating Procedures (SOPs). An important and (for employees) potentially distressing class of problems arises when the nominal defences -- the formal structures, policies, and procedures to which employees and/or managers pay lip service -- do not accord with the system's everyday working realities. An example of such a situation is described in Neil Johnston's discussion of the Clapham Junction crash:[19]

> The reality was that the concern for safety was allowed to co-exist with working practices which were positively dangerous... A concern for safety which is sincerely held and repeatedly expressed but, nevertheless, is not carried through into action, is as much protection from danger as no concern at all. (pp. 668-9)

The difference between the nominal and the actual policies and practices of an organization may be a crucial factor in determining both the level of employee stress and the probability of certain classes of system failures. (In fact, it is often the conjunction of these two factors that gives rise to 'whistle blowers' -- individuals who are sufficiently troubled that they draw attention to discrepancies, often with even more distressing consequences to themselves.)

There is accumulating evidence that the primary danger to a system's defences does not spring from the failure of individual components, be they electronic or mechanical devices (within the purview of software or hardware engineering), or even from human performance errors (within the purview of traditonal human factors). Rather, the main threat comes from the steady piling-up and proliferation of *latent* human failures within the organization -- of 'accidents waiting to happen'.

Bugs in the system: organizational pathogens

James Reason has likened these dormant failures to pathogens resident in an organism.[37] It is well understood in medicine that certain pathogens such as the opportunistic retroviruses (for example, herpes simplex, the virus responsible for cold sores) may lie unsuspected in the body until activated by an event or confluence of events that stresses the organism: fatigue, shock, emotional crisis, injury, or another disease. Similarly, organizations inevitably contain some 'pathogens' or latent failures -- managers more interested in corporate image than substance, supervisors who turn a blind eye to regulations, workers who override ESDs, and so on. These have been termed the 'routine sins' of organizations.

Reason argues that the more of these latent failures there are, the greater the chance that an accident will be 'triggered' by some unexpected confluence or coincidence of failures. Where an organization constitutes a tightly coupled and complex system, such as an aircraft or a nuclear power station, such a triggering event is quite capable of initiating a very rapid chain reaction of deterioration. The more complex and tightly coupled a systemis, the less tolerant it is of latent failures. Routine sins, in Perrow's[36] pithy phrase, can lead to very nonroutine results (p. 10).

There are several corollaries to this concept. One that brings the fate of Downeast Flight 46 back to mind is Reason's[37] observation that the "higher a person's position within the decision-making structure of the organization, the greater is his or her potential for spawning pathogens" (p. 885). And, of course, the more an organization is under stress, the more the power of decision is likely to centralize in just those senior personnel,

Hawaii, November, 1990: a VFR (visual flight rules)-only sightseeing company on a tour flight around the Hawaiian islands. In midchannel on the way to Upolo Point, I could see that the Hiamakua coast had a massive rain cell. I got within five miles of the showers and turned around due to low visibility. I tried going around the cell and south with no success. I decided to return to Honolulu via the south shore of Maui and Molokai. However, unforecast weather had moved in, causing me to get trapped between the islands of Maui, Kahoolane, Molokini, and Lanai. Unable to continue VFR, I filed an IFR (instrument flight rules) flight plan into OGG, although I had no IFR charts on board the aircraft. Nevertheless, I had no trouble until the radio/interphone switch jammed in the 'on' position.

I am current and qualified IFR but the operation is legally VFR only. The Director of Operations advised that in future I was to go 'bandit IFR' and not tell anyone. I consider that unsafe in the extreme and bordering on criminal. Other factors in the incident included changing aircraft three times that morning, as I couldn't get the first two to work. Thus there was inadequate time to preflight check the aircraft for charts. Also inadequate training is a factor. The company has been sold and is in bankruptcy, so there is no fiscal responsibility and therefore they don't care about safety.

-- NASA Aviation Safety Reporting System (Accession No. 164040)

irrespective of their competence. The phenomenon of centralization of authority is reviewed in Chapter 4 in the section on group decision making; while that discussion focusses on the behaviour of small teams, the same phenomenon has also been observed in larger organizations.[42] (It is even evident at the level of national politics: an analysis by Hertzler[17] determined that throughout recorded history, totalitarian dictatorships have almost invariably arisen in countries undergoing some kind of severe hardship or emergency.)

Another corollary is that while local triggers are all but impossible to spot beforehand (not least since they often stem from a coincidence of events), pathogens, the latent failures in the system, are at least potentially identifiable in advance. For example, no one could have predicted that in 1979 the crew of an Antarctic sightseeing flight would punch the wrong numbers into their inertial navigation system, that a fog bank would form, obscuring Mount Erebus (ironically, Latin for 'hell'), or that their Antarctic guide would leave the flight deck just in time to allow the crew to fly into the mountain (see sidebar). On the other hand, low level sightseeing is a notorious killer, and the longstanding practice of low flying in that tricky environment was a clear 'pathogen' that could, in theory, have been eliminated before instead of after the accident occurred.

We say 'in theory' because it is instructive at this point to run a thought experiment. Imagine yourself as an employee of a similar airline faced with the task of persuading management to stop low level 'photo opportunity' flights -- among the most popular, profitable, and apparently successful operations conducted by the company. You are in the position of arguing

---

At midday on November 28, 1979, Air New Zealand Flight 901, a DC-10 with 257 people on board, flew into the side of Mount Erebus in the Antarctic. There were no survivors. The aircraft had been flying VFR (that is, by visual references) at the low altitude of 1,500 feet on a sightseeing tour. The snow covered terrain apparently blended visually with the sky and clouds to 'white out' the surrounding scene. The government's Accident Investigation branch found that the probable cause of the accident was pilot error -- flying at low level in an area where visibility was compromised and position uncertain.

However, doubts about the pilots' culpability by (among others) New Zealand's airline pilots' association led to a Royal Commission of Inquiry. The airline allegedly went to some lengths to suppress information inconsistent with the original verdict, and some documentation, for example the captain's briefing notes, disappeared. However, it was determined that the company had positively encouraged crews to descend to low levels on these sightseeing trips and had even published approving accounts of them in the company newspaper. Moreover, the company had provided inertial navigation system (INS) coordinates to the crew of Flight 901, numbers which included a flight plan change of which the crew were unaware -- a course to Mount Erebus. The report of the Commission exonerated the crew, blamed the airline for the INS change, and suggested that a company conspiracy had attempted to conceal the truth. (Upon appeal it was confirmed that company personnel had indeed lied, although the conspiracy allegation was rejected on technical grounds.)

-- Condensed from Stanley Stewart's account in *Air Disasters*[43]

with your own senior management. 'Source type' latent failures are those generated by those at the top of the organization's hierarchy.[30,37] They have the most global and systemic effects within the organization, but at the same time are the most risky to identify and denounce. The prospect of this can give rise to troubling moral conflict and cognitive dissonance among employees, who, like the pilots of Downeast Airlines, may be seen either as 'can do' team players or as disloyal troublemakers.

Rituals, roles, and anxiety

Most organizations have, to a greater or lesser extent, hierarchies and formal structures. In the world of aviation, for example, there is a continuum of formality along which lie air forces, airlines, flying schools, air taxi services, and 'bush pilot' operations. While no two organizations are alike, a number of features are typical, certainly of the larger organizations. For example, there is customarily a certain degree of distance -- psychological, social, and sometimes even physical -- between managers and the people they manage. Another common characteristic of organizations is that they tend to make considerable use of formal modes of communication such as memoranda, impersonal posted notices, and scheduled meetings. Considerable resources may be devoted to external or 'presenting' features of the organization, that is, with appearances, image, and corporate ritual (or 'bull', in military parlance). This includes the wearing of uniforms (including 'cultural' uniforms such as business suits), the specification of grooming standards (e.g., particular hairstyles), an emphasis upon logos, company colours, and the use of titles, drills, and other ritual procedures. Some organizations place such a high value on homogeneity, especially of appearance, that manifestations of individuality may be regarded as a form of deviance to which sanctions must be applied. Recently, for example, certain US airlines were in the news for their controversial enforcement of weight limits for female cabin crew (see sidebar). Yet another feature of some organizations is an emphasis on strict compliance with the letter (more than the spirit or purpose) of formal rules and legal requirements. This may be carried to such an extreme that the problems the rules are intended to address may be ignored altogether. Pilots frequently complain, for example, that the regulations relating to fatigue and rest are (mis)used in this way.

However, formalities and rituals do have an important role to play in organizations. They have the effect of minimizing entropy, that is, the

Flight attendants still have weight limits on many airlines. If you are fat, you get fired. Only what passes for fat is average to you or me. Sue Liebling of Seattle is 44, stands 5 feet 4, weighs 144 pounds and wears a size 10 dress. Each year she has to complete an emergency training course, keeping current on all those crash contingencies we passengers don't like to consider at 30,000 feet. But if she doesn't get back down to 135 on schedule, twenty-four years of experience at United Airlines is down the drain.

This small cul-de-sac of institutional stupidity reflects a larger problem with consumer services in America. If airlines talked to their customers about their concerns, I suspect the size of the flight attendants would be far less important than the size of the seats. For many of us, the most attractive kind of flight attendant is one who can get you on that inflated slide and out of the airplane fast if it's on fire. The official United explanation for weight limits has to do with 'professional appearance'. In other words, svelte equals professional. But those who work within the flight attendants' unions think the restrictions have an uglier purpose, that they combine a yen for the 'fly me' era with the more contemporary corporate yearning to junk older, more experienced workers for younger, less costly ones.

-- Condensed from an editorial by Anna Quindlen, *Chicago Tribune*, May 13, 1993

tendency to become disorganized, and they can reduce uncertainty and anxiety. This is particularly useful where uncertainty is an occupational hazard. There is, of course, reassurance value in predictability and in the clear signalling of roles and responsibilities. Ritual has in fact been shown to reduce physiological arousal.[3] Certainly it preserves the status quo and the hierarchy of rank, privilege, and status. Orderliness can also be important to efficiency and safety, and can help foster group identity and social cohesion -- itself a powerful antidote to stress (see Chapter 7).

On the negative side, it may be observed that while ritual and 'bull' seem to counter disorderliness, in fact they may do so only superficially, and actually conceal functional disorderliness behind ceremonial order. Moreover, superficial or token orderliness may become an end in itself, particularly for individual managers; in addition to absorbing energy and resources, this is likely to divert attention from the substantive goals of the organization, or even undermine them outright. The question may then well be asked, "Whose anxiety is being reduced -- the workers', or only their managers'?"

The point may also be made that the traditional (even Dickensian) corporate climate and management style that still prevails in many airline organizations, with its top-down, nonconsultative lines of authority, contrasts very markedly with what pilots are now being taught as appropriate team behaviour in the cockpit. Modern cockpit resource management principles stress consultation and integration of all available evidence and the collective appraisal of risk; while the captain still bears the ultimate responsibility for decision making, he or she is expected to be receptive to input from other crew members, and, indeed, proactive in eliciting such

---

"Robineau," Riviere had said one day, "you must cut the punctuality bonus whenever a plane starts late."

"Even when it's nobody's fault? In case of fog, for instance?"

"Even in case of fog."

Robineau felt a thrill of pride in knowing that his chief was strong enough not to shrink from being unjust. Surely Robineau himself would win reflected majesty from such overweening power!

"You postponed the start till 6:15," he would say to the airport super-intendents. "We cannot allow your bonus."

"But Monsieur Robineau, at 5:30 one couldn't see ten yards ahead!"

"Those are the orders."

"But Monsieur Robineau, we couldn't sweep the fog away with a broom!"

The pilot who damaged a plane lost his no-accident bonus.

"But supposing his engine gives out when he is over a wood?" Robineau inquired of his chief.

"Even when it occurs above a wood."

Robineau took to heart the ipse dixit. *"I regret," he would inform the pilots with cheerful zest, "I regret it very much indeed, but you should have had your breakdown somewhere else."*

"But Monsieur Robineau, one doesn't choose the place to have it."

"Those are the orders."

The orders, thought Riviere, are like the rites of a religion; they may look absurd but they shape men in their mold.

-- Antoine de Saint-Exupery, *Vol de Nuit (Night Flight)*

input. Aircrew increasingly schooled in this style of leadership may find it difficult to see how a more authoritarian attitude on the part of their superiors can be justified within a company management. The management system, after all, makes decisions under risk, too -- macroscopic decisions, to be sure, but which may nevertheless influence the balance of safety, efficiency, and profit just as surely as flight deck decisions.

In addition to the management of human resources, there is another area in which company realities tend to clash with those of the flight deck: the *de facto* reward (or penalty) structure. Organizations such as airlines or regulatory agencies sometimes operate within a general climate of anxiety, bureaucratic ultraconservatism, or both. This can come about for reasons of financial instability, cutbacks, poor industrial relations, or the political culture of the organization. Whatever the causes, it is frequently the case in such contexts that the costs of error are greater than the rewards for success. Fear of failure, of being singled out or noticed, can have a stultifying effect upon managerial decision making. Under such circumstances being ultraconservative, or, indeed, doing nothing at all, may seem preferable to any kind of decisive action.

Indeed, there is a whole vocabulary that acknowledges this. Employees in many occupations talk about having to 'look over their shoulders', 'keep their heads down', and 'not stick their necks out'. The imperatives of 'keeping your nose clean' and 'not rocking the boat' can effectively preempt other objectives. In safety terms, however, this is rarely the case on the flight deck of an aircraft, where almost any positive decision is generally preferable to inaction, not least where unusual circumstances, incidents, or emergencies must be coped with. Many flight students have heard their flight instructors intone wearily "do something, anything, but do *something!*"* In other words, flight safety favours a psychological environment in which decisiveness is valued and rewarded while inaction is frowned upon and penalized. Many pilots promoted to 'flying a desk', especially in the military services, appear to find this a frustrating and stressful change of role, and strive to return to flying duty even if it means exchanging one set of stresses for another -- as is often the case in wartime, when a return to flight status may mean combat operations. Although anecdotal, this is compelling suggestive evidence for the importance of role and self image in generating stress, and it is certainly worth examining the research findings for empirical evidence.

---

*As we saw in Chapter 4, expert pilots tend to be less concerned about finding the one best decision than about putting into prompt effect any *adequate* course of action.

Conflict, role ambiguity, and insecurity

> This is the heart of the professional pilot's eternal conflict. Into one ear the airlines lecture, "Never break regulations. Never take a chance. Never ignore written procedures. Never compromise safety." Yet into the other ear they whisper, "Don't cost us time. Don't waste our money. Get your passengers to their destination -- don't find reasons why you can't." (Wilkinson,[49] p. 84)

There is certainly evidence that conflict or ambiguity in job role are important factors both in job satisfaction and in the aetiology of stress and stress related disorders. Both discontent at work and job related tension have been found to relate to role conflict; moreover, the higher up the management hierarchy is the source of the conflicting or ambiguous expectations the more dissatisfaction is found.[21] Reported role conflict has been shown to predict mean heart rate in office workers, and has also been linked to coronary heart disease.[1,10,39] By the same token, dentists who experience difficulties with their dual role as 'inflictors of pain' and as 'healers' have been shown to suffer more from elevated blood pressure.[5]

Of course, responses to conflict may vary considerably from one person to another. Perhaps surprisingly, the most vulnerable individuals appear to be of the introverted, flexible type, as opposed to extroverted, rigid types of persons.[11,22,40] It has been suggested that responsibility for other people, particularly for their safety and well-being, may be a specific source of stress in certain occupations,[26,40] and there is some evidence that these responsibilities do 'up the ante' for aircrew. For example, emergency medical evacuation services, which airlift critically ill or injured persons to hospitals, have increasingly adopted a policy of not providing the pilots with any personal or medical details about the patients they are tranporting, as emotional involvment in the situation has been found to lead to inappropriate risk taking and other impairments likely to endanger everyone on board.

For the most part, of course, these demands are reconciled well. Where they are not, airlines tend to err on the side of safety. In commercial aviation, accidents are rare, bankruptcies are common. As a chronic stressor, therefore, layoffs and unemployment probably loom larger than the possibility of injury or death for most pilots. The investment in time and money that pilots make to become pilots is, of course, very great. Recalling Hobfoll's resource investment view of stress discussed in Chapter 1, it is scarcely surprising that job insecurity and the prospect of a forced career change are deeply threatening to pilots.[18] As one TWA captain put it, "The feeling prevails that their job is a lifetime investment not easily transferred. Aviation skills, so specialized, rarely adapt to nonaviation employment" (Gunn,[14] p. 664).

The threat does not have to be as extreme as unemployment, however. In the US Navy, even slow promotion, 'status incongruence', and low pay raises have been associated with reduced military effectiveness, as well as with increased psychiatric disorders.[9] However, we need to be cautious in assuming that straightforward issues such as promotions or pay raises are the direct *causes* of discontent, even where unhappy employees cite such specifics.

> From researches in industrial psychology it has become abundantly clear that, for the workers in any large organization, physical health and mental well-being (and, as a result, productivity) depend rather more upon workers *feeling* that they are being cared for by an interested and benign management than upon such tangibles as large wage-packets. (Dixon,[7] p. 276)

Sex discrimination

No discussion of conflict and insecurity can be considered complete without a consideration of the problem of sexism in the workplace. Aviation, particularly at the professional level, has traditionally been very much a male bastion. Until quite recently, women who wanted to fly with the airlines were largely relegated to serving as cabin staff (a role which, especially in the past, was itself peculiarly sexualized and trivialized; see sidebar on p. 343). As recently as 1986, a demographic study of nearly 450 British airline pilots included not one single woman.[40] Now, however, airlines are beginning to recruit more women as pilots; in fact, some women recruited as first officers are now finding their way into the captain's seat alongside male subordinates. Similarly, women are increasingly finding their way into military aircraft, including front line combat aircraft.

It is a fact, however, that by no means all male pilots have adjusted fully to the presence of female crew members. Indeed, it is clear that some (presumably insecure) male pilots find the presence of women on the flight deck irritating, challenging and, in some sense, stressful. The prejudice and harassment that these pilots occasionally mete out to their female colleagues, however, is truly stressful by any measure. Of course, discriminatory behaviour is always distressing, in any vocational context. However, there are at least three reasons why such prejudice is particularly stressful and undesirable in aircraft cockpits.

Tijuana, Mexico, September, 1992: As a copilot I wasn't responsible for the weight and balance, but the captain wasn't going to do it so I had to. I asked the captain (who is also our Chief Pilot, "How much fuel do we have?" He answered, "We have as much fuel as we need to be legal." I answered him back with, "What is that supposed to mean?" The captain answered, in a very degrading voice, "Add up the passengers and baggage and I will tell you how much fuel we have."

I didn't want to argue with the captain and I thought we must be OK since he said we were. I finished up the weight and balance and he told me we had 1000 pounds of fuel. Once we were in the air, realized that we had more fuel than the captain had told me -- and we were 600 pounds overweight. I was pretty upset. I realized that the captain must have known because he signed the flight log going from Los Angeles to Burbank and back that morning with another pilot, burning only 322 pounds of fuel. In Tijuana I told the captain that we would be 600 to 800 pounds overweight. He told me we were going anyway. I realized he didn't care. Other people had told me that the captain and company people didn't like female pilots -- we were taking all the jobs, etc. Another company pilot on board the aircraft told me they were going to fire me and would have flown anyway. I was scared and intimidated by the captain, so we went to Los Angeles 600 to 800 pounds overweight. Next time I'm not going.

I reported this to the company. They tried to cover it up, so I had to prove it. The captain tried to deny it, saying he didn't know the aircraft was overweight and hiding the fuel slip. But he'd signed the flight log, flown with another pilot earlier, lied to me about the fuel in Los Angeles, and I told him (about the overweight condition) in Tijuana. So he flew two trips in a row overweight and he knew. I was terminated because I am a female pilot who reported the captain to the company.

[Callback conversation with reporter revealed the following information: the reporting pilot was fired two days after the incident. She reported the incident to the company and had no job when she came to work the next time. Her former company has no union. She reported the incident to both the Equal Employment Opportunity Commision (EEOC) and the FAA. Other 'girls' (her word) have been fired by this company and have reported this to the EEOC. The Chief Pilot, the man the reporter was flying with, was formerly the Director of Maintenance for this company. He had been in trouble with the FAA for his procedures previous to this incident.]

-- NASA Aviation Safety Reporting System (Accession No. 222442)

San Francisco, June, 1989: The captain who sexually harassed me had a long history of this behavior at my company. His misogyny was well known. When this individual and I were assigned to fly together other pilots came up to me and said things like, "You're flying with XXX? Better bring some mace or a baseball bat." Then they would walk away shaking their heads. I pressed them for details but they would not elaborate. We flew together during June of 1989. The harassment started soon into the month. He had listened to a female controller. When he got done talking to another aircraft he said "Bitch!" He didn't key up the mike and directly call her that but he felt that he should express his opinion of her. He would frequently say, "I hate women". According to him, "All women are bitches". Needless to say, I was getting scared of him; I didn't like being around him. He let me know that he didn't like having to fly with a woman. While flying, his way of asking me to get the ATIS [Automatic Terminal Information Service] was to say, "Get the ATIS, asshole". When I would try to deal with him as an adult and say that I did not like being treated that way and that he was not to do it again, he would smirk at me. Then, when we were on the ground he would say, "Check the gear doors, bozo".

On our last flight he threw a temper tantrum in the plane to scare me. However, it also scared the passengers. We were on final to 28 Left at San Francisco. I landed, intending to turn off at taxiway Echo, and waited for him to make the '80 knot' call so we could go into reverse thrust. (This is an FAA required call). After what seemed like a few seconds past when he should have called it out, I looked over at him. He looked at me and then screamed at me as he grabbed the controls. He pushed the power levers up so quickly and unevenly that we swerved 10 feet off the runway centerline. By this time taxiway Echo was rapidly approaching. He slammed the power levers back into beta and the aircraft swerved back across the centerline and 10 feet over onto the other side. We exited and taxied to our gate. After he shut the engines down he pulled his headset off and yelled at me in front of the passengers. He blamed me for his unprofessional and dangerous behavior, even though I had done a good landing. The passengers had no clue as to who was at fault: they had no idea that he had freaked out. Naturally, I tried to get off his schedule. The San Francisco Chief Pilot said that was impossible. That's not the shocking part. He next said that the captain had a history of grabbing the female rampers' butts, but it didn't count as they were just rampers. The last and most disturbing problem: both management and my union felt that what I had experienced was not sexual harassment.

-- NASA Aviation Safety Reporting System (Accession No. 212929)

First, a pilot subjected to such treatment cannot walk away from a flight deck colleague who is behaving badly. She cannot leave the coffee machine, go down the corridor and shut her office door like a company executive could. She is 'trapped' on the flight deck and must continue to interact with the other crew member -- all day and for several consecutive days in some cases. Neither can she easily change the crew rostering and avoid conflict that way. Since she can neither change her sex nor her colleague's attitudes, she is in the position of having little or no control over the aversive situation in which she finds herself. As we have noted elsewhere, perception of control is a powerful antidote to stress, and, by the same token, lack of control is a powerful stress booster.

Second, as we noted earlier, pilots have few transferrable skills. They cannot switch careers, or even change airline jobs very easily. Women pilots, no less than male pilots, have invested huge resources to become professional aviators. This investment is threatened when their competence and legitimacy as aircrew is denied, directly or indirectly. As Hobfoll's model of stress emphasizes, stress may be generated not only when losses are incurred but when due return on resources invested is threatened. This, of course, may well be the situation faced by a female pilot having to decide whether to report a captain's misconduct to her (largely male) management.

Finally, flight decks are not insurance offices or factory floors; on the flight deck conflict, stress, and poor communication from any source can cost a great deal more than lowered morale or lost productivity. Sexism is bad cockpit resource management and a threat to public safety.

Management relations and stress

Airlines, unions, and corporate instability

In the late 1980s Eastern Provincial, a medium sized Canadian airline, was involved in a lengthy and intense labour dispute with its own pilots. The dispute covered issues relating to working conditions and salaries. The course of the dispute was a depressingly familiar one: repeated layoffs and callbacks of pilots, refusal of many pilots to return to work, the hiring of nonunion pilots, and the resultant picketing of the airline by union pilots. A number of pilots were dismissed by the company. Of those union pilots who did return to work, many were demoted from the left seat to the right seat -- that is, from captain to first officer status, with a corresponding reduction in salary. These pilots found themselves running the gauntlet of the union pickets to fly as subordinates to the newly hired and inexperienced nonunion pilots.

In an attempt to determine the effects of stress on the health and well-being of pilots involved in the dispute, University of Ottawa investigators[12] administered psychometric tests to the pilots and conducted semistructured interviews. Three tests were given, the Eysenck Personality Questionnaire (EPQ), the Health Opinion Survey (HOS) and the Symptom Check-List 90 (SCL-90). These were used to assess personality, general mental health, and psychiatric symptoms, respectively. Twenty-six pilots volunteered to participate, representing about a quarter of the union pilots in the company. To help counter possible effects of sample bias, the assistance of a further twelve pilots was solicited, and eleven agreed to join the study. No significant differences were found between the two pilot groups on the EPQ, HOS and SCL-90 tests, and EPQ scores overall were unremarkable. However, this was not the case with the HOS results: about a quarter of the pilot sample were found to have elevated scores which classified them as 'psychologically at risk'. This proportion is about twice the incidence found in norms derived for other occupational groups, such as managers, technicians, or senior executives. Moreover, it was determined that if the criteria of the US Navy Medical Neuropsychiatric Research Unit had been applied, the absolute values of the scores were such that two of the pilots would have been categorized as 'unfit for duty', and one would have been recommended for discharge.

The SCL-90 results were consistent with this, also. In general, the pilots involved in the dispute exhibited marked symptoms of paranoia and anger/hostility at levels more normally associated with psychiatric outpatients. The 'at risk' subgroup also exhibited obsessive-compulsive symptoms involving forgetfulness, failure to 'take in' information, checking and rechecking actions, and slowed performance. Moreover, these symptoms were not linked to any of the personality variables measured, and thus could not be ascribed to any particular 'stress sensitivity'. (Norman Dixon[7] has observed that "under threatening conditions normal individuals behave like compulsive neurotics" (p. 192).)

The sample pilots also reported feelings of anxiety, depression, and anger over their treatment by the management, a management which they neither liked nor trusted. They complained of being spied upon, both on and off duty. In addition, stress at work and loss of pay and self esteem

Chicago, March, 1992: On the fourth day of five in a row, the atmosphere around air carrier operations had become one of suspicion and distrust. During the previous three days as many as ten line pilots (captains and first officers) had been taken 'off line' by management personnel for reasons ranging from aborted takeoff, for EFIS (electronic flight information system) computer problems, to cookie crumbs found in critical document envelopes. A line captain was taken 'off line' after stumbling across two management pilots in the tower cab. The two were allegedly monitoring aircraft movements and writing down names and flight numbers of company aircraft taxiing at speeds they felt were not acceptable to the company, etc. At present, then, the union and the air carrier are locked into a serious contract battle. That sets the stage.

While taxiing out I discovered that the captain's directional gyroscope and my RMI had frozen at a heading better than 120 degrees from our magnetic compass, my DG, and our known heading reference and taxiway position. I asked the captain if he wished to return to the gate or call company maintenance. He replied, "No, they wouldn't like that. Let me try this", and furiously began resetting circuit breakers. Just prior to takeoff, after making several distracted taxi maneuvers and repeatedly letting go of the tiller, the problem corrected itself temporarily. His DG was mostly inoperative over the next day and a half. Each time I asked him to call maintenance his response was one of fear: that if he reported a discrepancy he'd be taken 'off line' or even lose his job. Our flight attendant also asked him to call maintenance over a few things such as the emergency lights which were burned out, but he refused to put anything in writing in the maintenance log, expressing the same fear.

On the second to last leg I was at the controls, and I realized that with maximum throttle the right engine was still 400 pounds below its rated power. The captain again fiddled with the lever furiously but to no avail. He hesitated calling the company for some 15 minutes trying to justify the conditions. At this point I told him that I would not fly the aircraft out if we continued to our destination. Only after this did he call despatch and make the half-hearted choice to return to O'Hare.

The atmosphere here is one of survival over safety. I fail to understand why the administrators of the ATC facility would jeopardize the sterile environment of the control tower for such subversive activities. These actions have shattered the sense of shelter each pilot feels with his relationship to the FAA. We need to know that the FAA and NTSB are there to help promote safety, regardless of pressure from management or other corporate sources.

-- NASA Aviation Safety Reporting System (Accession No. 204009)

sometimes spilled over into domestic life, and marital problems ensued. Many of the pilots also reported fatigue from such sources as picket duty or the need to watch over the newly hired, less experienced replacement pilots. On the flight deck, the union pilots followed a policy of silence, refusing to speak with their nonunion colleagues, except for vital communications such as checklist challenges and responses. The pilots who flew in this abnormally strained atmosphere reported that it posed palpable risks to safety. The demoted union pilots even reported that they did not always intervene when errors were made by newly hired captains: sometimes they would permit a faulty approach to continue and then step in at the last moment to 'save the landing'. One researcher actually observed a fist fight break out on the flight deck.[13]

As a sort of paradoxical counterweight to the bad atmosphere on the flight deck, the 'mixed crew' (union and nonunion) arrangement tended to lead to an increase in crew arousal (and, one would presume, more alert functioning). However, this effect reportedly 'rebounded' once an all-union crew was operating together. That is, complacency set in and arousal went down in all-union crews, to the detriment of attention and vigilance. This became apparent in increased violations of altitude limits -- a dangerous and common correlate of pilot stress and fatigue, as a review of ASRS reports reveals.

While the results of this study provide compelling evidence of the prevalence of organizational pathogens and the effect of poor management relations on aircrew stress levels, it is instructive to examine the same issues in less strained corporate contexts. If the raw conflict characterizing the operations of Eastern Provincial is, as we would hope, not ubiquitous in the airline industry (even in these straitened times), corporate instability certainly is. In one such study, researchers from the Virginia Polytechnic Institute[28] distributed Gaffney's Symptoms of Stress Questionnaire to over 800 pilots from airlines with both stable and unstable corporate backgrounds. (The Symptoms of Stress Questionnaire lists eighteen putative symptoms of stress or markers of depression, including such items as feeling hopeless about the future, decreased attention, crying, loss of interest in sex, being accident prone, having migraine headaches, and sleeplessness. Subjects respond on a five point scale of incidence, ranging from 'almost never' to 'almost always'.) Responses showed no differences between pilots based upon age, rank, marital status, education, or even proportion of family income derived from flying for the airline. However, significant differences were found between pilots from stable and unstable

> *Detroit Metro, April, 1988: A Boeing 727-231 was taxiing for takeoff.*
> *However, while the aircraft was taxiing, the air conditioning pack*
> *became overheated and smoke entered the passenger cabin. A male*
> *passenger became alarmed and started to panic, shouting "Open the*
> *door!" The lead flight attendant mistook this call as an instruction*
> *coming from the cockpit. As a result she opened an exit door. The*
> *passengers interpreted her action as clearance to open another door and*
> *began to evacuate the aircraft. A total of twenty-one passengers evacu-*
> *ated before the captain intervened. Two flight attendants were on strike*
> *at the time and the flights were being staffed by supervisors and newly*
> *hired personnel. Thus, the lead flight attendant on this flight was a*
> *supervisor with no recent day to day cabin experience.*
>
> *-- National Transportation Safety Board brief of incident, file no. 5025*

airlines on twelve of the eighteen stress symptoms. As anticipated, it was the pilots from the unstable carrier who reported more symptoms, and it was the more educated pilots from this group who reported the most symptoms of all.

The authors of the report link this finding to the results of the US Navy study cited on p. 347.[9] That is, it is speculated that the better educated employees of the unstable airline were suffering disproportionately from 'status incongruence' and underpromotion. Age did not apparently interact with employment in the unstable airline to produce greater symptoms, in contrast to results reported by Cooper and Sloan in which older pilots who worried about their futures were found to be at increased psychiatric risk.[6] Some of the largest differences between the questionnaire responses of the pilots from the stable and unstable airline groups related to rather broad attitudes of mind. Pilots from the struggling airline, for example, were far more likely to report general dissatisfaction (28 percent versus 8 percent), pessimism (27 percent versus 6 percent), and feelings of hopelessness about the future (18 percent versus 2 percent). Admittedly, these are symptoms which can act as markers for potentially severe psychiatric disorders such as endogenous depression and related affective illnesses.[27] However, an important element in these disorders is that the feelings may vary independently of the objective realities of the individual's circum-

> *Newark International Airport, New Jersey, June, 1992: Our company just announced to us in our mailboxes that we were to take a $1,000 per month pay cut to assist the company out of bankruptcy. However, the employees are helping to finance the present management's 'golden parachute' for another investor's buyout of the company. Our attention was not on the business of flying an airplane. No matter how conscientious we tried to be, we still missed two very important items. I even announced while taxiing out that our attention has been seriously diverted, that we need to be very careful and attentive to what we are doing. We received a PDC from the company gate agent which indicated the Newark 4 Departure with an ended climb clearance to maintain 2,500 as opposed to the standard 5,000 feet. We did not see the amendment. Under certain emotional strain and stress a pilot should be able to disqualify himself from a flight without reprisal from the company or management (as would be the case in our airline).*
>
> *-- NASA Aviation Safety Reporting System (Accession No. 214452)*

stances. Given the circumstances of these pilots and the prevailing employment climate (where many airlines were going out of business), these attitudes do not appear to be irrational or unjustified. Other reported symptoms are more easily recognized as dysfunctional, for example, crying easily, sleep disorders, anger and irritability, lowered attention, and lowered libido. Pilots from the unstable airline reported a significantly higher incidence of these symptoms also. Nevertheless, the differences in absolute terms tended to be far less than those found for the overall attitude items. For example, crying was reported by 0.5 percent of the control group and by 4.7 percent of the pilots from the unstable airline; the analogous figures for inability to concentrate were 3.2 percent and 9.4 percent, respectively.

Air traffic control: management or workload stress?

Air traffic control is a highly technical vocation in which carefully selected, trained, motivated, and generally well-paid professionals provide a crucial 'life and death' service to the public. In some ways it resembles the medical profession. It is difficult to imagine eight out of ten physicians simply leaving their surgeries and hospitals, walking 'off the job' and into permanent unemployment or underemployment. However, as related in Chapter 10, in 1981 11,500 American air traffic controllers did just that.

The controllers, whose demands included both higher pay and shorter working hours, maintained that the conditions under which they worked were creating intolerable levels of psychological stress. They also stated that this situation was exacerbated by the autocratic management style of many of their supervisors, which, among other things, hindered communication and prevented them from exercising their professional judgment.

Very different opinions were expressed by middle and senior management within the FAA, however. A government task force appointed afterward to determine the roots of the conflict interviewed a large number of managers at a variety of locations; these individuals had generally positive views concerning the working climate in ATC facilities. While they conceded that workplace tensions had been widespread prior to the strike, these problems were blamed on the strikers themselves: with those 'problem' individuals out of the way, employee morale was now quite good. The strike itself was attributed to such factors as excessive expectations on the part of the controllers (in other words, greed), extreme peer pressure, and an undisciplined attitude toward authority.

Other, more general factors commonly cited included the military background and authoritarian style of most ATC managers, the limitations placed on collective bargaining by the fact that the controllers were government employees, and the notion that frequent intrusions by Congress hampered the effectiveness of managers. The point was also made that collective bargaining units are primarily equipped to address straightforward economic issues such as wages, benefits, and working conditions; elements such as managerial style and organizational climate do not lend themselves nearly as readily to union negotiation. When employee complaints stem more from the latter type of factor, this dissatisfaction may find expression within the more traditional areas of union activity, such as demands for pay increases.

In view of these circumstances, David Bowers, a psychologist with the University of Michigan Institute for Social Research, initiated a research effort aimed at assessing the organizational climate within which the controllers operated.[2] A standardized questionnaire, the Survey of Organizations (SOO), was administered to working and striking controllers at twenty-eight ATC facilities across the United States as well as to staff at FAA Headquarters. The questionnaire covered organizational climate, teamwork, and motivation, along with leadership, peer relationships, stress, and 'burnout'. The survey results were compared with national norms and an effort was made to throw light on the relationships between stress, burnout, and autocratic management.

Bowers was able to form several conclusions concerning the organizational frictions leading up to the strike. First, he affirmed that employee morale was indeed quite poor (contrary to the more positive picture painted by managers interviewed), and that workplace stress was endemic. This he attributed to a clash between the Theory X* beliefs and practices typical at the management level, and a more collaborative set of values favoured by the controllers and technicians, who tended to represent a younger generation of workers. Bowers suggested that managers who continue to insist on autocratic, 'top-down' supervision with today's workforce do so at their own risk and the risk of their organization, and concluded by noting that "a less directive, less bureaucratic organizational style would have buffered the problem. A participative or collaborative style would have solved it. A 1930s workforce would have prevented its emergence in the first place" (p. 12). As Spring[41] has observed,

> A sense of elitism is encouraged by managers and supervisors who were themselves once the controllers manning the various positions. They are attempting to bolster the morale of the hard pressed controllers. The result is a mixed bag of condescending arrogance versus subtle envy. It makes for a somewhat confused cultural environment marked by competition within the organization for recognition and compensation. (p. 489)

Concluding comments

Of all the sources and manifestations of distress that we have considered in this book, stress and fatigue linked to organizational factors have emerged as among the most ubiquitous and pernicious in aviation. This is necessarily a judgement insofar as there is, of course, no single common metric with which to compare, for example, life stress with flight phobia, or acute reactive stress with organizational stress. Nevertheless, the importance of organizational pressures is suggested by both the quantity and nature of the evidence. This includes the high level of complaints from pilots and from

---

*A term used to refer to a management attitude which assumes workers to be basically lazy, unreliable, and uncommitted, and in need of strong control, close supervision and direction.

air traffic controllers, the frequent reference to institutional pressures in incident and accident reports, the history of industrial disputes in aviation, and the disturbing nature of observations made by researchers. Certainly, we would be impressed with the apparent impact of life events had 11,500 controllers abandoned their careers because of (say) marriage problems and domestic tribulations, rather than organizational problems. If divorce and bereavement had many times led to long bitter disputes in the airlines, fist fights on the flight deck, the systematic violation of regulations, and threat to the livelihoods of aircrew, we would certainly acknowledge the importance of life events. In such a context, we would regard it as significant to find that life events were cited repeatedly (rather than, occasionally, as they in fact are) in incident and accident reports.*

Admittedly 'organizational factor' is a broad category and covers many phenomena, which accounts, in part, for the term's apparent ubiquity. However, the category 'life stress' is hardly narrower, yet, as we concluded in Chapter 5, the impact of life events upon aviation operations remains difficult to gauge. Certainly, for every stress related ASRS incident report which cited a life event, an acute reactive response, or some other stress or fatigue factor, we seemed to find two or three which contained words such as "Our company has just gone into Chapter 11 bankruptcy ..." (Needless to say, no statistical claims are being made here -- see the Preface for caveats concerning ASRS reports.)

These observations map onto the increasing realization among many human factors practioners that the preeminent problems in transportation and industrial safety may be best addressed by the study of human-machine systems in a broad, collective, institutional sense. Traditional human factors psychology, experimentation with individuals in test booths, has provided an important database and some vital insights into human capabilities and limitations. It helps us to better design cockpits, computer interfaces, and control gear. Such research does not, however, tell us much about the effects of real institutional pressures on the performance of shifts, crews, and teams where decision making is distributed between pilots, controllers, managers, and dispatchers. Events have redirected interest in this direction, however -- events such as the tragic downing of an Iranian A320 by the USS Vincennes, the Challenger debacle, Bhopal, Zeebrugge, Chernobyl, and others. It is a fact that in recent years the increased scrutiny of the organizational precursors of stress and failure has

---

*Life events apparently figure more prominently in certain subsets of incident reports, such as those relating to EMS (emergency medical services) operations.

been led, not by the prescience of researchers, but by catastrophe; however, the insights that these investigations have brought also have wide applicability to the more commonplace tribulations of working life.

References

1. Beehr, T.A., Walsh, J.T., and Taber, T.D. (1976), 'Relationship of stress to individually organizationally valued states: higher order needs as a moderator', *Journal of Applied Psychology,* vol. 61, pp. 41-47.

2. Bowers, D.C. (1983), 'What would make 11,500 people quit their jobs?' *Organizational Dynamics,* Winter, pp. 5-19.

3. Carr, A.T. (1970), *A Psychophysiological Study of Ritual Behaviours and Decision Processes in Compulsive Neurosis,* unpublished doctoral thesis, University of Birmingham.

4. Chase, W., and Simon, H. (1973), 'Perception in chess', *Cognitive Psychology,* vol. 4, pp. 55-81.

5. Cooper, C.L., Mallinger, M., and Kahn, R. (1978), 'Identifying sources of occupational stress among dentists', *Journal of Occupational Psychology,* vol. 51, pp. 227-34.

6. Cooper, C.L., and Sloan, S. (1985), 'Occupational and psychosocial stress among commercial aviation pilots', *Journal of Occupational Medicine,* vol. 27, pp. 570-6.

7. Dixon, N.F. (1976), *On the Psychology of Military Incompetence,* Futura Publications, London.

8. Einhorn, H.J., and Hogarth, R.M. (1986), 'Judging probable cause', *Psychological Bulletin,* vol. 99, pp. 3-19.

9. Erickson, J.M., Pugh, W.M., and Gunderson, K.E. (1972), 'Status congruency as a prediction of job satisfaction and life stress', *Journal of Applied Psychology,* vol. 56, pp. 523-5.

10. French, J.R.P., and Caplan, R.D. (1970), 'Psychosocial factors in coronary heart disease', *Industrial Medicine*, vol. 39, pp. 383-97.

11. French, J., and Caplan, R. (1972), in Marrow, A.J. (ed.), *The Failure of Success*, Amacon, New York, pp. 31-66.

12. Girodo, M. (1988), 'The psychological health and stress of pilots in a labor dispute', *Aviation, Space, and Environmental Medicine*, vol. 59, pp. 505-10.

13. Girodo, M. (1992), personal communication.

14. Gunn, W.H. (1991), 'Airline deregulation: impact on human factors', *Proceedings of the Sixth International Symposium on Aviation Psychology*, Ohio State University, Columbus.

15. Hancock, P.A. (1986), 'Stress, information-flow, and adaptability in individuals and collective organizational systems', in Brown, O., Jr. and Hendrick, H. (eds.), *Human Factors in Organizational Design and Management, II* (Second International Symposium on Organizational Design and Management), North-Holland, Amsterdam.

16. Hartley, L.R., Morrison, D., and Arnold, P. (1989), 'Stress and Skill', in Colley, A.M. and Beech, J.R. (eds), *Acquisition and Performance of Cognitive Skills*, John Wiley, Chichester, pp. 265-300.

17. Hertzler, J.O. (1940), 'Crises and dictatorships', *American Sociological Review*, vol. 5, pp. 157-69.

18. Hobfoll, S.E. (1988), *The Ecology of Stress*, Hemisphere Publishing Corporation, New York.

19. Johnston, N. (1991), 'Organizational factors in human factors accident investigation', *Proceedings of the Sixth International Symposium on Aviation Psychology*, Ohio State University, Columbus.

20. Kahn, A. (1991), 'Behavioral analysis of management actions in aircraft accidents', *Proceedings of the Sixth International Symposium on Aviation Psychology*, Ohio State University, Columbus.

21. Kahn, R.L., Wolfe, D.M., Quinn, R.P., Snoek, J.D., and Rosenthal, R.A. (1964), *Organizational Stress,* Wiley, New York.

22. Kasl, S.V. (1973), 'Mental health and the work environment: an examination of the evidence', *Journal of Occupational Medicine,* vol. 15, pp. 506-15.

23. Klein, G.A. (1989), 'Recognition-Primed Decisions', in Rouse, W. (ed.), *Advances in Man-Machine Systems Research,* vol. 5, JAI Press, Inc., Greenwich, Conecticut, pp. 47-92.

24. Klein, G.A., Calderwood, R., and Clinton-Cirocco, A. (1986), 'Rapid decision making on the fire ground', *Human Factors Society 30th Annual Meeting,* Human Factors Society, Santa Monica, CA.

25. Kletz, T. (1988), *Learning from Accidents in Industry,* Butterworths, London.

26. Kroes, W.H. (1976), *Society's Victim -- the Policeman. An Analysis of Job Stress in Policing,* Charles C. Thomas, New York.

27. Link, B., and Dohrenwend, B.P. (1980), 'Formulation of Hypotheses about the True Prevalences of Demoralization in the United States', in Dohrenwend, B.P. (ed.), *Mental Illness in the United States: Epidemiological Estimates,* Praeger, New York, pp. 114-32.

28. Little, L.F., Gaffney, I.C., Rosen, K.H., and Bender, M.M. (1990), 'Corporate instability is related to airline pilots' stress symptoms', *Aviation, Space, and Environmental Medicine,* vol. 61, pp. 977-82.

29. Mackie, J.L. (1974), *The Cement of the Universe: A Study of Causation,* Clarendon Press, Oxford.

30. Mintzberg, H. (1979), *The Structuring of Organizations,* Prentice-Hall, New Jersey.

31. Moray, N. (1989), 'Human factors research and nuclear safety', *Human Factors Society 33rd Annual Meeting,* Human Factors Society, Santa Monica, CA.

32. Moray, N., personal communication.

33. Nance, J.J. (1986), *Blind Trust: How Deregulation Has Jeopardized Airline Safety and What You Can Do About It,* William Morrow & Company, New York.

34. National Transportation Safety Board, Report NTSB-AAR-80-5.

35. Norman, D., and Bobrow, D. (1975), 'On data-limited and resource-limited processing', *Journal of Cognitive Psychology,* vol. 7, pp. 44-60.

36. Perrow, C. (1984), *Normal Accidents,* Basic Books, New York.

37. Reason, J. (1990), 'Types, tokens and indicators', *Proceedings of the Human Factors Society 34th Annual Meeting,* Human Factors Society, Santa Monica, California, pp. 885-889.

38. Rochlin, G.I., La Porte, T.R., and Roberts, K.H., 'The self-designing high-reliability organization: aircraft carrier flight operations at sea', *Naval War College Review,* vol. 40, pp. 76-90.

39. Shirom, A., Eden, D., Silberwasser, S., and Kellermann, J.J. (1973), 'Job stresses and risk factors in coronary disease among five occupational categories in Kibbutzim', *Social Science Medicine,* vol. 7, pp. 875-92.

40. Sloan, S., and Cooper, C. (1986), *Pilots Under Stress,* Routledge and Kegan Paul, London.

41. Spring, E. (1991), 'The human element in air traffic control (ATC), *Proceedings of the Sixth International Symposium on Aviation Psychology,* Ohio State University, Columbus.

42. Staw, B.M., Sandelands, L.E., and Dutton, J.E. (1981), 'Threat-rigidity effects in organizational behavior: a multi-level analysis', *Administrative Science Quarterly,* vol. 26, pp. 501-24.

43. Stewart, S. (1988), *Air Disasters,* Arrow, London.

44. Stokes, A.F., Belger, A., and Zhang, K. (1990), *Investigation of Factors Comprising a Model of Pilot Decision Making: Part II. Anxiety and Cognitive Strategies in Expert and Novice Aviators,* University of Illinois Aviation Research Laboratory, Savoy.

45. Stokes, A.F., Kemper, K., and Marsh, R. (1992), *Time-Stressed Flight Decision Making: A Study of Expert and Novice Aviators,* University of Illinois Aviation Research Laboratory, Savoy.

46. Weick, K.E. (1991), 'The Vulnerable System: An Analysis of the Tenerife Air Disaster', in Frost, P.J., Moore, L.F., Louis, M.R., Lundberg, C.C., and Martin, J. (eds.), *Reframing Organizational Culture,* Sage Publications, Newbury Park, London.

47. Wickens, C.D. (1984), *Engineering Psychology and Human Performance,* Charles E. Merrill, Columbus, Ohio.

48. Wickens, C.D., Stokes, A.F., Barnett, B., and Davis, T. (1987), *A Componential Analysis of Pilot Decision Making,* University of Illinois Aviation Research Laboratory, Savoy.

49. Wilkinson, S. (1994), 'The November Oscar incident', *Air & Space,* February/March, pp. 80-7.

12 Automation and boredom

Absence of occupation is not rest.
A mind quite vacant is a mind distressed.
                          -- William Cowper, *Retirement*

It's a depressing thought to a pilot who prides himself on his skill and ability that he is allowed by law to land his aircraft as long as the visibility is more than about 600 metres, but has to relinquish the job to a collection of wires and microchips if it is less.
                          -- Ken Beere, *Bluff Your Way on the Flight Deck*

In the concluding section of Chapter 10, 'Stress in Air Traffic Control', we discussed some of the changes to ATC work brought about by recent innovations in computerized automation technology. We also observed that the highly intelligent automated systems sometimes proposed for future ATC networks may bring about substantive changes in the controller's role, changes that could create new kinds of occupational stress for ATC personnel. This chapter will consider the place of automation in aircraft, as well as its effects on the pilots who operate them. In particular we will be looking at issues in automated flight deck design, the pilot's changed role, and the problem of monotony and boredom.

Consider the following exchange between Luton Approach and an aircraft on short final -- a Monarch Airlines Airbus 320, a highly automated 'glass cockpit' aircraft (see sidebar):

A320: "It's going around!"
Tower: Roger, Monarch 053, what are your intentions?"
A320: "Go with it, I think ... "[28]

More than any technical description, the nonchalantly detached humour of this exchange makes the point: pilots and computers now share control over the aircraft they fly. The electronics in the highly automated aircraft introduced in the 1980s -- among them the McDonnell Douglas 80, the Boeing 767, and the Airbus 320 -- perform a wide range of functions that were once the exclusive province of human operators. In so doing they

The Glass Cockpit

The glass cockpit cleaned up the general appearance of the flight deck but at first sight doesn't impress half as much. It is equipped with computer screens rather than individual instruments -- screens capable of displaying more information than the pilot would have to know to build the aircraft from scrap.

*Instead of the pilot scanning a large panel of individual instruments, almost all the information he needs to fly the aircraft efficiently is displayed on the screens in front of them [sic]. The design philosophy of the Boeing 747-400 ensures that neither of the two pilots ever needs to turn away from the front panel; all vital information, including failures, appear[s] automatically on the screens and advise[s] him of any action that's required. The central one, the **primary flight display** (PFD) tells him just what the aircraft is doing -- its speed, attitude, altitude, rate of climb or descent -- the full list is enough to make your head ache. The **navigation display** (ND) is less esoteric and much more interesting and is the one most proudly shown off to visitors. On this, a map of the route, radio beacons, the weather, nearby airfields, their runways and probably a moving picture of the chief training captain wagging his finger in astonishment, can be displayed after selection.*

*Above the central console, instead of the conventional engine instruments is another screen displaying a working picture of the conventional engine instruments. Its called the **EICAS** and not one pilot in ten can tell you what it stands for. Below it, the **monitor** writes messages to tell the pilots that, say, number four engine has failed, or worse, that number three tea-urn has sprung a leak.*

It's all very seductive, unless all the screens go blank and the pilots find themselves airborne in a small bare room. Happily, the aircraft designers insist there are so many backup systems that this cannot happen.

-- Ken Beere, *Bluff Your Way on the Flight Deck*

have in many ways made the pilot's task easier. For example, maps displayed on CRT screens can be adapted to fit the needs of the moment (e.g., by selecting only certain categories of information); they can also display information that was previously unavailable in this format, such as colour coded weather radar data. Automated flight decks also provide predictive course information that could previously be obtained only by mental calculation -- for example, the aircraft's future trajectory, or the precise map position at which the desired altitude will be reached. Other functions performed by today's automated flight decks will be discussed in the body of the chapter (although space limitations inevitably preclude a full enumeration).

These developments are, as suggested in Chapter 10, in part technology driven (with particular thanks to the microchip). However, other factors, including market forces, have also played a significant role in stimulating further innovations: in the airlines, deregulation, the general economic climate, and dramatically rising fuel costs have all made it imperative to streamline operations in every way possible, and automation technology has made substantial contributions to this goal. For example, automated throttle control systems regulate power inputs more precisely than a human operator could, thereby minimizing fuel wastage. Fuel is also conserved by computer aided navigational systems, which keep the aircraft more closely on course. In addition, automation has created savings by reducing personnel costs: many aircraft, even wide body jets, are now able to fly with two rather than the traditional three crew members. Obviously, design features such as these can assume no small significance when aircraft manufacturers are competing for contract bids with airlines.

Another factor that has contributed to the development of flight deck automation is that of safety. Machines are, in general, considerably more reliable and less error prone than the humans who operate them. They do not become tired or stressed; they do not become distracted or suffer vigilance decrements; they do not forget procedures. Some automated safety features have been implemented in response to specific types of accidents: for example, the ground proximity warning system (GWPS) has dramatically reduced the incidence of controlled-flight-into-terrain accidents.[21] Indeed, some systems have even been implemented by legislative mandate, not always with the benefit of comprehensive evaluation by human factors specialists: examples include both the ground proximity warning system and the emergency locator transmitter.[43]

One benefit often attributed to automation is that of workload reduction. This, it is assumed, should reduce pilot stress, fatigue, and error. Experience with conventional (that is, earlier generation) aircraft is often consistent with this belief. For example, the analysis of events leading up to the crash of Avianca Airlines Flight 052 (see sidebar) illustrates the contribution that loss of automated support can make to workload and fatigue, not least on a flight already stressed due to a variety of adverse factors.

Cove Neck, New York, 25 January, 1990: Avianca Flight 052 was a scheduled passenger flight from Bogota, Colombia to Kennedy Airport via Medellin, Colombia. Facing both low fuel and bad weather (including wind shear conditions), the crew of the Boeing 707 attempted an ILS [instrument landing system] approach to JFK. The approach failed, and although critically low on fuel the crew accepted vectors fifteen miles out for a second attempt. On the return leg the aircraft crashed due to fuel exhaustion. Of 158 persons aboard, 73 were fatally injured. While the wind shear conditions were a factor in the poorly flown ILS, they do not fully explain it. Other factors, both psychological and physiological, help to explain not only the crew's performance on the approach but its lack of anticipation of the wind shear and failure to discuss the need to land on the first approach as a result of fuel state.

Aircraft maintenance records indicate recurrent problems with the autopilot, including the altitude hold function. Additionally, the captain had problems with the flight director in the approach mode. These factors, as well as the approach itself, led the safety board to believe that the aircraft might have been flown manually from Medellin to JFK and that the ILS was flown using raw data, i.e., without the aid of a flight director. The hours of manual flying, combined with the ever-increasing criticality of the crew's situation, are consistent with increasing fatigue and adverse stress reactions. This situation is most evident in the captain's decreasing ability to timeshare multiple tasks. The captain, with limited English language skills, was dependent on the nonflying copilot to communicate with ATC. During the initial radar vectoring, the captain followed the copilot's ATC instructions and on occasion responded to ATC instructions without translation to Spanish. However, from the time that the airplane was on the final vector until the missed approach, there were nine distinct incidents of the captain asking for instructions to be repeated or for confirmation of the airplane's configuration. Additionally, the captain asked the copilot to speak louder.

These stress conditions are evident not only in the crew's performance on the ILS approach but in their failure to consider that they could not allow a missed approach. Moreover, when they did have a missed approach they did not take control of their situation and request the shortest path back to the airport. The safety board concluded that the flight crew's performance -- their inability to maintain a position on the glideslope -- was attributable to a combination of the wind shear conditions, fatigue resulting from a long flight, possibly flown without the benefit of an operable autopilot, and stress aggravated by their concern about the remaining fuel.

-- Condensed from NTSB report AAR-911/04

However, the complex issue of workload is arguably made rather more complex when truly advanced automation is considered. It has often been noted, for example, that radical reduction of pilot workload may, at least in some flight segments, result in marked 'underload', boredom, vigilance decrement, and the like, and thus need not necessarily represent a change for the better.

Second, the very premise that workload is reduced may be simplistic and subject to question. Automation undoubtedly relieves the pilot of certain tasks at certain times. However, it may tend to replace them with other tasks, perhaps at other times (an example being the need to monitor the automated systems, check modes, and so forth while in busy terminal airspace). Thus, one way of viewing flight deck automation would be to say that it changes the *nature* of pilot workload; it may or may not change the *amount* of it. One by-product of automation, of course, is that some human operators may be eliminated entirely; in such cases remaining crew members may find that their own net workload is not significantly reduced in any practical sense.

Design issues in automation

Functional categories

Traditionally, the kinds of automated systems that have been implemented in flight decks have differed somewhat, in functional terms, from those used in air traffic control. The ATC automated systems we discussed in Chapter 10 consisted mainly of computer assisted status displays whose purpose was to supply up-to-date information about the airspace, for interpretation by the human controller. (Mention was also made of future expert systems capable of assuming actual control and decision making functions.) Flight deck automated systems also display status information of various types; however, they have also already assumed the functions of control, decision making, and monitoring.[46]

The former, which include, for example, inertial navigation and auto-throttle systems, are essentially concerned with the physical maneuvering and guidance of the aircraft; as such they are designed to supplement the pilot's own manual control skills. Monitoring systems, as the term suggests, provide warnings, alerts, and other information about the status of the flight. The human functions they assist (and some fear, supplant) include vigilance, scanning, and situational awareness. In a sense the aircraft 'watches over' the pilot. Examples of this category of automation include stall warning systems, collision avoidance systems, and the ground proximity warning system.

Levels of automation and the pilot's role

One way to evaluate and classify automated systems is, as we have seen, by the types of human functions that they replace. However, automation can also be said to exist at various *levels*. Some systems, for example, are designed merely to assist the human operator, while others replace him outright. Likewise, in some cases the human operator controls the automated system, while in others the system dictates the actions of the human. These variables are likely to have considerable relevance to issues of automation and stress.

One important distinction, for purposes of the present discussion, concerns the extent to which the capabilities of the automated system exceed those of the human.[40] Some functions, for example, can if necessary be performed quite adequately by the human but are automated simply to reduce workload. For example (to cite a couple of everyday examples), automobile drivers do not need to explicitly signal to those behind them when they are decelerating, because brake lights are coupled to the brakes themselves and come on automatically. The same is true of the auditory warning given by trucks and vans when the vehicle is set in reverse. The presence of such features lightens the workload placed on the driver, freeing him to concentrate on other, perhaps more challenging tasks such as navigation. (Also, of course, it eliminates the danger that the procedure will be omitted accidentally).

At the second level of automation, the functions performed by machines can, in principle, still be carried out by humans, although perhaps not as precisely or efficiently. The throttle control systems referred to above come under this category, as do most guidance and navigation systems. Systems at this level of automation can generally be disengaged and over-ridden at the pilot's discretion; thus, the pilot retains the ultimate control over events.

The most advanced level of automation involves functions that are beyond the capabilities of human operators. An example would be the hypothetical (and futuristic) air traffic control systems discussed in Chapter 10, involving extensive computations and the manipulation of multiple situational variables. In systems of this sort the human may be incapable of intervening; as such he or she may be, in practical terms, 'out of the loop'.

What functions should be automated, and how?

As the available technology becomes increasingly sophisticated, the issues surrounding human-machine system design also become more and more com-plex.[32,40,46] Thus, an important task confronting the designers of modern aircraft is to determine which operational functions should be automated and which should be reserved for the crew. Humans and computers obviously have different capabilities to contribute in this respect, as well as different weaknesses.

For example, humans have a quite amazing ability to recognize patterns (for example, terrain features, instrument indications, weather trends, even patterns of events). We seem to be able to do this even when the patterns are ill-formed, partial, or 'fuzzy', and, within limits, even when we are tired or under stress. Even if we could haul the world's most powerful supercomputer on board an aircraft, we would find it remarkably primitive in this respect. This, of course, is the standard argument for manned (as opposed to robotic) space flight. On the other hand, even the most intelligent and highly trained pilots are relatively poor at performing calculations, monitoring systems, and storing detailed information. Pilots can tire, become less vigilant, and lose track of details. Even rather simple computers perform better than humans can on these sorts of tasks -- and, as we have noted, never suffer from stress or fatigue.

The traditional wisdom with respect to automated system design has stipulated that machines assume the more 'mindless' and repetitive aspects of a task, leaving the human operator with more attention to devote to the executive functions of planning, decision making, and intervening in the automated system when needed.[18] Modern automated flight decks have gone well beyond this level of human-machine interface, however: indeed, pilots of these aircraft have experienced something of a role change, becoming less 'hands-on operators' and more 'system monitors' -- as is evidenced in the radio exchange on the opening page of this chapter.

This development has had both positive and negative repercussions. On the one hand, pilots can indeed devote more attention to the tasks for which they are still responsible, such as monitoring the airspace for other aircraft. On the other hand, the assumption of more and more functions by machines can lead to a certain passivity on the pilot's part. There are also certain pitfalls inherent in allocating monitoring and vigilance tasks to humans, as these functions are rather easily disrupted by, for example, fatigue, boredom, or 'underarousal' (see Chapter 3).

In this connection it is worth recalling Fitt's Principles, a set of automation guidelines drawn up as early as 1962.[9] These were general in nature, but as applied to aviation would stipulate as follows:

1. The tasks that pilots are expected to do should be intrinsically motivating.

2. The pilots' tasks should provide activity.

3. The computers should monitor the pilots, rather than the pilots monitoring the computers.

Many aspects of flight deck automation, as it currently exists, appear to fly in the face of all three of these 'principles', leaving pilots sitting on their hands, figuratively speaking (some pilots put it more colourfully), watching the computers fly the aircraft. Knowing what we do of pilots' active, self-reliant, and controlling personalities, as well as the great investment they make in becoming pilots, it is not surprising that the prospect of this fate is not always 'intrinsically motivating' to them. Of course, automation has not yet sidelined the crew entirely, and many pilots actually prefer advanced technology automated 'glass cockpit' aircraft to the older, 'clockwork'* flight decks. Nevertheless, it is an irony that automation, one of the newest technologies to have a major impact upon flight deck design, risks compromising some of human factors' most established system design principles.

Automation and decision making

Jens Rasmussen has pointed out that there are, in a sense, not one but three decision makers in an automated flight system. First, there is the system design team, whose input comes via the stored rules, computer programs, and procedural specifications of the automated system. Second, there is the system itself, responding to inputs from sensors but constrained by its design parameters. Third, there is the cockpit crew or, in the case of an

---

*A pilots' tongue-in-cheek expression for traditional electromechanical instrumentation. Other terms that have been applied to traditional aircraft include 'steam gauge', 'rope start', and 'pterodactyl'.[45]

ATC system, the controllers. Human input also constrains or enables the automated system in various ways.[29] This 'tripartite decision maker' has one particularly positive aspect: only one of its components, the crew, is susceptible to acute reactive stress. It is possible, of course, that the humans involved at the design stage may be subject to chronic stress connected with organizational factors or life events. However, any decisions they make have the benefit of relatively unhurried team consideration, analysis, and review.

Consider, for example, the stressful situation arising when two opposing fighters are closing and each pilot must decide when to fire his air-to-air missile. Each pilot is are acutely aware that if he fires too soon he may miss and fall victim to his opponent's better timing. If he leaves it too late, on the other hand, his adversary's weapon is already locked on and streaking toward him. However, the fire decision can be made long before the pilot finds himself in any such harrowing circumstances. When he does, the second decision maker (the sensors and circuitry on board the aircraft) can ensure that the design team's plan is executed faithfully irrespective of stress effects upon the pilot (e.g., distraction, time distortions, attentional narrowing, or even 'frozen pilot' syndrome -- see Chapters 3 and 7).

Given this, however, there is no escaping the fact that automation, while holding out the opportunity to reduce stress created by workload, diffuses responsibility and thus has the potential to complicate decision making by the crew or controller team. Foushee[10] points out that there is a very real risk that high levels of automation may, in addition to removing workload from the flight crew, create a "psychological sense of loss or diffusion of responsibility" (p. 7). He also observes that investigations suggest that in these circumstances human operators often experience a decrease in vigilance and become slower to respond to emergencies. Alternatively, they may fail to recognize genuinely dangerous or threatening situations, redefining them as essentially nonthreatening.

For designers, then, the challenge is to provide for 'graceful degradation' in automated system malfunctions. It is naturally a potential source of anxiety for aircrew to believe that an automated system, should it fail, will fail 'clumsily', that is without providing trend information or alerting and diagnostic assistance (see sidebar). If the system does malfunction the pilot may find himself in the very stressful situation of having to intervene without any 'feel' for what the problem is or what the aircraft is doing.

It has been suggested that whereas minor abnormalities should be corrected by the automated system (providing due feedback to the crew), more

Kagis, September, 1991: We took off in heavy rain -- typhoon conditions. Approaching Kagis we got our first (of many) EICAS caution messages. It indicated a bleed or nacelle overheat on the No. 1 engine. It was followed by more messages in rapid succession. I was flying the airplane. First officer was in the right seat and handled all ATC communications, emergency checklists, etc. Extra captain sat behind me and did most of the public announcements and communications with flight attendants, as well as helping with all phases of the emergency. Extra first officer was in the right hand jumpseat. He handled company calls, helped first officer go through the procedures, and assisted each of us in many aspects of the emergency.

The stick shaker activated several times as the high speed and low speed red lines came together and merged into one solid red line. It stayed like this for much of the flight. I believe the cabin altitude reached 13,000 feet before we caught it on the way down to 10,000 feet. Fuel dumping took about forty minutes. After we landed the tower informed us that we had a fire in our No. 1 engine. While we were fighting that fire the tower called again to say that there was a fire on our right wing. Door 3R was not used as an exit for this reason. Then the tower called again to say that the No. 2 engine was on fire and we should evacuate passengers out of the right side.

The word came from downstairs that the flight attendants couldn't get the doors open -- we were still pressurized. We looked out the right side and saw passengers running away from the aircraft, so we knew they had managed to open the doors. Over 40 injuries occurred going down the wet chutes. Days later we learned there was a fire in the wing forward of the forward spar inboard of No. 2 engine caused by a fuel leak. The fire melted and shorted numerous wires giving all our EICAS messages. We never got a fire indication.

I would commend the entire flight crew for doing an excellent job of handling this potentially disastrous emergency situation. Company procedures were followed to the greatest extent possible. Despite the high techology, two-pilot 'glass cockpit' design of the aircraft, two pilots could not adequately deal with this particular scenario. It took the maximum effort of four pilots here to successfully handle the situation. Despite the sophistication of the EICAS, it was giving us all the wrong indications. It was telling us everything except what the real problem was!

-- NASA Aviation Safety Reporting System (Accession Nos. 189759 and 188985)

important problems should prompt the automated system to bring the pilot into the control 'loop' in a very explicit way. On the other hand, it has also been suggested that the pilot's available decision options be restricted as much as possible, on the theory that as difficult situations are likely to be stressful, the opportunities for defective human judgement should be minimized.[3]

Specific problems with automated flight decks

Mode confusion

Many modern electronic devices may be operated in several, often many, configurations or functional states. These operating 'modes' can be remarkably opaque or hidden, as many owners of digital watches and VCRs know only too well. It is not surprising, then, to find that in aircraft featuring sophisticated electronic aids, pilots occasionally experience difficulty with the various modes that their flight deck equipment supports. This is true even for the older 'clockwork' flight decks (see for example the sidebar on the Avianca crash on p. 367). In highly automated aircraft, however, there is much more opportunity for pilots to make mode related errors, especially errors involving the selection of an inappropriate interface mode.

One classic (and tragic) example of a mode error surfaced in an investigation of an accident involving an Air Inter A320 on a nonprecision approach at Strasbourg in June, 1992. Although nonprecision approaches do not, of course, provide a glideslope, the A320 permits a flight path angle to be entered into its Flight Control Unit. In this case the crew selected a flight path angle of 3.3 degrees. Unfortunately, however, the guidance unit was not in flight path mode at the time, but in vertical speed mode. Thus, 3.3 selected a 3,300 feet per minute descent rate. Although the mode was displayed in at least three places the crew failed to check and correct it; the aircraft crashed, killing eighty-seven of the ninety-six persons on board.

It may be significant that the crew of the A320 had transitioned directly from one of the most venerable 'clockwork' airliners still in service (the 1960s technology Caravelle) to one of the world's most advanced airliners.[34] Automation may require special indoctrination and training over and above normal transition training.

Training for automation

A great many flight students today are very largely trained on cockpit equipment that has changed little since their grandparents learned to fly. These students then move on to the airlines having had little opportunity to develop a 'feel' for highly automated systems. Of course, the airlines will train them to operate the automated systems that they will use, in the sense of teaching which buttons to press and so forth; however, there are dangers in treating the sophisticated integrated computer systems of advanced automation simply as an additional 'box of tricks' to be mastered.

Advanced automation represents a qualitative change in the flight deck, a change in which the notion of 'mastery' doesn't quite strike the right note. In some respects, an advanced automation system is not so much a piece of flight deck equipment as an electronic copilot that will share in the decision making and control of the flight. Students, however, generally receive little specific indoctrination in how to 'live with' automation in this wider sense, and may experience difficulty in determining how much faith and reliance to place in automated systems. Uncertainty, as we have discussed in earlier chapters, is an important source of stress, and this may contribute to the development of unease and a suspicious distrust of automation. Some airlines are now addressing this problem by creating a special, pre-ground-school seminar for pilots preparing to transition from conventional to automated aircraft.[45]

Having made these points, it is important to note that to attribute fault to pilots and to call for improved training is no substitute for rectifying design flaws in the aircraft. The so-called 'blame and train' response is inadequate. As Earl Wiener[45] has put it, "When well trained, well motivated, well standardized pilots are still confused about the implications of the autoflight modes they have selected, it is not a training problem; it is an interface problem" (p. 3).

Automation complacency

Automation is by no means always viewed with suspicion by pilots; it is also possible to err in the opposite direction. Automation complacency, as this tendency is known, consists of overconfidence in automated systems leading to the temptation to 'let the aircraft get on with it'. Chapters 6 and 7 discussed a variety of psychological defence mechanisms, including rationalization, denial, invulnerability, and belief in the benign power of authority and institutions to provide protection. (This issue is discussed further in Chapter 7, pp. 224-225). Manufacturers wouldn't install equipment that could not be depended on, would they? (Or so the feeling goes.) Airlines and regulatory agencies wouldn't permit it anyway, right? So (the complacent crew is apt to feel), automation can presumably be trusted implicitly.

This sentiment is all the more understandable in the light of the remarkable safeguards that automation really can provide (for example, protection from errors and from inadvertently exceeding the aircraft's design limits). This can lead to exaggerated feelings of security and a heightened sense of invulnerability on the part of the crew. Indeed, automation complacency has been cited in connection with the loss of a highly automated Airbus 320 at Mulhouse-Habsheim in 1988, and the destruction of another A320 at Bangalore, India in 1990. As the sidebar on the first of these accidents suggests, complacency has real risk: automation does not necessarily compensate for poor pilot judgement.

Situational awareness

A further danger of overdependence upon automated systems is that the pilot's mental model of the situation may lag behind events; in other words, the crew may lose what air traffic controllers call 'the picture'. 'The picture' refers to the cognitive overview of the airspace, traffic movements, systems status, intentions, and probable future states that permits informed judgements to be made. In a well designed system with properly trained pilots, situational awareness should actually be enhanced: after all, automated displays have the capability to convey far greater amounts of information than conventional instruments, and to do so in a more readable format.[45]

However, if the system is configured such that there is no easy way to break into an automated sequence once the computers have switched into that mode, the pilot may find herself involuntarily 'locked out' of the control and information loop during a critical segment of the flight. If this occurs, no amount of vigilance or conscientiousness will be of much use. It goes without saying that this could be a source of anxiety and frustration even where there is no system failure or emergency to contend with. As Boeing engineering psychologist Rolf Braune[3] has put it, "labeling the pilot as a systems' monitor introduces the risk of perceiving the pilot as a simple back-up factor to improve the reliability equation" (p. 12).

Mulhouse-Habsheim, 26 June, 1988: An Airbus A320 was making a televised overflight of the airfield. It was intended to be a low and slow demonstration of the aircraft's remarkable handling qualities. In connection with this the aircraft was to be flown at the maximum alpha permitted by the automated flight control system. ('Alpha' refers to the angle of attack or nose high attitude.) The system controls both power and pitch to maintain maximum alpha at a safe speed (some 110 knots) for level flight.

Inbound from Basle-Mulhouse, the captain spotted Habsheim late and found himself high and fast. He closed the throttles, extended undercarriage and flaps, and descended. At 100 feet, the planned fly-by altitude, the aircraft was still too fast at 151 knots. The descent continued at 600 feet per minute down to thirty feet above the ground, whereupon the aircraft leveled out at 123 knots.

The throttles were still at idle. The first officer warned of pylons ahead and the captain said "don't worry", selecting full (take-off/go-around) power within four seconds. The engines began to spool up. The captain pulled his control stick fully back to command maximum pitch up. Before the engines reached maximum thrust, however, the rear fuselage struck the woods on the far side of the airfield. The engines began to ingest twigs and branches and the aircraft sank into the trees and was destroyed.

In the last twenty-two seconds before impact the automated flight control system (which was working perfectly) switched control laws several times. The system started in the en route mode, in which stick forces are kept around load factor 1 (that is, 'normal' g load). Triggered by radar altimeter height data it then switched to pitch-attitude control law as appropriate for final approach to landing. The system switched back to en route mode and then back to pitch-altitude mode again.

Four seconds prior to impact the system switched to 'Alpha Prot', the mode which 'protects' high angles of attack against stall by maintaining speed. As one account of the accident stated, "millions of television watchers saw the final seconds of A320 F-GFKC on their national news, and found slightly eerie the way in which the aeroplane was perfectly under control as it sank into the trees."

-- Condensed from accounts in *Aviation Week and Space Technology* and *Flight International*, April, 1990.

Loss of proficiency

Some pilots are indeed anxious that routine reliance on advanced automation (particularly of the 'control' type) will erode their 'stick-and-rudder'
flying skills. Such concerns may in fact be justified: it has been reported,
for example, that first officers on wide body aircraft who are promoted to
serving as captains on smaller, less automated aircraft sometimes find that
their manual control skills are no longer fully adequate to the task.[44] This
problem has a number of direct safety implications, which may themselves
be anxiety provoking.

Consider, for example, the following situation, which is not unknown:[3]
an aircraft's automatic systems are unintentionally disabled during a critical
flight phase, and the pilot, who is, perhaps, 'rusty' from lack of routine
hands-on control, and perhaps bored and out of touch with the developing
situation, is suddenly faced with having to fly the aircraft manually. It is
entirely conceivable that this combination of systems failure and abrupt
demand could, in some cases, be associated with acute reactive stress
which may further degrade performance. (Rasmussen, putting an apt twist
on the old cliche about the life of a soldier, has described the life of an
automated system monitor as 99 percent boredom and 1 percent terror.[29])

Loss of proficiency may be doubly significant in the case of reversion to
manual control, because aircraft designed for automated control are often
relatively unstable. Conventional aircraft are designed to have good natural stability characteristics. In automated aircraft, however, there are a
number of advantages to be derived from making (for example) tailplanes
or wings smaller than is optimal for manual control. Some of these advantages include reduced drag, increased speed, and greater fuel economy, all
of which add up to a more competitive airliner in the marketplace. Highly
automated 'fly-by-wire' (i.e. electronically controlled) aircraft have sophisticated computer sensing and continuous precise adjustment of control
surfaces which can compensate for this reduced natural stability. Pilots
know that in the event of loss of automatic control, the aircraft (particularly certain military aircraft) may be difficult (and in some cases, impossible)
to fly manually.

Pilots' concerns about loss of proficiency may also have a psychosocial
dimension, relating to the issue of threats to identity and self image discussed in Chapter 1. It will be recalled that according to the model proposed by Hobfoll, stress can arise when invested resources fail to 'pay
off'.[14] Pilots go to considerable trouble and expense to become pilots. For

these highly motivated and committed individuals 'pilot' is not merely a job description, it is who they are. Erosion of hard won skills may be threatening to this sense of identity. Moreover, pilots often tend to be active, interventionist, controlling types of individuals who may be uneasy when responsibility for the flight is under someone else's (or some*thing* else's) control.*

As a related issue, some authors have suggested that pilots working amid electronic systems may come to feel that their skills have been devalued, that they are 'cogs in an impersonal machine', so to speak.[46] Humans have always tended to be distrustful of new and unfamiliar technologies, of course, and concerns about social alienation represent one aspect of this. Thus far, however, while pilots have expressed a range of concerns about flight deck automation, there is little evidence to suggest that they find it dehumanizing. For example, a 1985 study of DC-9 crews transitioning to the (more highly automated) MD-80 reported that the predominant attitude was one of enthusiasm and pride at being given the opportunity to fly state-of-the-art aircraft.[42] Similar findings were obtained in a three-year opinion survey of aircrew flying the 'glass cockpit' Boeing 757. The survey included among its questions the statement, "Sometimes I feel more like a 'button pusher' than a pilot"; while attitudes to automation were somewhat mixed, most pilots did not express agreement with this statement.[44]

Increased monitoring load

The extra watchfulness required by automation implies an increased monitoring load. As we noted earlier, automation can reduce workload in some areas, but increase it in others, not least with respect to display monitoring. Keeping 'tabs' on the progress and status of the flight can be complicated by the fact that many processes or changes within an automated system may be 'occult', that is, hidden or only indirectly observable. Such processes require effort to monitor adequately. For example, in most aircraft, the throttle position constitutes an easy, intuitive, tactile, and visual indication of power setting. In the A320, however, computers can set power independently of the throttle positions, and further monitoring of instrumentation is necessary to avoid being misled.

Many other processes in highly automated systems are even more invisible. For example, multifunction displays (that is, computer screens which

---

*Many pilots, for example, will admit to making poor airline passengers.

can switch from one type of information display to another upon demand) require active control on the pilot's part; desired information does not appear automatically but must be sought out. Thus, system information that is not explicitly requested may not reach the pilot's attention. Looked at from another perspective, of course, this feature could be said to be at least partly consistent with Fitt's Principles, insofar as it 'provides activity'. More often, however, automation reinforces the role of the pilot as a *passive* monitor: the pilot watches over systems that fly the aircraft, rather than flying the aircraft himself or herself. Some additional implications of this change in the pilot's role will be addressed in the discussion of boredom that follows.

Workload reduction, passivity, and the problem of boredom

It is unlikely that boredom and monotony can ever be completely eliminated in any highly automated system.

-- Richard Thackray

We turn now to a fuller discussion of one particular problem often associated with workplace automation: the problem of boredom. A number of researchers have attempted to define and explain the phenomenon of boredom as it occurs in the workplace; it has been attributed at various times to monotony (i.e., the performance of repetitive tasks), to underload (not having a sufficient amount of work to do, or having work that is unchallenging[38]), or, more generally, to 'lack of stimulation'.

Work underload has often been associated with performance decrements. For example, a study at the RAF Institute of Aviation Medicine examined 149 military flying accidents in British forces, and found that a major cause of aircrew error was cognitive failure, that is, a type of error in which actions fail to match intentions (omissions or slips). These were more often said to be linked to under- rather than overarousal. Overarousal had an important impact upon error but via its role as a secondary factor arising out of a primary event such as a bird strike, a mechanical failure, disorientation, or 'mishandling' of the aircraft.[6]

Is boredom 'stressful'?

A study conducted at Old Dominion University examined the relationship between subjective workload and boredom in a vigilance task.[12] It was hypothesized that subjective assessments of boredom would be associated with overall workload scores, to the extent that high workload scores are, in fact, a function of the exertion required to maintain an 'optimum' level of 'arousal' (in its sense of wakefulness and alertness). Students were assigned to one of three groups, each of which undertook a sixty minute vigilance task using a video display. The groups differed in the rate at which events on the screen (critical signals) took place. In the slowest condition, for example, six events per minute took place, while in the fastest the rate was forty events per minute. The intermediate condition provided for an event rate of twenty-one per minute. It was found that a direct relationship linked event rate and subjective estimates of workload, that is, the faster the event rate, the greater the estimate of workload. The students reported increased boredom, sleepiness and irritation during the vigilance task, and their ratings increased with event rate. However, the effect may not have been genuine, as statistical analysis failed to show significance in the results. Finally, frustration was significantly and moderately strongly associated with boredom ($r = 0.45$).

There is little doubt that (for example) repetitive tasks that provide little variety or stimulation are often experienced as being boring and monotonous. Such tasks may be endured for financial reasons, but they are generally regarded as being neither rewarding nor fulfilling in the psychological sense. However, this is a far cry from saying that boredom and monotony are actual stressors, that is, factors detrimental to the individual and to individual performance. In the twentieth century, first production line manufacturing and more recently, automation, have been viewed as having brought increased efficiency at the price of an impoverishment of the role and contribution of the individual. It has been suggested that this underutilization of human potential may well be a 'stressor'.[4,11,17,30,39] This notion, if accurate, clearly has important implications for individuals working in highly automated (or otherwise monotonous) environments: as Thackray[36] has stated, "If understimulation is an important source of stress, then attempts to reduce excessive workloads through increased automation could have the ironic effect of replacing one sort of stressor with another" (p. 2).

Some theorists have attempted to explain the 'stress' of boredom in transactional terms: if, as the transactional model states, stress arises from an imbalance between (perceived) demand and (perceived) coping ability, this imbalance could operate in either direction. In other words, the imbalance could operate in the direction of task *underload* as well as task *overload.*[23] This proposition was investigated in a study by Harris and Berger, who monitored the reactions of students giving class presentations likely to have considerable impact on their final course grades. Since evidence of acute reactive stress was (not surprisingly) observed only in students who felt uncertain of their ability to perform satisfactorily, Harris and Berger concluded that task underload was not a 'stressor'. Of course, this study did not address monotony per se; nor did it consider the possible role of task underload in engendering chronic or psychosocial stress.[13]

Other researchers have addressed the issue of boredom not in terms of 'underload' but in terms of stimulation level. Levi, for example, posited a 'U-curve' relationship between stimulation and stress, arguing that under-stimulation is dangerous to well-being in the same way, and to the same degree, that overstimulation is.[19,20] Research on this question has tended to proceed, more or less implicitly, from physiologically oriented response based models of stress (see Chapter 1); thus, a number of studies have explored the relationship between stress and boredom by assessing levels of neuroendocrine activity or physiological arousal in individuals subjected to monotonous or low-stimulation conditions.[2,11,25,27,37] Such studies have generally failed to establish consistent biological markers for boredom,[33] although the most common response to monotonous conditions is for (presumably adrenergic) arousal to decrease.

One reviewer, Thackray, has concluded from this that understimulation should not, in itself, be regarded as a 'stressor'.[36] However, Thackray himself then goes on to point out (in a more transactional spirit) the importance of situational demand. Observing that since monotonous conditions generally lead to decreased vigilance and attentiveness,[22,35] he suggests that boredom and lowered arousal could become threatening in situations where it is crucial to remain alert. As he puts it, "The coupling of repetitive, monotonous work with requirements for high alertness, continuous and rapid decisions, and various penalties for any errors that occur, may well represent a combination that is quite stressful" (pp. 173-4). He cites, for example, a Swedish study conducted on sawmill workers operating hazardous, high speed machinery under monotonous and repetitive conditions; urinary adrenalin output, illness records, and self reported tension levels were significantly higher in these workers than in a control group performing self paced maintenance tasks.[17] Air traffic controllers, too, he notes, could easily become stressed in the absence of adequate stimulation, given the high degree of vigilance that their work entails; this might particularly be the case for controllers who feel ill at ease with automated systems.

This view was echoed in a 1981 paper by O'Hanlon, who theorized that the boredom of long drawn out and repetitive work creates stress because of the need to maintain an adequate degree of arousal in circumstances more likely to lower arousal.[26] This notion has since been extended and formalized in Apter's Reversal Theory,[1] as discussed in Chapter 2. A similar dynamic is likely to occur with passive monitoring tasks, although few studies have addressed this issue directly. Passive monitoring tasks are known to be associated with increased error rates when compared with active involvement,[8,41] and it is easy to imagine how troubling it could be to be engaged in a vital but soporific vigilance task, such as scanning a naval radar screen for a rare but deadly threat (an incoming Exocet missile, perhaps). It is plausible that such an operator with 'nothing to do' for long hours might nevertheless rate his workload as being high.

Despite such theoretical considerations, it may still seem difficult to accept that passive monitoring of systems really can, in practice, be stressful in the same sense that high workload and time pressure can be. However, an unusual and interesting field study reported by a University of Stockholm researcher in 1989 addressed precisely this issue using a transactional, cognitive appraisal based approach to stress assessment.[16] The subjects of the study were control room operators involved in industrial process control. One group (for convenience, termed the 'underload' group) supervised stable continuous processes which predominantly involved passive monitoring. These operators were required to intervene actively only when production problems or disturbances arose. A second group of operators (the 'active' group) coordinated production, planning, and control in a steelworks. These individuals were subject to considerable time pressure and high workload, directing labor and materials to appropriate parts of the plant at appropriate times. One of the researchers noted that to the outsider the job appeared hectic and stressful.

The results of the study showed that *both* groups of operators excreted significantly more adrenalin at work than in nonwork hours. (The 'active' group appears to have a much greater increase over nonwork baseline values, but no group by condition interaction statistics are provided). Subjective assessments of mood and alertness tell a very different story, however. The 'active' operators rated their work as significantly more enjoyable and stimulating (especially at night) than did the passive monitors of the 'underload' group. Feelings of mastery, control, and confidence were reported by the 'active' operators, whereas the 'underload' group reported vague uneasiness during night shifts. The researchers concluded that passive monitoring with continuous action readiness represents an underload associated with subjective perceptions of strain and effort. That adrenergic arousal possibly increased less for the passive than for the active operators would also be in keeping with Apter's predictions, to the extent that arousal level may have been less than the passive monitoring group felt desirable -- a source of unease in its own right.

In conclusion, boredom associated with increased monitoring load appears to be a good example of a task fitting Apter's model of stress. 'Tension stress' may be incurred as a result of the discrepancy between the level and type of arousal preferred by the pilot and the underload often associated with routine monitoring activities. In addition, 'effort stress' may be incurred in trying to maintain interest in a task which is not intrinsically interesting, however important it might be to some remoter or less immediate goal.

Summary and conclusions

Earl Wiener[45] has described the 1980s growth in flight deck automation in the following terms: "suddenly cockpit technology was running in fast-forward, but the human factors profession was not" (p. 2). The human factors profession has made some progress, however -- one aspect of which has been an increased appreciation of the problems of boredom and underload.

As we noted earlier, in the early years of human-machine system design the prevailing philosophy dictated that mechanistic tasks be assigned to the (mindless but reliable) machines, and that human operators retain the role of executive decision maker.[18] This type of configuration made a certain amount of sense as long as humans were the most 'intelligent' components in the system. Eventually, however, advances in automation made it possible to considerably expand the range of tasks that could be defined as 'mechanistic', and it was then that the pilot's role began to shift (in some aircraft and on some flight segments) from one of active decision maker to passive monitor. Many of those who witnessed this development, both psychologists and pilots themselves, became increasingly uneasy at the prospect of captains and first officers having little to do but watch the aircraft fly itself and intervene (or try to) if anything went wrong. Thus, there is now a renewed interest in ensuring that human operators, whatever their specific duties, remain cognitively 'in the control loop'.

These insights notwithstanding, it has to be conceded that much of the existing knowledge base remains somewhat speculative. While we are aware of some of the problems that *may* arise with today's automated flight decks, there is still little in the way of specific, empirical data.[31] One way of approaching the subject has been through retrospective analyses of accidents and incidents.[7,24] These can certainly provoke interesting questions, but they are, of course, biassed in the direction of worst case scenarios. Nor do they allow us to predict when, how, or to whom future accidents are most likely to occur. Other researchers have undertaken attitude surveys of pilots;[15,42,44] these, too, can be quite informative, but the data thus obtained are, of course, subjective.

In Chapter 10 the point was made in connection with air traffic controllers that experimental approaches to automation, performance, and stress have often (necessarily) examined modest, incremental, evolutionary changes in automated support for controller duties -- duties which remain similar now to what they have been in the past. Is extrapolation to the near future possible using this approach? Certainly, on the basis of developments in present day electronics it is possible to broadly predict the technical capabilities of advanced, radical automation. In contrast, however, the human consequences of radical automation (among them changes in roles and the redefinition, if not actual renaming of operator duties) largely remain the realm of speculation. The effects of systemic, radical automation upon human performance, job satisfaction, anxiety, fatigue, and so on, cannot be so easily gauged by extrapolation from present day experience, not even by reference to the most advanced of current ATC equipment. An analogous problem characterizes automation on the flight deck.

The most automated airliners today still need a crew, individuals who can and must talk with each other and with ATC personnel. The crew still sees the external world through a windshield, can still 'hand-fly' the aircraft,* and still retains a great deal of discretionary power over the flight. Consider, however, the following. Even with today's technology it is possible for GPS (Global Positioning System) satellites to track an aircraft with uncanny accuracy and to differentiate the position of the aircraft's wingtips, nose, and tail, such that aircraft attitude can be monitored. These data can be passed to an automatic ATC facility whose computers

---

*Design studies at Boeing have even included plans for a 'no glass' cockpit, in which the crew of a supersonic transport sees the external world solely via remote sensors. The British Aerospace HOTOL project envisaged a near space airliner with no flight deck crew at all.

can issue advisories and instructions via data link to the aircraft's computers. Plans in hand today call for such transmissions to be displayed to the crew. However, the aircraft's computer could act on such instructions without the need of human intermediaries -- navigating globally, avoiding conflicting traffic, turning the aircraft inbound to its destination airport, initiating the descent, and carrying out the landing.

What will be the role of aircrew, then, in such a system? At one time, perhaps in the days before cockpit resource management (CRM) training, many captains were notorious for 'hogging' all the hands-on flying. First officers' duties sometimes seemed to be confined to little more than making cabin announcements and radioing for wheelchairs to meet elderly passengers, and they often resented and chafed under this role. In this context there was a hackneyed old pilots' joke: "What is the difference between a first officer and a duck?" The answer was, "Ducks sometimes get to fly." It would be an irony indeed if the future were to revive the old joke and make it apply to the entire crew (perhaps a crew of one -- the captain). It is doubtful if today's captains would want to retain such a job. At least, different personalities would be needed.

We are confident that no such drastic changes of role are likely to occur in the near future. Nonetheless, as researchers Clark and Herlehy have observed, flight deck automation is likely to lead to significant changes in the ways in which pilots are selected and trained.[5] It is anticipated, for example, that commercial air transport operations of the future will increasingly make use of sophisticated, perhaps supersonic or hypersonic aircraft that will depend more than ever on computer technology for their safe operation. In such an environment, the kinds of selection criteria in use today may well prove inadequate: as Clark and Herlehy put it, the 'right stuff' of today and the 'right stuff' of tomorrow may turn out to be rather different things.[*]

Many authorities in this field contend that the pilot training programs of the future will probably attach rather less importance to manual control and perceptual-motor abilities, and more importance to higher level cognitive and management functions such as planning, prioritization, communication -- and, of course, the ability to work well with computer systems. While the notion that traditional piloting skills are about to become obsolete is a debatable one, it is clear that technological developments in aircraft design are likely, in the long term, to have a profound effect on the nature of the

---

[*]The same authors cite one (anonymous) expert as stating that "Chuck Yeager would not qualify for flight training today".

pilot's task, as well as on the types of individuals who become pilots. By extension, such developments will necessarily affect the nature of stress and fatigue as it influences performance.

References

1. Apter, M.J., and Svebak, S. (1989), 'Stress from the Reversal Theory Perspective', in Spielberger, C.D., Sarason, I.G., and Strelau, J. (eds.), *Stress and Anxiety,* vol. 12, Hemisphere Publishing Corporation, New York, pp. 39-52.

2. Barmack, J.E. (1939), 'Studies on the psychophysiology of boredom: part I. The effect of 15 mgs. of benzedrine sulfate and 60 mgs. of ephedrine hydrochloride on blood pressure, report of boredom, and other factors', *Journal of Experimental Psychology,* vol. 25, pp. 494-505.

3. Braune, R. (1987), 'Summary of the workshop on cockpit automation in commercial airplanes', *Proceedings of the Fourth International Symposium on Aviation Psychology,* Ohio State University, Columbus, pp. 9-15.

4. Caplan, R.D., Cobb, S., French, J.R.P., Harrison, R.V., and Pinneau, S.R. (1975), *Job Demands and Worker Health,* Department of Health, Education, and Welfare, National Institute for Occupational Safety and Health Report No. NIOSH 75-160.

5. Clark, R.E., and Herlehy, W.F., III (1993), 'Commercial flight crew selection for automated flight decks', *Proceedings of the Seventh International Symposium in Aviation Psychology,* Ohio State University, Columbus.

6. Chappelow, J.W. (1989), 'Causes of aircrew error in the Royal Air Force', *AGARD Proceedings 458, Human Behaviour in High Stress Situations in Aerospace Operations,* NATO, Neuilly-sur-Seine.

7. Eldredge, D., Dodd, R.S., and Mangold, S.J. (1991), *A Review and Discussion of Flight Management System Incidents Reported to the*

Aviation Safety Reporting System, Volpe National Transportation Systems Center, Columbus, Ohio.

8. Ephrath, A.R., and Young, L.R. (1981), 'Monitoring vs. Man-in-the-Loop Detection of Aircraft Control Failures', in Rasmussen, J. and Rouse, W.B. (eds.), *Human Detection and Diagnosis of System Failures*, Plenum Press, New York and London.

9. Fitts, P.M. (1962), 'Function of men in complex systems', *Aerospace Engineering*, vol. 21, pp. 34-9.

10. Foushee, H.C. (1981), 'The role of communications, socio-psychological and personality factors in the maintenance of crew coordination', *Proceedings of the First Symposium on Aviation Psychology*, Ohio State University, Columbus, pp. 1-11.

11. Frankenhaueser, M., Nordheden, B., Myrsten, A., and Post, B. (1971), 'Psychophysiological reactions to understimulation and overstimulation', *Acta Psychologica*, vol. 35, pp. 298-308.

12. Fulop, A., and Scerbo, M.W. (1991), 'The effects of event rate on perceived workload and boredom in vigilance', *Proceedings of the Human Factors Society 35th Annual Meeting*, Human Factors Society, Santa Monica, California.

13. Harris, J.H., and Berger, P.K. (1983), 'Antecedents of psychological stress', *Journal of Human Stress*, June, pp. 24-31.

14. Hobfoll, S.E. (1988), *The Ecology of Stress*, Hemisphere Publishing Corporation, New York.

15. James, M., McClumpha, A., Green, R., Wilson, P., and Belyavin, A. (1991), 'Pilot Attitudes to Flight Deck Automation', paper presented at the meeting of the Royal Aeronautical Society, London.

16. Johansson, G. (1989), 'Stress, autonomy, and the maintenance of skill in supervisory control of automated systems', *Applied Psychology: An International Review*, vol. 38, pp. 45-56.

17. Johansson, G., Aronsson, G., and Lindstrom, B.O. (1978), 'Social psychological and neuroendocrine stress reactions in highly mechanized work', *Ergonomics,* vol. 21, pp. 583-99.

18. Kelly, C.R. (1968), *Manual and Automatic Control,* Wiley, New York.

19. Levi, L. (1973), 'Stress, distress, and psychosocial stimuli', *Occupational Mental Health,* vol. 3, pp. 2-10.

20. Levi, L. (1974), 'Psychosocial Stress and Disease: A Conceptual Model', in Gunderson, E.K., and Rahem R.H. (eds.), *Life Stress and Illness,* Charles C. Thomas, Springfield.

21. Loomis, J.P., and Porter, R.F. (1981), 'The performance of warning systems in avoiding controlled-flight-into-terrain accidents', *Proceedings of the First Symposium on Aviation Psychology,* Ohio State University, Columbus.

22. Mackworth, J.R. (1970), *Vigilance and Habituation,* Penguin Books, Baltimore.

23. McGrath, J.E. (1976), 'Stress and Behavior in Organizations', in Dunnette, M.D. (ed.), *Handbook of Industrial and Organizational Psychology,* Rand McNally, Chicago.

24. Norman, D.A. (1990), 'The "problem" with automation: inappropriate feedback and interaction, not "over-automation"', *Philosophical Transactions of the Royal Society of London,* B327.

25. O'Hanlon, J.F., Jr. (1965), 'Adrenaline and noradrenaline: relation to performance in a visual vigilance task', *Science,* vol. 150, pp. 507-9.

26. O'Hanlon, J.F. (1981), 'Boredom: practical consequences and a theory', *Acta Psychologica,* vol. 49, pp. 53-82.

27. O'Hanlon, J.F., Jr., and Horvath, S.M. (1973), 'Interrelationships among performance, circulating concentrations of adrenaline, nora-

drenaline, glucose, and the free fatty acids in men performing a monitoring task', *Psychophysiology,* vol. 10, pp. 251-9.

28. *Pilot* magazine, February 1994, news item.

29. Rasmussen, J., Pejtersen, A.M., and Goodstein, L. (1991), *Cognitive Engineering: Concepts and applications, Vol. 2: Applications* Working Paper.

30. Reighard, H.L. (1976), *Aviation Medicine,* FAA Office of Aviation Medicine Report No. AM-76-8.

31. Sarter, N.B., and Woods, D.D. (1992), 'Pilot interaction with cockpit automation: operational experiences with the flight management systems', *The International Journal of Aviation Psychology,* vol. 2, pp. 303-21.

32. Sheridan, T.B., Fischoff, B., Posner, M., and Pew, R.W. (1983), 'Supervisory Control Systems', in National Research Council, *Research Needs for Human Factors,* National Academy Press, Washington, DC.

33. Smith, R.P. (1981), 'Boredom: a review', *Human Factors,* vol. 23, pp. 329-40.

34. Strauch, B. (1994), personal communication.

35. Stroh, C.M. (1971), *Vigilance: The Problem of Sustained Attention,* Pergamon Press, New York, 1971.

36. Thackray, R.I. (1980), *Boredom and Monotony as a Consequence of Automation: A Consideration of the Evidence Relating Boredom and Monotony to Stress,* FAA Office of Aviation Medicine Report No. FAA-AM-80-1.

37. Thackray, R.I., Bailey, J.P., and Touchstone, R.M. (1977), 'Physiological, Subjective, and amd Performance Correlates of Reported Boredom and Monotony While Performing a Simulated Radar Control

Task', in Mackie, R.R. (ed.), *Vigilance: Theory, Operational Performance, and Physiological Correlates,* Plenum, New York.

38. Welford, A.T. (1965), 'Fatigue and Monotony', in Edholm, O.G. and Bacharach, A.L. (eds.), *The Physiology of Human Survival,* Academic Press, London, pp. 432-60.

39. Welford, A.T. (1973), 'Stress and performance', *Ergonomics,* vol. 16, pp. 567-80.

40. Wickens, C.D. (1992), *Engineering Psychology and Human Performance* (2nd ed.), HarperCollins, New York.

41. Wickens, C.D., and Kessel, C. (1981), 'Failure Detection in Dynamic Systems' in Rasmussen, J. and Rouse, W.B. (eds.), *Human Detection and Diagnosis of System Failures,* Plenum Press, New York and London.

42. Wiener, E.L. (1985), *Human Factors of Cockpit Automation: A Field Study of a Flight Crew in Transition,* NASA Contractor Report No. 177333, Moffett Field, California.

43. Wiener, E.L. (1988), 'Cockpit Automation', in Wiener, E.L. and Nagel, D.C. (eds.), *Human Factors in Aviation,* Academic Press, San Diego.

44. Wiener, E.L. (1989), *Human Factors of Advanced Technology ("Glass Cockpit" Transport Aircraft,* NASA Contractor Report 177528, Ames Research Center, Moffett Field, California.

45. Wiener, E.L. (1993), 'Life in the second decade of the glass cockpit', *Proceedings of the Seventh International Symposium on Aviation Psychology,* Ohio State University, Columbus.

46. Wiener, E.L., and Curry, R.E. (1982), 'Flight-deck Automation: Promises and Problems', in Hurst, R., and Hurst, L. (eds.), *Pilot Error: The Human Factors,* Granada, London.

Name and author index

Subject index